KILLING

IN THE NAME OF

HEALING

KILLING

IN THE NAME OF

HEALING

Confronting Medical Holocausts Past and Present

WILLIAM C. BRENNAN

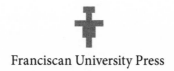

Franciscan University Press

Franciscan University Press
1235 University Boulevard
Steubenville, OH 43952
740-283-3771

Distributed by:
The Catholic University of America Press
c/o HFS
P.O. Box 50370
Baltimore, MD 21211
800-537-5487

ISBN 978-1-7339889-8-8.

Library of Congress Cataloging-in-Publication Data
available from the Library of Congress

Cover Image: used with permission of iStock.com
Printed in the United States of America.

CONTENTS

KILLING
IN THE NAME OF
HEALING

INTRODUCTION

In this account, the sanctity-of-life ethic intrinsic to the Judeo-Christian heritage serves as a prime basis for challenging the widespread exploitation of technology and distortion of language propagated under the cover of an exclusionary quality-of-life ideology responsible for fueling the medical destruction of human lives past and present, especially during the Nazi era and in contemporary American society. The involvement of medical doctors and health care professionals in every phase of the Nazi Holocaust encompassed not only the extermination of Jews, Gypsies, and others deemed unworthy lives, but also the expendable unborn inside the Third Reich and among the "surplus populations" of countries under Nazi occupation. Currently, the bulk of medical killing throughout the world is aimed at victims before birth, while increasing numbers of individuals after birth are likewise being afflicted.

Justice Byron White—one of the two dissenters in the 1973 US Supreme Court decisions in *Roe v. Wade* and its companion *Doe v. Bolton*, which legalized abortion—castigated the ruling as "an improvident and extravagant ... exercise of raw judicial power."[1] He neglected to mention it was largely the "exercise of raw medical power" directed against the unwanted unborn that made this possible. Long before *Roe* and *Doe*, physicians were performing abortions in violation of the law and could be found heading up campaigns aimed at legitimizing their destructive practices. Similarly, German doctors began agitating for legalizing the extermination of the unwanted before and after birth decades prior to the enactment of numerous laws, ordinances, and decrees against these groups in the Third Reich.

A key phenomenon underpinning these findings is that of medicalization—an unwarranted, overreaching intrusion of medicine into areas of human experience where it too often results in the infliction of serious harm, thus vesting an inordinate amount of illicit power and control in the medical profession. Ivan Illich's 1976 scathing analysis of medicalization in modern industrial societies, *Medical Nemesis: The Expropriation of Health*, concludes that "the medical profession has become a major threat to health," producing "a new kind of anesthetized, impotent, and solitary survival in a world turned into a hospital ward."[2] The participation of German physicians in the destruction process perpetrated by the Nazi regime ranks among the most extreme cases of medicalization in history. My critique documents the extent to which medicalization also provides an essential perspective for revealing how extensively similar destructive practices under medical auspices are being repeated in present-day society against the unwanted unborn and vulnerable born.

When I first began exploring this topic several decades ago, I did so with the utmost caution. The climate then, as now, was not favorable to making any associations between the Nazi atrocities and today's assaults on individuals before or after birth. Those opposed to making these comparisons commonly assert that no reasonable connections can be possibly drawn between offering women the option of pregnancy termination in contemporary reproductive health clinics and the extermination of Jews and others in Nazi death camps. They also maintain it is ludicrous to morally equate such entities as pregnancy tissue, protoplasmic masses, fertilized eggs, zygotes, embryos, and fetuses in the practice of abortion with the horrendous plight of actual human beings in the Holocaust who possessed distinctive names, identities, and personalities. Furthermore, contemporary proponents of physician-assisted suicide and euthanasia typically portray their procedures as compassionate acts of caring on behalf of the most seriously afflicted patients, in contrast to the doctors of the Third Reich who perverted medical skills as a means of doing away with disabled human lives considered devoid of value.

But a closer examination of the wording utilized in opposition to making comparisons between what is happening today and what occurred in Nazi Germany reveals the widespread existence of a highly biased lexicon in which euphemistic rhetoric and degrading concepts are designed to conceal the reality of killing today's unwanted unborn and vulnerable born, while forthright terminology is relied upon to expose the actuality of exterminating victims in the Holocaust. This book will challenge such diverse uses of language by revealing the extensive similarities between medical-induced destruction now and in times past, many of which have been rarely touched upon, let alone examined in depth. Such an approach is in close accord with prolific author Rabbi Jacob Neusner's characterization of "mass abortion" in contemporary Israel as comparable to the "mass murder of Jewish children in Hitler's Germany" facilitated by the definition of abortion as "a perfectly ordinary medical procedure" constituting the removal of "mere protoplasm."[3]

Immersing oneself in the literature of past and current medical-induced destruction is an especially sobering and eye-opening experience replete with profoundly disturbing revelations. What emerges with striking clarity and persistence is a multitude of legitimate comparisons between medical killing in the Third Reich and medical killing in contemporary society. And even more alarming, the horrendous practices uncovered are, for the most part, not the creation of incompetent butchers who *accidentally* kill their patients because of surgical errors or slipshod procedures, but rather the handiwork of skilled practitioners who *deliberately* and *proficiently* destroy unwanted human beings before and after birth.

After having remained silent for more than six decades following the end of World War II, the German Medical Association, on May 23, 2012, finally issued a public acknowledgment of and an apology for the significant role that "outstanding representatives of renowned academic medical and research institutes" played in organizing and carrying out the Holocust.[4] Equally prominent medical practitioners and scientists today are continuing the legacy of medicalized destruction against unborn and born human lives within American and international hospitals and university medical centers.

A prime ingredient underlying the killing in the Third Reich and

in today's world is the horrendous nature of the destructive procedures employed. Mutilation and chemical asphyxiation comprised
some of the methods utilized to carry out the wholesale destruction
of European Jews and others. Even contemporary proponents of experimenting on the doomed unborn—Drs. Willard Gaylin and Marc
Lappe—provided a similar characterization of abortion procedures as
"unimaginable acts of violence" that "subject the fetus to dismemberment, salt-osmotic shock or surgical extirpation."[5]

An additional characteristic common to Nazi Germany and today's society is the enormous scope of the destruction process. During
the twelve years of the Third Reich, the Holocaust consumed some six
million Jews, five million non-Jews, more than 275,000 people afflicted with disabilities, and countless numbers of unborn discards. Ever
since the US Supreme Court legalized abortion in 1973, more than sixty million unborn lives have been extinguished in America alone.

Some leading abortion proponents are nonetheless dissatisfied
with the numerical output; they actually believe the figures should be
higher! As far back as 1975, a prominent compiler of abortion statis-
tics, Dr. Christopher Tietze, lamented, "The shocking fact is that …
most of the unmet abortion needs end up in the cradle."[6] The latest
proliferation of Planned Parenthood mega abortion centers built adjacent to low-income communities are intended to take up the slack
by fulfilling what are considered the perennial unmet abortion needs,
particularly among poor and ethnic minority groups.

Another central feature of past and present programs of destruction involves abolition of the word "kill" and the transformation of
killing into a minor medical procedure performed on victims perceived as nothing more significant than indiscriminate masses of
subhuman expendables. Today, increasing numbers of individuals are
being defined as less than human and devoid of value and respect.
Once any group, born or unborn, is deemed unworthy of the designation human, the pernicious precedent is established for declaring
them stateless and bereft of human rights, including the most basic
right, that of life itself.

Although the preponderance of findings in this study is taken up with focusing on these and other parallels between medicalized killing in Nazi Germany and in today's world, they are not confined to these two periods. Some substantial comparisons will also be derived from the early through the middle decades of twentieth-century America, a time when the medical advocacy of abortion, assisted suicide, and euthanasia was already underway, helped along by a growing eugenics movement funded by wealthy corporations such as the Rockefeller Foundation and the Carnegie Institute.[7]

Part I, "The Technology of Exterminative Medicine," examines the technological factors powering the medicalization of destruction, past and present. Chapter 1 focuses on unvarnished accounts of surgical mutilation, poisonous gases, toxic chemicals, imposed starvation and dehydration, lethal injections, and deadly pills as the major methods of extermination resorted to during the Third Reich and in contemporary society. The emphasis in chapter 2 is on the medical perpetrators' unwavering commitment to perfecting procedures that destroy quickly, proficiently, and decisively. Chapter 3 discloses the protocols instituted for averting destructive technology's most dreaded complication: the presence of temporary survivors. Chapter 4 analyzes the techniques employed in erasing the evidence of extermination through disposal of the victims' remains in huge ditches, crematoriums, incinerators, body grinding devices, and garbage receptacles. Chapter 5 explores the psychological responses relied upon to justify participation in the destruction process, ranging from temporary discomfort to emotional detachment to a sense of professional pride. The focus in chapter 6 is on a range of experimental procedures imposed on the doomed subjects before, during, and after their demise. Chapter 7 examines the establishment of antiseptic medical fronts for covering up the dirty work of medicalized killing.

The long-standing dictum—when war comes, the first casualty is the truth—functions as a basic precept underpinning part II, "Rhetoric in the Service of Medical Mayhem," which highlights the quality-of-life ideology generating the corruption of language and thought so instrumental in advancing historical and contemporary assaults on undesired human lives inside and outside the womb.

Chapter 8 stresses how the dogma of human inequality furnishes the overriding ideological justification for doing away with individuals who fail to meet increasingly elitist criteria of worth. Chapter 9 highlights a 1970 California Medical Association editorial that proposed a linguistic strategy of lying dubbed *semantic gymnastics* (defining the victims as *something other than human* and what is done to them as *something other than killing*) for promoting abortion, euthanasia, and other assaults on human life put forth under the "socially impeccable auspices" of organized medicine.[8]

The remaining chapters in part II reveal how the strategy of semantic gymnastics spawned by the lives-not-worth-living creed has resulted in a litany of dehumanizing and benign expressions for expediting the perpetration of both historical and contemporary forms of medicalized killing. Chapter 10 draws attention to the relegation of victims to the degrading designations "subhuman," "nonperson," "lower animal," "parasite," "vegetative existence," "waste matter," and "research material and specimens." The major concern of chapter 11 stresses the transformation of killing into mainstream medical procedures under the guise of such clinical sounding classifications as "treatments," "procedures," and "operations" performed on victims reduced to "disease entities." Chapter 12 accentuates the freedom-laden and autonomy-ridden slogans "choice" and "selection" designed to obscure what specifically is chosen or selected: the destruction of unwanted human lives. Chapter 13 indicates how the rhetoric of evacuation camouflaged racial genocide as "the evacuation of Jews to the East" and masks contemporary feticide as "the evacuation of products from the womb." Chapter 14 concentrates on the widespread portrayals of past and present perpetrators as decent practitioners who endow their destructive procedures with the utmost benevolence.

The book's final section—part III, "Challenging Destructive Medical Rhetoric"—presents some resolutions for overcoming killing in the name of healing. Chapter 15 underscores the formidable power of graphic verbal and pictorial images for challenging the Nazi media's blackout on the Holocaust atrocities and the contemporary mainstream media's attempts to obscure today's medical destruction of millions before birth. In chapter 16, the radical contradiction uncovered between the nineteenth-century crusade against abortion, led by physicians of the American Medical Association (AMA), and the current AMA policy in support of abortion reveals a dire need for waging a revitalized doctors' campaign against killing. Chapter 17 probes the significance of the Hippocratic Oath, the assaults on its do-no-harm and sanctity-of-life provisions by Nazi doctors and contemporary medical practitioners, and a movement among some medical groups to restore its healing ethic as an indispensable philosophical foundation for waging a long-overdue physicians' campaign against all forms of killing before and after birth.

The findings in this study are based on a diverse array of sources, including correspondence, memoranda, and conference notes compiled by medical and nonmedical perpetrators; war crimes trials testimony and documents; concentration camp survivors' accounts; medical policy statements; media coverage; books on various facets of past and present destruction processes; contemporary judicial decisions on abortion, physician-assisted suicide, and euthanasia; and material on bioethical issues published in medical, legal, philosophical, sociological, and bioethical journals. A segment at the end of chapter 15 comparing photos of Holocaust and contemporary aborted unborn victims illustrates how some of history's most horrific atrocities are being directed against today's least visible and most vulnerable individuals. All of the other chapters in the book conclude with tables summarizing the main parallels linking the destructive practices and semantics of the past with those of the present.

The reader of this book needs to be cognizant of the fact that making connections between medicalized killing today and during the Third Reich is likely to result in considerable opposition, especially from those who view the Nazi extermination of Jews and others deemed unworthy lives as so barbaric and unconscionable that it cannot possibly be comparable to any other atrocity. And anyone who dares make such comparisons is viewed as harboring the most extreme form of anti-Semitism. All the more reason for the reader to avoid presenting today's medical assaults as constituting a full-scale holocaust exactly comparable to everything the Nazi doctors did to their victims. Nevertheless, the linkages made in this book between medicalized extermination now and in the Third Reich are numerous, perfectly valid, and backed up by solid documentation.

PART I

THE TECHNOLOGY
OF EXTERMINATIVE
MEDICINE

CHAPTER 1

The Methods of Medicalized Killing

Nazi doctors pioneered the perversion of medicine for malevolent purposes on a massive scale. In a radical reversal of their professional role as healers, they distorted the very skills and instruments on behalf of patients as a means of exterminating Jews, Gypsies, handicapped people, and other lives deemed not worth living residing in concentrations camps, euthanasia institutions, nursing homes, hospitals, and children's institutions. Some contemporary physicians are continuing this same legacy, the main difference being that it is now directed primarily against the unwanted unborn, but it has also spilled over to engulf increasing numbers of vulnerable individuals in the postnatal phases, especially infants born with disabilities and cognitively impaired adults. Doctors of both eras have developed a comparable array of destructive procedures against their respective victims, including surgical mutilation, poisonous substances, imposed starvation and dehydration, lethal injections, and deadly pills.

Surgical Mutilation

Although not employed as often as mass gassing, the Nazis resorted to dismemberment as one of their most sadistic methods of extermination. Upon liberation of the concentration camps in 1944 and 1945, the allied forces came across numerous scenes of mutilated corpses. At the Maidanek camp, a correspondent reported on the existence of "mass graves containing the mutilated bodies of men, women, and children."[1] Another account featured the sight of broken bodies, strangled women, and mutilated prisoners encountered at the Maidanek and Auschwitz camps.[2] German villagers who were forced to tour Buchenwald viewed exhibits of lampshades derived from "tattooed human skin" and "shrunken heads [used] as trophies and paperweights."[3]

Female Polish prisoners at the Ravensbrueck concentration camp were subjected to a series of barbaric operations in which they were partially dismembered. Before the Nuremberg War Crimes Trials Court in 1947, Dr. Zdenka Nedvedova-Nejedla, a physician prisoner who survived Ravensbrueck, furnished an eyewitness account of the mutilating operations. "Parts of long bones, as much as 5 centimeters (fibulae and tibiae), were removed and in some cases replaced by metal or left without connection," she testified. "High amputations were performed; for example, even whole arms with shoulder blade or legs with osiliaca were amputated. These operations were performed mostly on insane women who were immediately killed after the operation by a quick injection of evipan."[4]

Additional information on the dismembering process was furnished by another Ravensbrueck survivor, Dr. Sofia Maczka:

The following were carried out: (a) bone breaking; (b) bone transplantation; and (c) bone grafting:
a. On the operating table, the bones of the lower part of both legs were broke into several pieces with a hammer, later they were joined with clips or without clips and were put into a plaster case....
b. The transplantations were carried out in the usual way, except that whole pieces of the fibula were cut out, sometimes with periosteum, sometimes without periosteum....
c. Bone grafting.... During the preparatory operation two bone splints were put on the tibia of both legs; during the second operation such bone splints were cut out together with the attached bones.[5]

Gustawa Winowska, who survived several mutilating operations, recalled an incident involving a healthy young Ukrainian woman who was forcefully taken to the Ravensbrueck operating room, "where one of her healthy legs was amputated" and "later on was given a lethal

injection." Winowska also remembered that "under similar circumstances another Ukrainian girl had her arm and shoulder girdle removed. She was also killed by injections."[6]

Today, dismemberment is the most frequently utilized method for
destroying the unwanted unborn. This destructive procedure involves
mutilating the preborn human inside the uterus and then removing
the dismembered body parts with sharp instruments or through the
force of a suction machine.

Dr. Richard Ough, who stopped performing abortions in 1975, provided revealing details about the dismemberment process associated
with the performance of the D&C (dilation and curettage) procedure:
"Under direction from a senior colleague, I dismembered the living
foetus, and with my instruments extracted the tiny parts—arms, legs,
torso and finally the head, which came out reluctantly, as its firm
roundness tended to slip from the forceps' grasp. The patient had
scarcely missed her second period, yet the tiny feet and hands were
almost perfectly formed."[7]

D&E (dilation and evacuation) has emerged as the method of
choice for abortions performed in the second and third trimester. It
employs the same tools of disintegration used in early abortions—
sharp-edged instruments, forceps, and suction curettes—but they
need to be larger and more powerful in order to carry out the task
of mutilating the bodies of bigger and studier victims. In D&E, the
abortionist inserts the forceps into the uterus, grasps an arm, a leg, or
other body part, and, with a twisting motion, rips it from the unborn
human's body and yanks it out of the womb. This is repeated until all
of the mangled body parts are removed.

During the proceedings of a 2004 abortion case held in the federal
court of New York, Dr. Timothy Johnson, a University of Michigan
Medical School professor, furnished a detailed description of the challenge involved in extracting from the womb a fetal head that becomes
severed during the D&E abortion dismemberment process:

> So one of the common technical challenges of a dismemberment
> D&E is what is called a free-floating head or a head that becomes
> disattached and needs to be removed.... In the situations that I have

observed ... they [the physicians] all used a crushing instrument to deliver the head, and they did it under direct observation.[8]

After listening to this rendition, presiding jurist Richard C. Casey decided it was an opportune moment to ask Dr. Johnson some additional questions about the crushing instruments used to remove the amputated head:

> THE COURT [JUDGE CASEY]: What did they utilize to crush the head?
>
> THE WITNESS: An instrument, a large pair of forceps that have a round, serrated edge at the end of it, so that they were able to bring them together and crush the head between the ends of the instrument.
>
> THE COURT: Like the cracker they use to crack a lobster shell, serrated edge?
>
> THE WITNESS: No.
>
> THE COURT: Describe it for me.
>
> THE WITNESS: It would be like the end of tongs that ... you use to pick up salad.... The instruments are thick enough and heavy enough that you can actually grasp and crush with those instruments as if you were picking up salad or picking up anything with—
>
> THE COURT: Except here you are crushing the head of a baby.
>
> THE WITNESS: Correct.[9]

Soon after the death of former abortionist Dr. Ulrich Klopfer on September 4, 2019, authorities found 2,246 medically preserved remains of aborted babies at his home in Illinois. By the middle of October, an investigation by the Will County Sheriff's Office revealed the discovery of additional numerous fetal remains stored in an outdoor gated lot owned by Dr. Klopfer. Dr. Geoffrey Cly, who knew Klopfer, speculated that he kept the babies' remains as some sort of grisly trophy.[10]

Poisoning the Environment

Asphyxiating individuals with lethal chemicals became the premier method for doing away with the expendables of the Third Reich. The first gas chambers were used to exterminate German mentally ill and handicapped patients in six euthanasia institutions: Bernburg, Brandenburg, Grafeneck, Hadamar, Hartheim, and Sonnenstein. Doctors served as the technical executioners for the entire gassing process. According to instructions issued by euthanasia administrators Dr. Karl Brandt and Victor Brack, only doctors were allowed to turn on the gas tap, releasing the deadly flow of carbon monoxide. Dr. Johann Paul Kremer testified that "all SS doctors in the camp health service took part in these gassings, each in his turn."[11]

Mass gassing was transported to the Nazi-occupied eastern territories for the more monumental task of racial genocide. Special gas vans holding as many as one hundred victims were constructed to exterminate Jews, Gypsies, and Russians after the German army invaded the Soviet Union in June 1941. Carbon monoxide from engine exhausts was directed to the interiors of the vans, which were crammed with victims. Dr. Zalman Levinbuck, a survivor of the Minsk ghetto, furnished details about how the gas vans operated: "They were poisoned on the way with gas and exhaust fumes, which resulted from the combustion of gasoline in the engine. These exhaust fumes were introduced into the van through a special hose, instead of being released into the air as is normal, and so people were killed by the carbon monoxide."[12]

Personnel with experience in the construction and management of the euthanasia gassing facilities were sent to eastern Poland, where their expertise was put to use in building stationery gas chambers on the grounds of concentration camps. From 1942 to 1943 at the Maidanek concentration camp, "The carbon monoxide, which was in steel bottles, was introduced through a system of ducts leading from an anteroom located in front of one of the small gas chambers. From this anteroom the gas flow was regulated by means of a hand-operated valve, and the gassing process could be observed without danger through a little window in the wall."[13]

Josef Kramer, commander of the Natzweiler-Struthof death camp, concocted a solution of water mixed with salts to asphyxiate female inmates in the gas chamber. In testimony during the Nuremberg Doctors' Trial, he explained how he carried out this procedure:

> I told these women that they were going into a disinfection room, without letting them know that they were going to be asphyxiated.... As soon as the door was closed, they started to scream. Once I had closed the door, I placed a fixed quantity of the salts in a funnel attached below and to the right of the peephole. At the same time I poured in a fixed amount of water, which flowed, mixed with the salts, into a pit made inside the gas chamber under the peephole....
>
> I illuminated the chamber's interior by means of a switch located near the funnel, and I observed what was happening inside the chamber through the outside peephole.... I found the women stretched out lifeless in their excrement.[14]

One of the major contemporary methods developed to destroy humans before birth during the middle trimester of pregnancy and later—the instillation of a poisonous saline solution or sodium chloride (mixture of salt and water) into the amniotic sac enclosing the unborn victim—possesses some destructive qualities in common with the infusion of poisonous gas and other toxic solutions into the chambers enclosing the Nazi victims. The saline profoundly contaminates the intrauterine environment, leading to severe salt poisoning, shock, and death. Thus the uterus—once considered a sanctuary exquisitely suited for nurturance, growth, and development—is transformed into a type of death chamber polluted by the invasion of lethal substances that defy the most fundamental laws of ecology and humanity.

A study designed "to assess the morphologic effects of hypertonic saline solution on the fetus in the hope of gaining an insight into the actual mechanism of death" was conducted during autopsies performed on 143 fetal bodies aborted by saline at the Columbia University College of Physicians and Surgeons. The researchers compared their findings on "severe fetal dehydration" to "those described in acute salt poisoning of infants":

> Finally the possibility must be considered that fetal shock may actually constitute the most important intermediary mechanism of fetal death during saline abortion, as well as in other instances of acute salt poisoning....
>
> In conclusion, the evidence suggests that the infusion of hypertonic saline solutions into the amniotic cavity directly results in

acute salt poisoning of the fetus. Development of fetal hypertonicity (hypernatremia) leads to widespread vasodilatation, edema, congestion, hemorrhage, shock, and death.[15]

A preliminary hearing before a California municipal court on April 18, 1977, was conducted to determine whether there was sufficient evidence to bring abortionist Dr. William Waddill to trial for the strangulation death of a newborn girl who survived a saline abortion. In the process of trying to impress upon the court that it was the saline that killed the baby and not him, Dr. Waddill furnished unusually frank observations about the lethal impact of saline:

> Hypertonic saline causes tremendous basal dilatation of the blood vessels. In other words, the vessels just dilate and just stay dilated and with the extreme dehydration that occurs throughout the baby through the lungs, the gastrointestinal tract, the kidneys, through the vasculature, the cardiovascular system inside the baby, and the blood vessels of the baby, the brain is, I'm sure, destroyed from lack of blood supply.... It is such a caustic and tremendously bad and hostile environment for the baby that it just creates an enormous destructive process.[16]

Carbon monoxide poisoning is not just a relic of the past confined to the Nazi extermination process; it also comprised a central component of Dr. Jack Kevorkian's serial assisted-suicide spree that claimed some 130 individuals during the 1990s. His suicide machine, dubbed "the mercitron," functioned as a device for releasing the lethal gas. A partial description of its operation was posted on the Internet: "Carbon Monoxide: 1. A cylinder of the deadly gas is connected by a tube over the person's nose and mouth. 2. A valve must be released to start the gas flowing."[17]

Imposed Starvation and Dehydration

Enforced starvation became a prime method of killing in the Nazi euthanasia program after the discontinuation of gassing. One of the earliest programs of mass starvation took place at the Eglfing-Harr state hospital, where starvation diets were imposed on "useless eaters" (patients with disabilities and individuals incapable of engaging in productive work). Those subjected to these diets were isolated in dwellings that became known as "hunger houses." Eglfing-Harr director Dr. Hermann Pfannmueller was so totally committed to this method of extermination that several times a week he tasted the "food" to make sure no unauthorized protein supplements had been added: "We'll keep them without fats or proteins and then they'll die of their own accord."[18]

By November 17, 1942, at a conference held in the Ministry of the Interior in Munich, the heads of Bavarian asylums met to consider the implementation of a "special diet" for certain categories of patients. According to a conference participant, Kaufbeuren-Irsee Asylum director Dr. Valentin Faltlhauser promoted a gradual starvation diet: "Those patients who were incapable of working, or hopeless cases, would be given a fat-free diet, consisting for example of vegetables cooked in water. The effect would be the slow onset of death after a period of about three months."[19]

The children of foreign workers under Nazi rule deemed unfit were likewise subjected to death by gradual starvation. They were dispatched to a network of homes where they expired on a starvation diet. An inspector's report on one such institution revealed that "the home receives only a pint of milk and a piece and a half of sugar per day per baby. With these rations the babies are sure to die of malnutrition in a few months."[20]

At the Auschwitz extermination camp, death by starvation and dehydration was a daily occurrence. Prisoner survivor Dr. Miklos Nyiszli recalled the plight of the "living-dead" upon admission to the camp hospital: "For the most part they were living skeletons: dehydrated, emaciated, their lips were cracked, their faces swollen.... Within a few days their already weakened organisms had disintegrated entirely.... Fifty or sixty deaths a day was normal. Their last days were spent in indescribable suffering."[21]

Imposed starvation and dehydration—especially withholding or withdrawing nutrition and hydration from cognitively disabled patients—is also becoming a standard component of today's mainstream medicine. One of the most highly publicized cases of enforced starvation involved "Infant Doe," a boy born on April 9, 1982, in a Bloomington, Indiana, hospital. The child had two afflictions, Down syndrome and a malformed esophagus, which prevented food from reaching the stomach. His parents denied permission for the life-saving surgery and for intravenous feeding. A "Do Not Feed" sign was taped on the infant's crib. Two days later, stomach acids began corroding his lungs, and he started spitting blood. When the hospital nurses threatened to walk out, he was transferred to another part of the hospital, and private-duty nurses were hired to keep the death watch. It took him six days to expire. An attorney involved in trying to save the child reported that Infant Doe cried uncontrollably during the last four days of his life.[22]

The following year, an article published in *Pediatrics*, the journal of the American Academy of Pediatrics, disclosed that over a five-year period (1977-82) twenty-four infants born with spina bifida at the Oklahoma Children's Memorial Hospital were denied life-sustaining treatment and nourishment. In a manner echoing the plight of victims in the Third Reich who starved to death in "hunger houses" and other facilities, "all 24 babies" were placed in "a children's shelter" where "the age of death has ranged from 1 to 189 days, with a mean of 37 days."[23] Nurses and aides who worked at this "intermediate nursing care facility" called it an "overcrowded ... unsanitary ... charnel house."[24]

A variation on the contemporary practice of imposed starvation and dehydration—the removal of feeding tubes from adults with disabilities—was supported by a 1986 American Medical Association policy sanctioning the withdrawal of nutrition and hydration from comatose or terminal patients.[25] The best-known case of this type is that of Terri Schiavo, who on the morning of March 31, 2005, succumbed to imposed starvation and dehydration in a Florida hospice almost two weeks after her feeding tube had been removed. Terri's brother, Bobby Schindler, recalled his sister's horrific condition on the night before she died:

The sight of Terri was awful. Her skin was discolored, and there was
blood pooling in her eyes, which were darting wildly back and forth.
Her cheeks were hollowed out, and her teeth were protruding. She
looked like a skeleton from a horror movie.[26]

Lethal Injections

Lethal injections were often resorted to as another means of killing concentration camp victims. Buchenwald survivor Eugen Kogon
testified regarding Dr. Waldemar Hoven's method of doing away with
inmates he considered dangerous—"Air was injected into the heart so
that air embolisms occurred."[27]

Injections in the heart became a mainstay for killing twins at
Auschwitz. According to a deposition submitted by prisoner pathologist Dr. Miklos Nyiszli, Dr. Josef Mengele "felt for the left ventricle
of the heart and injected 10 c.c. of chloroform. After one little twitch
the child was dead.... In this manner, all fourteen twins were killed
during the night."[28]

Auschwitz medical orderly Josef Klehr performed many intracardiac injections of phenol in a medically impeccable fashion. At the
Auschwitz Trial in 1964, he testified that because their veins were hard
to find, "the phenol was injected directly into the hearts of the prisoners." Klehr introduced several ways of making the cardiac area more
readily accessible by having the victims raise their left arms and place
their hands over their mouths "so he could get to the heart and inject
without difficulty."[29]

Prisoner survivor Dr. Czeslaw Glowacki provided the Auschwitz
tribunal with details about the more than one hundred children from
the Polish city of Zamosc who were killed by phenol injections administered directly into their hearts. He stated that "when the children of
Zamosc put their thin arms across their mouths, the poison needle
jabbed between their skinny ribs, and they fell down like cut blades
of grass and were dragged out to the other victims, to make room for
those who were still playing outside."[30]

Today's physician abortionists have come up with needle-admin-
istered destructive procedures that bear a disquieting resemblance

to the intracardiac injections of the Third Reich. In June 1981, Mount Sinai School of Medicine (New York) faculty members Drs. Thomas Kerenyi and Usha Chitkara announced they had pierced the heart and drained out almost half the blood from an unwanted unborn twin with Down syndrome. In what was heralded as an extremely challenging technological accomplishment, "the needle had to hit a moving target [the heart] less than an inch across." An ultrasound scan and a videotape helped increase "the chance that they had found the right target [the abnormal twin]."[31] This procedure—closely resembling a precision military action against an enemy—was hailed as a scientific breakthrough and "a very gratifying experience."[32]

Unusually candid testimony on the medicalized killing of the unborn with lethal intracardiac injections was presented at an abortion case heard in 2004 in California. During the questioning, Planned Parenthood medical director and University of California, San Diego, clinical faculty member Dr. Katharine Sheehan was asked whether she ever used "a chemical agent to cause fetal demise." She replied, "We administer the digoxin with a needle" and "We are aiming to get it into the fetal heart, or at least into the fetal thorax."[33]

American physician abortionists have also come up with a counterpart to the deadly air embolisms produced by the injection of air into the hearts of Buchenwald concentration camp inmates. Dr. Mitchell Goldbus and colleagues at the University of California, San Francisco, Medical Center employed "cardiac puncture with air embolization" (placement of a needle into the fetal heart followed by the rapid injection of air) as one of the techniques for the "selective termination of multiple gestations." According to this protocol, "a 20 gauge needle was sonographically guided into the fetal heart ... and then air was injected rapidly through a sterile millipore filter directly into a cardiac cavity."[34]

The injection of deadly substances into the heart is a method of medicalized killing not confined to unborn children but has expanded to engulf vulnerable victims after birth. By 1998, Dr. Jack Kevorkian moved beyond assisting the patient in administering poisonous solutions when he directly injected Thomas Youk, a fifty-two-year-old man suffering from Lou Gehrig's disease, with lethal chemicals. His videotape of this destruction process was featured on November 21, 1998, on the CBS News program *60 Minutes* for the purpose of challenging the law against physician-induced euthanasia. The tape shows Kevorkian administering Seconal for inducing sleep and a muscle relaxant to "paralyze the muscles" so that Youk could no longer breathe. The climax occurred when Kevorkian told host Michael Wallace, "Now I'll quickly inject potassium chloride to stop the heart," and he then pointed out that a straight line on the cardiogram indicates "the heart is stopped."[35]

A 2002 study titled *Angels of Death* uncovered the existence of a euthanasia underground of health professionals who provided revelations about the methods devised for killing their patients, one of the most prominent being injections of deadly substances. Russell, a doctor who worked in a hospital unit with a widely shared "intention to hasten death," indicated that the main method employed was overdoses of intravenous narcotics. A community nurse acknowledged he had injected air into a patient's veins. A "cosmopolitan and cappuccino-drinking" doctor named Gary said with a bizarre theatrical flair, "*At high noon*, I just went around [and] ... I just injected him."[36]

Deadly Pills

In addition to fatal injections, another method of killing utilized in the Third Reich consisted of administering death-inducing medication in the form of tablets and pills to patients. At the Hadamar Euthanasia Trial, Hadamar medical director Dr. Adolf Wahlmann testified he "had to hand out medications" to his chief nurses and emphasized, "That was my task, and without medications death would not have set in."[37]

Hadamar chief nurse Heinrich Ruoff identified lethal overdoses of chloral hydrate in tablet form as one of the main regimens applied to bring about many of the patients' deaths. "Concerning the tablets," Ruoff testified, "we had a large amount of those. They were in the house pharmacy, and one could get from it what one needed." He claimed that tablets, rather than injections, constituted the most frequently applied method of "putting aside [killing]" patients. "We mostly gave tablets, and it was only in those cases when some of them did not want to take the tablets because they were bitter that we gave injections.... We did quite a bit of work with tablets."[38]

Killing vulnerable human beings with deadly pills and tablets did not go away with the fall of the Third Reich; instead, it has become embedded in contemporary mainstream medical practice as a prime method for destroying the unborn early in pregnancy (principally during the first forty-nine to sixty-three days of gestation). An extensively employed drug is the abortion drug RU 486, a two-pill combination that initiates a complex destruction process and works its deadly effects over an extended period of three office visits. During the first visit, the woman is "handed three mifepristone [the generic name for RU 486] tablets." This powerful synthetic drug blocks the action of progesterone, the hormone responsible for maintaining the uterine environment protective of early pregnancy, and thus deprives the unborn human of essential life-sustaining nourishment by breaking down the uterine lining. On the second office visit two days later, the woman ingests the prostaglandin misoprostol to stimulate uterine contractions that expel the emaciated, shriveled body of the dying or dead individual. A third office visit a week later is required to confirm the completion of the abortion.[39]

Another lethal drug combination directed against the unborn in the early stages of development involves the use of methotrexate and misoprostol. Methotrexate—a highly toxic medication that has been in use since the early 1950s to treat cancer and severe cases of arthritis and psoriasis—is administered intramuscularly in the abortion doctor's office. It acts to destroy the proliferating tissue (trophoblast) surrounding and providing nourishment to the developing human in utero. Three to seven days later, the misoprostol tablets are self-administered orally or vaginally for the purpose of expelling the emaciated victim within. After another week, a follow-up ultrasonic examination is conducted to make sure that all the components associated with pregnancy are ejected from the womb. New York Mount Sinai School of Medicine gynecologist abortionist Dr. Richard Hausknecht claimed credit for employing the methotrexate-misoprostol protocol in successfully aborting 171 of 178 women up to sixty-three days of gestation.[40]

The uterus—once considered a private sanctuary suited for nurturance, growth, and development—has been transformed into a deadly environment polluted beyond belief by the invasion of lethal instruments and substances that defy the most fundamental laws of ecology and humanity.

Table 1 highlights the close similarities between some of the destructive medical procedures perpetrated in the Third Reich and those performed in contemporary American society.

TABLE 1. DESTRUCTIVE MEDICAL PROCEDURES

The Third Reich	The United States
SURGICAL MUTILATION	
"High amputations were performed ... even whole arms with shoulder blade or legs ... were amputated."	"I dismembered the living foetus, and with my instruments extracted the tiny parts—arms, legs, torso and finally the head."
(Affidavit of Ravensbrueck concentration camp survivor Dr. Zdenka Nedvedova-Nejedla, 1946)	*(Description of D&C abortion by Dr. Richard Ough, who no longer performs abortions, 1975)*
"Mass graves containing the mutilated bodies of men, women, and children" and "shrunken heads [used] as trophies."	"Authorities find more bodies of aborted babies on property of abortionist who kept 2,246 as trophies."
(Accounts of dismembered victims compiled during the allied liberation of the Nazi concentration camps, 1944–45)	*(The discovery of dismembered aborted remains preserved by Dr. Ulrich Klopfer, October 2019)*
POISONING THE ENVIRONMENT	
"They were poisoned on the way with gas and exhaust fumes, which resulted from the combustion of gasoline in the engine."	"The infusion of hypertonic saline solutions into the amniotic cavity results in acute salt poisoning of the fetus."
(Ghetto survivor Dr. Zalman Levinbuck on the asphyxiation of victims in gas vans, 1942)	*(Columbia University physicians' findings on the effects of saline abortions, 1974)*
"The carbon monoxide, which was in steel bottles, was introduced through a system of ducts" and "the gas flow was regulated by means of a hand-operated valve."	"Carbon monoxide: 1. A cylinder of the deadly gas is connected to a mask over the person's nose and mouth. 2. A valve must be released to keep the gas flowing."
(Maidenek concentration camp gas chamber, 1942–1943)	*(Dr. Jack Kevorkian's assisted suicide device, 1990s)*
IMPOSED STARVATION AND DEHYDRATION	
"With these rations the babies are sure to die of malnutrition in a few months."	"The age at death has ranged from 1 to 189 days, with a mean of 37 days."
(Inspector's report on the fate of "unfit" children subjected to starvation, 1944)	*(The fate of "disabled" children denied nourishment, 1977-82)*
"They were living skeletons: dehydrated, emaciated, their lips were cracked, their faces swollen."	"Her cheeks were hallowed out, and her teeth were protruding. She looked like a skeleton from a horror movie."
(Auschwitz survivor Dr. Miklos Nyiszli's characterization of concentration camp victims, 1944–45)	*(Bobby Schindler's portrayal of sister Terri Schiavo's condition on the night before her death, 2005)*
LETHAL INJECTIONS	
"Air was injected into the heart so that air embolisms occurred."	"Air was injected rapidly ... [and] directly into a cardiac cavity."
(The killing of Buchenwald inmates, 1943–44)	*(The killing of unborn humans, 1988)*
"The phenol was injected directly into the hearts of the prisoners."	"Now I'll quickly inject potassium chloride to stop the heart."
(Auschwitz medical orderly Josef Klehr's method, 1943)	*(Dr. Jack Kevorkian's euthanasia procedure, 1998)*
"He felt for ... the heart and injected 10 cc."	"We are aiming to get it into the fetal heart."
(Dr. Josef Mengele's chloroform injection of twins at Auschwitz, 1945)	*(Dr. Katharine Sheehan's description of the digoxin injection abortion procedure, 2004)*
DEADLY PILLS	
"We mostly gave tablets.... We did quite a bit of work with tablets."	The woman "is handed three mifepristone tablets."
(Fatal doses of chloral hydrate pills administered to Hadamar patients, 1944–45)	*(RU 486 pills for aborting unborn humans during the first trimester of pregnancy, 1994)*

CHAPTER 2

Advances in Medicalized
Killing Proficiency

The mass extermination of human lives is a formidable project requiring destructive procedures up to the task of doing away with huge
numbers of individuals. Extensive participation of physicians, other
health professionals, and scientists in a project of such an enormous
magnitude facilitates the creation of measures for killing the victims
in a rapid, proficient, and conclusive manner while keeping their
plight hidden from public and sometimes even perpetrator view. An
additional component enhancing medicalized killing occurs when the
destructive procedures are defined as part of a natural process. All of
these factors constituted the technological hallmarks of large-scale extermination in the Third Reich. Today, they facilitate the wholesale destruction of the unwanted unborn and the growing assaults on those
declared expendable after birth.

Fatality of the Dosage Levels

An overriding matter extensively researched by the Nazi doctors
involved determining the amount of destructive substances required
to end the lives of the victims. Hadamar Hospital Trial defendants
furnished detailed information about the lethal dosages of morphine
and scopolamine administered to patients. Nurse Heinrich Ruoff asserted, "You have to judge that from the person. The smallest dose

was 2 ½ to 3 c.c. for children, up to 8 to 10 c.c. for adults."[1] Hadamar's chief physician, Adolf Wahlmann, testified about the maximum dosage necessary to bring about death: "If I have a very strong person, then I have to use more. If I have a person who is used to morphine, then I have to use very much. If I have a very weak person, then I need very little."[2]

When Dr. Herman Pfannmueller, former director of the Eglfing-Haar state hospital, was asked at the Nuremberg Doctors' Trial about how much luminal was used to administer "a mercy death" to sick people at his institution, he responded in a manner similar to that of Dr. Wahlmann:

> It varied greatly.... The maximum doses are arranged according to age. It is prescribed that for children up to a certain age we give a dose of luminal which is one-third as small as in the case of adults.... These maximum doses ... vary greatly and are always being revised.[3]

Doctors at Auschwitz developed a deadly recipe—an intracardiac injection of phenol—for the disposing of prisoners: "The injection (8 to 15 grams of phenol in 10 to 15 milligrams of concentrated water solution), administered by a long puncturing needle into the heart, caused death."[4] Regarding "the composition of the phenol injection" applied to kill the Buchenwald concentration camp victims, Dr. Erwin Ding told the Nuremberg tribunal that "as far as I can remember, it consisted of undiluted raw phenol, which was to be administered in doses of 20 cc." While only 5 cc's of phenol were usually sufficient to result in a deadly effect, 20 cc's were injected to maximize a fatal outcome. "The rest of the dose was injected as a precautionary measure," explained Dr. Ding, "although part of the injection would have been enough for the fatal result (I estimate 5 cc.)."[5]

Today's physician abortionists are likewise dedicated to developing the optimal dosage levels of poisonous solutions for doing away with the unwanted unborn. Contemporary medical journals are replete with detailed data on the comparative effectiveness of various amounts of saline, potassium chloride, digoxin, and other destructive substances to bring about the fatal effects. After a review of the medical literature and a detailed assessment of 143 saline abortions,

Dr. Robert Galen and colleagues at the Columbia University College of Physicians and Surgeons concluded, "The amounts of sodium chloride administered during most saline abortions far exceed the lethal dosage as far as the fetus is concerned."[6]

An age-related regimen regarding the dosage of potassium chloride needed to destroy the "abnormal twin" detected in eighty-two twin pregnancies was specified by Dr. Yuval Yaron and associates affiliated with the Hutzel Hospital/Wayne State University in Detroit: "A 22-gauge needle was inserted transabdominally and manoeuvred into the fetal thorax. Potassium chloride (KC1) was inserted until cardiac asystole [cessation of heart contractions] was noted for at least one minute. The amount of KC1 required was usually 1 ml; however, at higher gestational stages, a larger amount would most often be needed (as much as 10 ml at 20 weeks)."[7]

Contemporary physician-assisted suicide and euthanasia practitioners have also become exceedingly adept at concocting a wide variety of deadly drug dosages for killing an increasing number and range of individuals after birth. In his *Final Exit: The Practicalities of Self-Deliverance and Assisted Suicide for the Dying*, Hemlock Society founder Derek Humphry includes a chart that rates a series of drugs according to the doses necessary for self-destruction. Nembutal (8 g) is rated "very lethal, the premier drug for self deliverance," while Seconal (8 g) is ranked "extremely lethal" and "close behind Nembutal as the best for self-deliverance." Morphine (200 mg) is considered "extremely lethal provided the patient has not acquired tolerance by previous use." Such drugs as Dalmane (3.0 g), Phenobarbital (4.5 g), and Valium (500 mg or more) are all viewed as "lethal" when used with "a plastic bag."[8]

Rapidity of the Destruction Process

The widespread medicalized destruction of human life perpetrated under the Nazi regime required methods of extermination that killed not only decisively, but also in the shortest time possible. In early January 1940, a demonstration of the relative merits of gassing (carbon monoxide) and lethal injection (morphine and scopolamine) was tested on patients at the former Brandenburg-Havel prison near Berlin, an institution transformed into a euthanasia facility. Gassing proved to be a superior method for destroying larger numbers of people in a shorter time span. Only "after a minute or two,"[9] according to chemist August Becker, did the gas have a fatal impact on the men led into the gas chamber, while those subjected to the lethal injections were "not dying rapidly enough" and therefore were also gassed.

Prominent Nazi hunter Simon Wiesenthal highlighted the preoccupation of medical scientists at the Hartheim euthanasia center with assessing how quickly assorted gassing combinations wreaked their deadly effects:

> Various mixtures of gases were tried out to find the most effective one. Doctors with stopwatches would observe the dying patients through the peephole in the cellar door of Castle Hartheim, and the length of the death struggle was clocked down to one tenth of a second. Slow-motion pictures were made and studied by the experts. Victims' brains were photographed to see exactly when death had occurred. Nothing was left to chance.[10]

The ultimate in rapid mass destruction was achieved at Auschwitz with the more powerful and quicker-acting hydrogen cyanide, also widely known as Zyklon B. Survivor Dr. Miklos Nyszli observed that Zyklon B was dropped into a gas chamber jam-packed with three thousand people, and "within five minutes everybody was dead."[11]

Although gassing in chambers proved to be the quickest method of exterminating huge numbers of victims, the Nazi doctors and their accomplices often resorted to lethal injections as a prime method for the rapid destruction of individuals. Dr. Erwin Ding disclosed that when Dr. Waldemar Hoven injected phenol into the arms of Buchenwald victims, "they died in an immediate total convulsion during the actual injection."[12] Auschwitz phenol technician Josef Klehr became so proficient at the rapid administration of lethal phenol injections that "he injected two prisoners at a time."[13]

On an overall basis, it was in the Nazi death camps where annihilation as a speedy assembly-line enterprise came of age. Holocaust scholar Raul Hilberg concluded, "A man would step off a train in the morning, and in the evening his corpse was burned and his clothes packed away for shipment to Germany."[14]

The rapidity with which the unwanted unborn are destroyed also comprises a dominant technological focus in the contemporary medical literature. This is especially the case regarding first-trimester vacuum aspiration abortion, which dismembers the unborn child by the suction force of a curette (a slender hollow tube) attached to an electric pump and a collecting bottle. A *Chicago Sun-Times* exposé of Chicago abortion clinic operations in the late 1970s profiled Dr. Ming Kow Hah's matchless record of vacuuming the victims to smithereens at a breakneck pace—six to eight abortions per hour, and twenty, thirty, forty per day. His reputation was further enhanced by a report that on several occasions he "performed two abortions simultaneously."[15]

The injection of cardiotoxic substances directly into the hearts of the unborn likewise works its deadly effects quickly. Doctors affiliated with the Mount Sinai Medical Center in New York described cases in which "irreversible cardiac arrest occurred almost immediately after injection of potassium chloride into the fetal heart."[16]

Physician abortionists have even become adept at rapidly performing the late-term, brain-disintegrating, destructive partial-birth abortion procedure. When Planned Parenthood medical officer and ob-gyn clinical professor Dr. Maureen Paul was asked at a 2004 abortion trial about how long it typically took to carry out this process, she replied, "I have had it happen in a minute or two."[17]

For the most part, today's medical perpetrators of assisted suicide and euthanasia prefer a fast-acting lethal drug overdose as the method of choice for targeting vulnerable patients. Those interviewed in Roger Magnusson's study of underground euthanasia practitioners talked freely about how speedily their deadly concoctions worked. Gary, a physician, revealed that a fatal injection he administered simply expedited the dying process: "This took a minute or two; to me that does not seem to be a huge problem since it's hastening things up only a little in the scheme of things." Josh, a general practitioner, discussed the ultra-swift effects of Lethabarb (pentobarbitone), a drug he obtained from a veterinarian: "It actually causes ... cardiac arrest pretty quickly, and certainly causes complete neurological desensitization and death within about a second."[18]

Of all the destructive procedures employed today against individuals before and after birth, the lunch-hour abortion closely epitomizes the rapid, assembly-line process of killing in the Third Reich. Thanks to the "walk-in walk-out" abortion service[19] pioneered by Marie Stopes International in England in 1997, today's "working woman" can enter an abortion clinic on her lunch hour and, by the time she returns to work, all the remains of her unborn baby's body and intra-uterine life support membranes are completely obliterated.

Remoteness of the Victims

The Nazis considered the gassing of human beings in huge permanent chambers the ideal method for mass extermination, not only because of the speed and decisiveness with which it dispatched millions to extinction, but also because of its capacity to conceal the horrendous plight of the victims, therefore rendering them and their fate invisible. They were killed inside the walls of gas chambers where their death agonies could not be seen or identified with. Aside from a technical expert or sadist who peered through a small window to observe how efficiently the machinery of destruction was operating, no one saw anyone being killed. The medical officer who dropped gas canisters into the chambers did not see the deadly impact of his action. Neither did those who herded the victims into the chambers; nor did those who removed the dead bodies out of the chambers. The sights and sounds of men, women, and children being suffocated and trampled to death were hidden behind the thick impenetrable chamber walls.

A plan for the annihilation of Jews and others in the eastern territories was reinforced by relegating them to insignificant and primitive masses. During a 1971 interview conducted with former Treblinka commandant Franz Stangl in his prison cell, a reporter asked him how was it possible to preside over the destruction of almost a million people. He responded, "They were cargo.... It had nothing to do with humanity—it couldn't have; it was a mass—a mass of rotting flesh.... It was always a huge mass."[20]

Like the ordeal of victims herded into gas chambers, the killing of those crammed inside gas vans in the Nazi-occupied territories of Eastern Europe occurred out of sight within airtight compartments. Although the pressure of the driver's foot on the accelerator activated the release of the lethal gas, he did not see the victims being killed; he was simply driving the vehicle. Those who removed the bodies at the end of the journey and dumped them into huge ditches did not see anybody being killed, either; they were merely involved in the task of corpse disposal. A top secret communiqué of June 5, 1942, on "technical changes" for these "special vans" used the references "pieces," "merchandise," and "the load" as a means of furthering the remoteness of the victims by reducing them to inanimate objects for proper disposal. One of the report's proposed changes included keeping the light on in the interior of the van during the beginning of the operation so that "the number of pieces," "the merchandise aboard," and "the load"[21] did not rush toward or push against the rear doors as they were being locked and darkness set in.

Contemporary abortion technology and Nazi gas chamber extermination methodology share a factor that facilitates the remoteness of the victims: concealment of the destruction process. In most abortion procedures, unborn lives are destroyed inside the uterus where the medical executioners do not see the victims being torn apart or poisoned. The uterine walls of today, like the gas chamber walls of the Third Reich, serve as a buffer to shield the perpetrators from having to view the horrendous consequences of their destructive actions. This is particularly the case during first-trimester abortions, when it is easier to deny the humanity and existence of unborn victims owing to their tiny size and lack of visibility.

Whether resorting to suction devices or other instruments, physician abortionists have become so proficient at obliterating the miniscule bodies inside the walls of the uterus that all they usually see is the inconsequential aftermath—indistinguishable "products" being scraped, sucked, or ejected from the womb. Even if some of the man-gled body parts appear in a somewhat intact condition, they are invari-ably too small and fragmented to have any appreciable impact. This situation aids the physician perpetrators in solidifying their view of abortion as a strictly technical task. A slew of references to the dismem-bered remains of abortions as "tissue," "contents," "masses," or "prod-ucts" are further intended to reinforce the remoteness of the aborted victims and expunge from them any potential vestiges of humanity.

In 1970, two psychiatrists were called into Hawaiian hospitals to help nurses upset by the sight of "fetal parts sucked or scraped out in the operating room" or "in the bed dead fetuses or pieces of limbs, fin-gernails and hair." They assured the nurses that "what is aborted is a protoplasmic mass and not a real, live, grownup individual."[22] Several years later, American ob-gyn Dr. William Sweeney's willingness "to abort a woman if that's what she wants" was based on a perception of the fetus before twelve weeks as "just an amorphous mass."[23]

By 1995, such terminology had become a prominent ingredient in physician abortionists' vocabulary of rationalizations. Dr. Suzanne Poppema likened an unborn human she tore apart and sucked out of the womb to "tissue" that "possibly resembles the residue that would approximate the color, texture, and volume of a single pureed straw-berry."[24] At the "Lovejoy Surgicenter" in Portland, Oregon, the prod-ucts of a suction abortion are referred to as "vacuumed contents" and "an unformed mass that resembles a red jellyfish."[25]

Thus the kind of destruction that occurred behind the gas cham-ber walls of the past and that is happening inside the walls of the uter-us today is unlimited because there are no perceptible victims. Tech-nology has the insidious effect of robbing killing of its most repulsive features and reducing it to the trivial level of a minor medical proce-dure conducted on invisible, remote, or insignificant entities.

A Natural Process

Despite the prolonged expenditure of time involved in implement-ing the enforced starvation deaths in the euthanasia institutions of the Third Reich, this method of killing was touted as having the advantage of giving the appearance of death by natural causes. In 1939, Eglfing-Harr Hospital director Dr. Hermann Pfannmueller revealed how the naturalness attributed to the process of gradual starvation imposed on children made it superior to such methods as poison or lethal injections. "Our method," he proclaimed, "is much simpler, and more natural, as you will see."[26]

An affidavit—signed by Dr. Gerhard Schmidt, the postwar head of Eglfing-Harr, and presented in evidence by the prosecution at the Nuremberg Doctors' Trial—indicated how enforced starvation served as a naturalistic phenomenon for covering up the extermination of "useless eaters":

> At the end of 1942 a conference took place in the Bavarian Ministry of the Interior ... about the procedure for starving such people to death. In this conference, the directors of the asylums were instructed that "useless eaters" who could not work very much, should be killed by slow starvation. This method apparently was considered very good, because the victims would appear to have died a "natural death." This was a way of camouflaging the killing procedure.[27]

Today, a similar characterization is commonly used in describing abortions performed early in pregnancy. Early Options (EO), an abortion center with outlets in Brooklyn and Manhattan in New York, calls the aspiration abortion procedure "the most natural abortion method." It is promoted as "a quick and simple procedure" that "provides gentle suction that naturally releases the pregnancy lining from the uterine wall."[28] Another feature intended to heighten its naturalness is the absence of disturbing suction noise, since the suction device employed does not rely on electricity but is hand operated.[29]

Defining the coerced starvation deaths of patients with disabilities as a "natural process" also persists in contemporary American society. A prime example is the 1998 case of Hugh Finn, a forty-four-year-old former news anchorman who was starved and dehydrated to death over eight days following the removal of his feeding tube, thanks to the Virginia Supreme Court ruling that "the withholding and/or withdrawal of artificial nutrition or dehydration from a person in a persistent vegetative state merely permits the natural process of dying and is not mercy killing."[30]

On *Larry King Live* on October 27, 2003, Michael Schiavo and his attorney, George Felos, relied upon this characterization to rationalize their unrelenting efforts to remove Terri Schiavo's feeding tube. "It's painless and probably the most natural way to die," proclaimed Michael Schiavo. "This is not euthanasia. This is not assisted suicide," insisted Felos. "This is letting nature take its course."[31]

In the technologically charged, highly competitive world of exterminative medicine—past and present—the controversy is not over killing per se; this is a given, an acceptable and noncontroversial way of professional life. What is at issue is the method of killing. The procedures that finally win out in the relentless race to destroy more and more human expendables are those that kill precisely, quickly, conclusively, inconspicuously, and, apparently naturally. The persevering dedication of health care professionals to perfecting these techniques is an alarming commentary on the deplorable state of medical ethics. Prospects for the survival of future generations—whether they be declared unfit, imperfect, unwanted, or inconvenient—are becoming exceedingly dim as the growing insensitivity to unmitigated violence spawned by destructive medical technology threatens to engulf increasing segments of society's most vulnerable members.

Table 2 summarizes some of the main similarities between the proficiency of historical and contemporary destructive procedures at the hands of medical professionals.

TABLE 2. THE CHARACTERISTICS OF PROFICIENT EXTERMINATION

The Third Reich	Contemporary Society
FATALITY OF THE DOSAGE LEVELS	
"The rest of the dose was injected as a precautionary measure, although part of the injection would have been enough for the fatal result (I estimate 5 cc.)." *(Dr. Erwing Ding on the Buchenwald killings, 1942)*	"The amounts of sodium chloride administered during most saline abortions far exceed the lethal dosage as far as the fetus is concerned." *(Columbia University surgeons' assessment, 1974)*
"You have to judge that from the person. The smallest dose was 2 ½ to 3 c.c. for children, up to 8 to 10 c.c. for adults." *(The dosage of morphine and scopolamine used to kill patients at Hadamar, mid-1940s)*	"The amount of KCl required was usually 1 ml; however, at higher gestational ages ... as much as 10 ml at 20 weeks." *(The dosage of potassium chloride needed to kill the unborn at various stages, 1990s)*
RAPIDITY OF DESTRUCTION	
"He injected two prisoners at a time." *(Phenol technician Josef Klehr's method of killing, Auschwitz Trial, 1964)*	"Two abortions simultaneously." *(Dr. Ming Kow Hah's method of killing, Chicago-Sun Times, 1978)*
"They died in an immediate total convulsion during the actual injection." *(Phenol injections administered to inmates at the Buchenwald concentration camp, 1942)*	"Irreversible cardiac arrest occurred almost immediately after the injection." *(Potassium chloride administered to unborn humans at Mount Sinai Medical Center, 1989)*
Only "after a minute or two." *(Chemist August Becker on how long it took to kill victims in the gas chamber, 1940)*	"I have had it happen in a minute or two." *(Dr. Maureen Paul on how long it takes to perform a partial-birth abortion, 2004)*
REMOTENESS OF THE VICTIMS	
"Pieces," "merchandise," "the load," "this primitive mass," "a huge mass." *(References to gassed victims, 1942)*	"Tissue," "contents," "products," "protoplasmic mass," "unformed mass." *(References to aborted victims, 1967–present)*
A NATURAL PROCESS	
"This method apparently was considered very good, because the victims would appear to have died 'a natural death.'" *(The rationale given to the directors of German mental hospitals to justify the imposed starvation deaths of patients, 1942)*	"The withholding and/or withdrawal of artificial nutrition from a person ... merely permits the natural process of dying." *(A Virginia court ruling allowing the removal of a feeding tube from a patient existing in a "persistent vegetative state," 1998)*
"Our method is much simpler, and more natural, as you will see." *(Dr. Hermann Pfannmueller's justification for favoring the use of imposed starvation over the injection and poisonous gas methods of killing, 1939)*	"A quick and simple procedure" that "naturally releases the pregnancy lining." *(The Early Options abortion center's justification for ranking the aspiration abortion destruction process as "the most natural method," 2011)*

CHAPTER 3

When Killing Goes Awry

*The Management of Breakdowns
in Destructive Technology*

Any technological enterprise, no matter how proficient, may contain some imperfections. When the purpose of the technology is to dispatch huge numbers of individuals to oblivion, it is bound to fail at least once in a while. The most vexing difficulty faced by Nazi medics and their accomplices was dealing with those who momentarily survived the administration of deadly drugs or toxic gasses. Today's abortion doctors and their associates experience a similar dilemma when the "products" of their destructive procedures take a longer-than-expected time to expire inside the uterus or are expelled alive into the extrauterine environment. Contemporary assisted suicide and euthanasia practitioners encounter a comparable situation when their victims continue to live despite being subjected to lethal drug overdoses or other terminal measures. How such stressful situations were handled in the past and how they are dealt with in the present demonstrate the triumph of extermination technology over humanity.

Resilient Temporary Survivors of the Destruction Process

The huge numbers of individuals who were so quickly and efficiently killed in the euthanasia institutions and concentration camps of the Third Reich attest to how successfully the technology actually operated. Nevertheless, even the most flawless destructive procedure broke down occasionally. The particular method employed did not always kill as swiftly as anticipated or did not kill at all. And the one thing the perpetrators wished to avoid was the sight of living victims moving and gasping for air.

In the Hadamar Hospital, injections of morphine and scopolamine usually killed most patients quickly. Periodically, the dosage was insufficient to accomplish this goal. Even overdoses sometimes failed to exterminate all of the victims. The drugs administered had reduced some of the patients' respiratory rates to such low levels that they appeared to be dead but were actually still alive.[1]

A patient at the Eichberg state hospital expired only after being subjected to four injections over several days. A male nurse who administered one of the injections remarked, "I'll be damned, but that fellow has a tenacious hold on life."[2]

Although the gas chambers claimed the greatest toll of victims in the most proficient manner, they too did not always live up to their destructive capabilities. This was especially the case when carbon monoxide gas was pumped into the chambers. More often than not, after the chamber doors were opened, many people were still breathing, moaning, or twitching. Use of the more powerful Zyklon B gas at Auschwitz left fewer temporary survivors, but there were more technological failures than acknowledged. Technicians had frequently economized too much on the amount of gas applied, and some individuals, owing to high natural resistances, took an inordinate amount of time to expire.[3]

Children comprised another segment of those stalwart individuals who momentarily survived the gassing. In 1944, Filip Müller—a prisoner forced to carry out the task of removing victims from the gas chambers—testified at the Auschwitz Trial, "Sometimes when members of the special detail removed the bodies, they would find that the hearts of some children were still beating."[4]

Today's sophisticated methods of destroying unborn humans usually work with a high degree of proficiency. Once in a while, however, something goes awry, and they do not always succeed in killing the victims either before or after expulsion outside the mother's body. Just how often technical malfunctions yield living babies will never be truly known. Such a disturbing state of affairs is not something physician abortionists are prone to personally acknowledge, let alone bring to public attention.

Even something as decisively destructive as the injection of lethal substances into the fetal heart does not always bring about immediate cardiac stoppage. During the mid- to late 1980s, doctors affiliated with the Mount Sinai School of Medicine in New York acknowledged that only minutes after having injected potassium chloride directly into the hearts of three unborn humans between nine and thirteen weeks' gestation, "ultrasound examination revealed that cardiac activity had resumed."[5] Dr. Richard Berkowitz and his team of Mount Sinai abortionists could not help but concede with a sense of almost grudging awe, "The fetal heart is extraordinarily resilient to insults in utero."[6]

During the early 1990s, a woman who had her multifetal pregnancy "reduced" by injections of "salt water into the fetal heart" at the Columbia Presbyterian Medical Center in New York City responded similarly after watching on the ultrasound screen the initial failure of a deadly injection to bring about its intended effect:

> With the first fetus ... [the doctor] tried but it didn't work. The heartbeat kept going on and on. And he had to leave it and come back to try again later. I said, "Maybe this poor baby wants to live. And we are killing it."[7]

Descriptions of the fate of temporary survivors from failed euthanasia attempts are incorporated in Roger Magnusson's study of health professionals operating in the euthanasia underground. When Chris, a hospital nurse, heard that the patient "had started breathing again" despite being overdosed with morphine and pethidine, he responded with exasperation, "When is this man going to die?" According to community nurse Michelle, patients with HIV/AIDS exhibit a pronounced tendency to withstand multiple euthanasia attempts because they are likely to have strong hearts unaffected by HIV: "Even if they've been sick for a long time, they're still young, relatively healthy young men with booming, bumping great 'Phar lap hearts' that are really hard to stop."[8]

Repeating the Original Killing Method

Most Auschwitz prisoners who were injected in the heart with phenol by medical assistant Josef Klehr died immediately, and those few who continued living after the first injection were injected again. At the Auschwitz Trial, witness Dr. Czeslaw Glowacki testified about the case of "a tall, strong, well-built man who sat down in the wash-room, although he had just been given an injection in the heart.... Then Klehr came and gave him a second injection and killed him."[9]

When some individuals momentarily survived the asphyxiating gas, additional doses of gas served as a prime method for doing away with them. A defendant at the Nuremberg Doctors' Trial revealed how he implemented this method:

> Q: In case the inmates would not have been killed following the introduction of gas done by you, would you have killed them with a bullet?
> A: I would have tried once again to suffocate them with gas, by throwing another dose into the chamber.[10]

During the 1970s, physician abortionists came up with what many of them considered a final solution to a rash of live births from prostaglandin-induced abortions: multiple injections of corrosive saline into the amniotic sac. Dr. Thomas Kerenyi and fellow abortionists in the saline induction unit at Park East Hospital in New York City, however, reported on one case in which the saline injection method resulted in the birth of two living survivors, at seventeen and twenty weeks' gestation. The medical staff therefore proceeded to develop a protocol for averting the recurrence of such an unintended outcome by conducting routine ultrasound checks for intrauterine fetal heartbeats at two-hour intervals after the infusion of saline. If after six hours the fetal heartbeat was still present, another injection of saline was administered.[11]

In the 1980s, Dr. Richard Berkowitz and associates at New York's Mount Sinai Medical School observed the resumption of "cardiac activity" on the ultrasound screen in three unborn humans who had been subjected to injections of potassium chloride into the heart. They were then "scheduled to undergo the procedure again one week later," and "in all three cases, the procedure was repeated successfully." On the basis of this outcome, it was "recommended strongly that whenever a termination attempt is unsuccessful, it should be repeated on the fetus until the objective [killing] has been achieved."[12]

Botched euthanasia attempts often occur when those administering lethal drugs miscalculate the doses required to kill the patient. In his underground euthanasia study, Magnusson was told about a common hospital procedure that allowed "nurses to give 'break-through' doses of morphine or other analgesics when existing doses, administered every few hours, are not having their intended [deadly] effect."[13]

Health practitioners who originally underestimated the dosages necessary to achieve death were frequently surprised by the large number of drug overdoses needed before the patient actually expired. Liz, a hospital nurse, revealed to Magnusson an episode regarding a nonvoluntary act of euthanasia committed "on an emaciated and demented patient in her unit." She expressed astonishment at his tolerance to "grams of morphine, not milligrams, [but] grams." He was "only 5 foot tall," but "it took about '13 bags of the cocktail to kill him.'"[14]

Resorting to Backup Methods of Killing

Medical executioners in the Third Reich were constantly on the lookout for methods of extermination that operated so decisively that none of the intended targets survived, even temporarily. If the original method failed to kill after repeated efforts, the perpetrators promptly resorted to completing the destructive task with more effective backup measures.

At the Treblinka death camp, a range of destructive strategies evolved to deal with situations in which the gassing technology failed to asphyxiate all of the victims. Treblinka escapee Jankiel Wiernik revealed that those still alive upon opening of the chamber doors were "finished off with rifle butts, bullets or powerful kicks." When the motor generating the gas was not operating, the victims were kept in the gas chambers overnight, during which numerous individuals perished as a result of overcrowding and lack of air. Nevertheless, Wiernik disclosed, many continued to survive, "particularly the children showed a remarkable degree of resistance. They were still alive when they were dragged out of the chambers in the morning, but revolvers used by the Germans made short work of them."[15]

Another alternative method of killing came into play following SS Dr. Alfred Trzebinski's lethal injections of morphine administered to twenty children on April 20, 1945, in an abandoned school at Bullenhuser Damm in Rothenburgsort, a section of Hamburg, Germany. According to a Nazi official's report, "those who still showed some signs of life after the injection were carried into another room. A rope was put around their necks and they were hung up on hooks like pictures on a wall."[16]

In their quest to avoid what has become widely known as abortion's most dreaded complication—"a live birth"—medical practitioners of abortion in contemporary society are ever poised to substitute backup methods of destruction when repeated applications of the original ones fail to bring about the deadly result intended. A prime example of what happens took place in 1977 when obstetrician Dr. William Waddill was brought to trial for the strangulation death of an hour-old infant who survived a saline abortion at the Westminster Community Hospital nursery in Westminster, California. According to the testimony of pediatrician Dr. Ronald Cornelson, Dr. Waddill considered three methods of dealing with what he called the "baby here that came out alive": strangulation, potassium chloride injection, and drowning in a bucket of water. Cornelson revealed that Waddill finally chose strangulation. "I saw him put his hand about the baby's neck.... I saw his pushing down with his hand and with his hand around the neck pushing down on the neck."[17]

A 261-page grand jury report released on January 14, 2011, by the First Judicial District of Pennsylvania charged abortionist Dr. Kermit B. Gosnell and his staff with utilizing an especially barbaric method of killing babies who survived illegal late-term abortions performed on mainly poor and black women at his abortion facility in Philadelphia, the Women's Medical Society. The method employed consisted of inducing the "labor and delivery of intact fetuses" and then "severing the spinal cords" of those who were still moving and breathing. According to the report of the grand jury:

> When you perform late-term "abortions" by inducing labor, you get babies. Live, breathing, squirming babies.... Gosnell had a simple solution for the unwanted babies he delivered: he killed them. He didn't call it that. He called it "ensuring fetal demise." The way he ensured fetal demise was by sticking scissors into the back of the baby's neck and cutting the spinal cord. He called that "snipping."[18]

Dr. Gosnell could not be prosecuted for most of these destructive operations because he had destroyed the telltale files. But the grand jury indicted him for the first-degree murders of seven infants aborted alive where evidence still existed. Staff member Kareema Cross provided testimony about the fate of one of these fully documented cases, that of Baby A:

> After the baby was expelled, Cross noticed that he was breathing, though not for long. After about 10 to 20 seconds, while the mother was asleep, "the doctor just slit the neck," said Cross. Gosnell put the boy's body in a shoebox. Cross described the baby as so big that his feet and arms hung out over the sides of the container. Cross said that she saw the baby move after his neck was cut, and after the doctor placed it in the shoebox. Gosnell told her, "It's the baby's reflexes. It's not really moving."[19]

Today's physician-assisted suicide and euthanasia practitioners have come up with their own assortment of lethal measures when previous methods fail to kill or take too long to bring about a fatal result. A 1994 Canadian study of botched suicides uncovered a variety of backup methods utilized by doctors, nurses, and other health professionals in finishing off patients: shooting with a handgun, slitting the wrists of an individual who had vomited his pills and fallen into a coma, multiple heroin injections, and smothering with cushions.[20]

A similar type of situation involved Daryl, a patient with an AIDS-related condition who was killed by his partner, Allen, with a plastic bag after the failure of numerous other attempts. The ordeal began in the afternoon when Daryl became unconscious following the ingestion of four sleeping pills and a dose of heroin. From then until ten o'clock in the evening, Allen tried a diverse array of concoctions: additional shots of heroin, more than sixty shots of liquid oral morphine, and ten injections of vodka. But nothing worked. "At ten," Allen revealed, "I slipped a plastic trash bag over his head and held it around his neck with my hands. It only seemed to take about four minutes before he stopped breathing."[21]

Establishing the Most Decisive Destructive Procedures

To the architects of destructive technology in the Nazi regime, the killing of victims by mass gassing became the most definitive method of extermination, culminating in the deaths of millions. According to historian and political scientist Raul Hilberg, "The gas-killing method had evolved through three separate channels, each more advanced than the previous one: first the carbon monoxide gas vans, then the carbon monoxide gas chambers, and finally the hydrogen cyanide (or Zyklon) combination units."[22]

Auschwitz commandant Rudolf Hoess pioneered the ultimate in the mass execution of lives considered devoid of value: combination killing units, each consisting of an anteroom, a gas chamber, and an oven for body disposal. He repeatedly boasted about the surefire destructive impact of Zyklon B. From his prison cell in 1946, he told American prison psychiatrist Dr. G. M. Gilbert, "I knew of not a single case where anyone came out of the chambers alive."[23]

Former Auschwitz prisoner Fred Wetzler's account of hydrogen cyanide gas chamber operations, published two years earlier by the US War Refugee Board, had likewise concluded, "So far, no instance has come to light of a single victim's having shown the least sign of life when the room was opened."[24]

Today, besides the destructive advantages that dismemberment dilation and evacuation (D&E) enjoys over labor induction as the procedure of choice for abortions beyond the first trimester, owing to its greater speed and purported safety, it possesses another indispensable destructive feature—the production of badly mangled body parts devoid of any life signs whatsoever. As early as 1981, a study of live-birth abortions recognized D&E as the only abortion method that "never, ever results in live births."[25]

During 2004, as part of their testimony before US district courts in California, Nebraska, and New York in opposition to laws banning partial-birth abortion, veteran abortion doctors furnished information about their heart-stopping methods for preventing the "live-birth abortion complication." Dr. Katharine Sheehan told the California court that starting at twenty-two weeks, "to prevent the eventuality of a live birth ... we administer the digoxin with a needle ... into the fetal heart."[26] Dr. Jill Vibhaker testified in the Nebraska case, "typically for induction terminations at 22 weeks or greater, my colleagues and I inject intracardiac KCL [potassium chloride] ... to prevent the birth of a living fetus."[27] Before the New York court, Dr. Marilynn Fredriksen disclosed, "Normally I would like to do an intracardiac injection of potassium chloride the day prior to doing the induction in an ultrasound suite where we assure the death of the fetus."[28]

Contemporary right-to-die proponents and practitioners tout lethal injections and smothering with a plastic bag among the most decisive methods for doing away with vulnerable individuals after birth. In a letter to the *New York Times* following passage of the assisted-suicide law in Oregon, Hemlock Society founder Derek Humphry wrote, "The only two 100 percent ways [of] accelerating dying are the lethal injection of barbiturates and curare or donning a plastic bag. I prefer the injection."[29]

Euthanasia practitioners are ever ready to utilize the most decisive techniques of destruction. According to a study of general practitioners and nursing home physicians in Holland during the 1990s, about two-thirds endorsed the following statement: "A physician who provides assistance with suicide should be prepared to administer a lethal dose if the suicide attempt fails."[30]

Table 3 accentuates the extraordinary closeness between the Nazi doctors' responses to eradicating the tenacious survivors of their lethal operations and the contemporary destructive practices directed toward eliminating the resilient survivors of today's destructive technology.

TABLE 3. COPING WITH BREAKDOWNS IN
DESTRUCTIVE TECHNOLOGY

Nazi Expendables	Unborn Victims	Postnatal Discards
RESILIENT TEMPORARY SURVIVORS		
"The hearts of some children were still beating."	"The heartbeat kept going on and on."	"Young men with 'hearts' that are hard to stop."
(The reactions of these Auschwitz victims after being gassed, 1944)	*(Unborn child's response to deadly injection attempt, early 1990s)*	*(Nurse's description of patients subjected to lethal injections, 2002)*
"I'll be damned but that fellow has a tenacious hold on life."	"The fetal heart is extraordinarily resilient to insults in utero."	"When is this man going to die" who "started breathing again?"
(Nurse's characterization of patient who momentarily survived multiple lethal injection attempts, 1940s)	*(Dr. Richard Berkowitz's explanation for lethal fetal cardiac injection failures, 1988)*	*(Nurse's exasperation with patient who was still alive after receiving lethal medication overdoses, 2002)*
REPEATING THE ORIGINAL KILLING METHOD		
"Then [medical assistant] Klehr came and gave him a second injection and killed him."	"If after six hours the fetal heart-beat was still present, another shot of saline was administered."	"'Break-through' doses when existing doses are not having their intended [deadly] effect."
(Testimony of Dr. Czeslaw Glowacki, 1945)	*(Report by Dr. Thomas Kerenyi, 1973)*	*(A study by Roger Magnusson, 2002)*
"I would have tried ... again to suffocate them ... by throwing another dose into the chamber."	"Whenever a termination attempt is unsuccessful, it should be repeated on the fetus."	Although he was "only 5 foot tall, it took about '13 bags of the cocktail to kill him.'"
(Nuremberg trial defendant, 1947)	*(Dr. Richard Berkowitz, 1988)*	*(Liz, a hospital nurse, 2002)*
RESORTING TO BACKUP METHODS OF KILLING		
To "those who still showed some signs of life after the injection ... a rope was put around their necks."	"I saw him [Dr. Waddill] ... put his hand about the baby's neck ... pushing down on the neck."	"I slipped a plastic trash bag over his head and held it around his neck with my hands."
(A report on the killing of children at an abandoned school, 1945)	*(Dr. William Waddill's method of dealing with a failed abortion, 1977)*	*(Assisted suicide death following a botched suicide, 1996)*
Upon opening of the chamber doors, those who were still living were "finished off with rifle butts or powerful kicks."	"The way he ensured fetal demise was by sticking scissors into the back of the baby's neck and cutting the spinal cord."	Botched suicides were dealt with by shooting, the slitting of wrists, heroin injections, and smothering with cushions.
(Treblinka escapee Jankiel Wiernik, 1942-43)	*(Dr. K. Gosnell's killing of infants aborted alive, 2011)*	*(A Canadian study of botched suicides, 1994)*
ESTABLISHING THE MOST DECISIVE DESTRUCTIVE PROCEDURES		
"I knew of not a single case where anyone came out of the chambers alive."	The D&E dismemberment method of abortion "never, ever results in live births."	"Two ways [of] accelerating dying are the lethal injection or a plastic bag."
(Rudolf Hoess on the effects of Zyklon B gassing, 1946)	*(Live-birth abortion research conducted in 1981)*	*(Hemlock Society Founder Derek Humphry, 1994)*
"So far, no instance has come to light of a single victim's having shown the least sign of life when the room was opened."	"To prevent the eventuality of a live birth ... we administer the digoxin with a needle ... into the fetal heart."	"A physician who provides assistance with suicide should be prepared to administer a lethal dose if the suicide attempt fails."
(Fred Wetzler on the impact of Zyklon B gassing, 1944)	*(Dr. Katharine Sheehan's use of lethal injections, 2004)*	*(Approval of this statement by Dutch physicians, 1990s)*

CHAPTER 4

Body Disposal

Erasing the Evidence of Destruction

In any large-scale killing operation, the perpetrators are not only intent on destroying the victims, but also on getting rid of their remains as quickly as possible. The presence of undiscarded corpses poses too great a threat for a destruction process whose very credibility depends on concealing the true nature of its activities from personal and public view. The Nazi body disposal squads had a challenging job because most of the bodies they dealt with were large and intact. Burying in mass graves and burning in huge ovens and open pits came to be the most common technological means of total annihilation. Although contemporary body disposers of aborted humans specialize in removing much smaller and less intact corpses, they still have the arduous task of making sure that all of the victims' body parts are removed from the womb. Their ultimate destination is sometimes burial, but far more often it is disintegration in a hospital, clinic, or city incinerators along with the garbage and trash.

Extracting Newly Destroyed Bodies

The killing of millions in the Nazi death camps usually proceeded quite smoothly, but the post-destruction phase was sometimes fraught with problems. According to Auschwitz commandant Rudolph Hoess, "The killing itself took the least time. You could dispose of 2,000 head in a half hour."[1] Dragging the enormous number of dead bodies out of the gas chambers, however, proved to be a more burdensome physical and psychological undertaking. Auschwitz survivor Dr. Miklos Nyiszli furnished a graphic report on the difficulties encountered by the body disposal squads:

> The bodies were ... piled in a mass to the ceiling. The reason for this was that the gas first inundated the lower levels and rose but slowly towards the ceiling. This forced the victims to trample one another in a frantic effort to escape.... The separation of the welter of bodies began. It was a difficult job. They knotted thongs around the wrists, which were clenched in a viselike grip, and with these thongs they dragged the slippery bodies to the elevators.... Again straps were fixed to the wrists of the dead, and they were dragged onto the specially constructed chutes which unloaded them in front of the furnaces.[2]

According to other eyewitness accounts, it was impossible to separate the compressed and entangled corpses because "in their hideous suffering, the condemned had tried to crawl on top of one another," and "some had dug their fingernails into the flesh of their neighbors." This necessitated the development of another corpse removal technique—"The Germans invented special hook-tipped poles which were thrust deep into the flesh of the corpses to pull them out."[3]

Comparable problems awaited those consigned to remove the bodies from the gas chambers at the Belzec extermination camp:

> The dead were still standing like stone statues, there having been no room for them to fall or bend over. Though dead, the families could still be recognized, their hands still clasped. It was difficult to separate them in order to clear the chamber for the next load. The bodies were thrown out blue, wet with sweat and urine, the legs covered with excrement and menstrual blood.[4]

Extracting the remains of today's aborted humans from the uterus is not nearly such a monumental task owing mainly to their small size. Nevertheless, the contemporary body removal process is plagued with some vexing obstacles. The major technological challenge involves removing all of the unborn victim's dismembered body parts.

Veteran abortion doctors view the postabortion fetal reconstruction process as an essential but not always foolproof approach toward guaranteeing the retrieval of all the butchered remains. In reply to questions posed during a 2004 New York abortion trial, Dr. Gerson Weiss supplied some specific details about the difficulties encountered in determining whether all the aborted body parts had been extracted:

> Q: Can you eliminate the risks of retained fetal tissue in a D&E [dilation and evacuation] involving dismemberment by counting the fetal parts at the end of the procedure?
> A: No, you can't. You can count roughly. You can count there is a limb here, I can see feet and hands, I can see skull fragments, I can see a trunk. But when you see little pieces, if there are small pieces left behind that are torn off, you can't fully reconstruct and you cannot fully count the small pieces.[5]

At the same trial, Dr. Timothy Johnson testified about the predicament involved in attempting to remove a dismembered fetal head during a late-term abortion: "So one of the common technical challenges of a dismemberment D&E is what is called a free-floating head or a head that has become dis-attached and needs to be removed.... Technically it is difficult to grasp the head; it is round, it slips out of the instruments that we generally use."[6]

The fact that some prominent abortion doctors are willing to acknowledge the problems associated with removing the bodies severed in the dismemberment D&E abortion procedure does not mean they are on the verge of abandoning this barbaric practice; they have simply added another brutal procedure to their repertoire—sucking out the brains of an almost-born child—and have promoted it as an "intact D&E," which increases the likelihood that no heads, arms, legs, hands, feet, torso, or any other fragments will be left inside the uterine walls since the method consists of pulling out the entire body, with the crumpled head still attached. Dr. Maureen Paul, an avid proponent of intact D&E, asserted: "I've extracted the whole fetus, and so the risks of having retained fetal parts or tissue is virtually eliminated."[7]

The Burial-Burning Controversy

During the summer of 1942, discussions centered on the relative merits of burying versus burning as the best means of dealing with the huge number of Holocaust victims. The most worrisome thing about the mass graves was the traces left of unprecedented extermination. Some Nazi ideologues were not bothered, because to them the graves provided concrete evidence about the awesome success of "the final solution." Nazi realists, however, grew increasingly uneasy about the existence of such evidence.

At one of these discussions in Lublin, Poland, Odilio Globocnik, an SS and police leader consumed with Nazi ideology, told visiting officials from Berlin that he supported not only continuing to bury the bodies, but also placing bronze plaques over the graves with the inscription, "It was we, we who had the courage to achieve this gigantic task." Enforced sterilization expert Dr. Herbert Linden, a realist, opposed mass burials. "But would it not be better to burn the bodies instead of burying them?," he asked. "A future generation might think differently of these matters." Globocnik replied, "But gentlemen, if after us such a cowardly and rotten generation should arise that it does not understand our work which is so good and so necessary, then gentlemen, all National Socialism will have been for nothing."[8]

Reality won out over idealism, and in June 1942, Paul Blobel, commander of the *Einsatzkommando 4a* mobile killing unit and an architect by profession, was put in charge of "Operation 1005," a project designed to obliterate all traces of mass murder by eradicating the mass graves.[9] By 1942, the exhumation and cremation of corpses was in full swing.

Questions regarding the fate of today's aborted humans—whether they should be buried or incinerated—constitute, in many respects, a replay of the burial-burning controversy over the destiny of the bodies of Holocaust victims. A burial-burning dispute erupted in March 1997 over the destiny of fifty-four fetal bodies found alongside a Chino Hills, California, embankment, stuffed inside five boxes sealed with duct tape. Members of an ecumenical Christian group, the Cradles of

Love, petitioned the San Bernardino Coroner's Office to give them the bodies for a religious burial after completion of the criminal investigation. The American Civil Liberties Union informed Coroner Brian McCormick that doing so would violate the doctrine of the separation of church and state. "It is more than just the appearance of the state sanctioning a particular religious belief," maintained ACLU Associate Director Elizabeth Schroeder. "Under California law there is only one way to dispose of this material ... that would be by incineration."[10]

On October 9, 1998, McCormick released the remains to a local mortuary, which donated them to the Cradles of Love. Despite another ACLU protest, no further action was taken to halt the highly personalized and reverential ceremonies, which involved the placement of the bodies in separate coffins, the names given to them by area church groups being engraved on the coffins and on a black granite grave marker, scriptural verses being read by clergy across denominational lines, the singing of religious songs, and the release of fifty-four doves symbolizing the spirit of each deceased child.[11]

Permitting secular or sacred burial rites for the remains of induced abortion is still far from the norm. Aborted humans are rarely granted even these minimal expressions of respect. Most of them are summarily consumed by the flames of an incinerator or disposed of along with the garbage and trash. One cannot help but conclude that individuals and organizations in the vanguard of today's war on the unwanted unborn—like those in the Third Reich who perpetrated the war against Jews and other vulnerable groups—prefer burning as the optimal method of body disposal, not because of any legal principle, but because it so conclusively disintegrates all traces of destruction. Burial—especially Christian burial—not only bestows upon the victims a transcendental value intolerable to abortion practitioners and apologists, but also highlights a disquieting reality they so vociferously attempt to deny: the existence of bona fide victims.

Obliterating the Remains

Erasing the evidence of widespread destruction in the Third Reich was carried out primarily by burning in crematory ovens and mass burial in huge ditches. Although burning large numbers of bodies reached its highest level of proficiency in the Nazi death camps, this method of disposal was actually pioneered in the German euthanasia institutions. In December 1939, stories about the destruction-disintegration process at the Hadamar Hospital began circulating among the townspeople:

> The arrivals are immediately stripped to the skin, dressed in paper shirts, and forthwith taken to a gas chamber, where they are liquidated.... The bodies are reported to be moved into a combustion chamber by means of a conveyor belt, six bodies to a furnace. The resulting ashes are then distributed into six urns which are shipped to the families. The heavy smoke from the crematory building is said to be visible over Hadamar every day.[12]

Burning in crematory ovens and huge pits eventually replaced mass burials as the premier method of obliteration in the extermination camps. At the Maidanek camp, a new crematorium with five furnaces was completed in the fall of 1943. An innovation designed to further increase their destructive capacity involved a pre-burning dismemberment procedure—"hacking off the extremities" of the victims so that a greater number of bodies could be placed in each furnace. After examining the structure of the furnaces, a group of technical experts concluded, "Four bodies with hacked-off extremities could be placed in one furnace at a time. It took 15 minutes to burn four bodies ... and so with all furnaces working round the clock it was possible to burn 1,920 bodies in twenty-four hours."[13]

Death camp survivor Olga Lengyel recalled that upon arriving at Auschwitz, "A cool wind carried to us a peculiar, sweetish odor, much like that of burning flesh. Although we did not identify it as that. This odor greeted us upon our arrival and stayed with us always."[14]

Burning in incinerators also constitutes a prime method of effacing the bodies of contemporary aborted humans. The infamous late abortionist Dr. George Tiller of Wichita, Kansas—a specialist in kill-ing preborn human lives during the second and third trimesters—dealt with the problem of body disposal by having a million-dollar in-dustrial crematorium installed in his state-of-the-art abortion center dubbed Women's Health Care Services. This ten-thousand-square-foot windowless facility, located on a busy street between two new car dealerships, resembled a warehouse for top-secret technologies. It was equipped with video cameras spanning the surroundings and had an armed security guard on duty to greet Tiller's customers. According to Troy Newman, director of the pro-life activist organization Operation Rescue, "One can observe and taste the putrid smoke billowing from the 10,000 square foot abortuary."[15]

At a 1995 conference sponsored by the Chicago-based Pro-Life Ac-tion League, Luhra Tivris, who once worked for Dr. Tiller, recalled her reaction to his on-site crematorium:

> My office manager had told me that's the crematorium in that room
> ... and she said it's a full size crematorium just like they have in
> funeral homes. And I couldn't ignore that machine any more.... I
> heard him [Dr. Tiller] fire it up. It's a gas-powered oven and the most
> horrible thing was I could smell those babies burning because I was
> just around the corner.[16]

A practice reminiscent of hacking off the extremities of victims prior to burning in the crematory furnaces of Nazi concentration camps took place at the Isesaki Clinic, a Japanese gynecological facili-ty located in Yokohama, south of Tokyo. In July 2004, it came to light that abortions were performed on "fetuses 12 weeks and older," and before they were dumped in the regular trash, "clinic staff reportedly snipped off their arms and legs with scissors to make it easier to throw them out in plastic bags." At first, clinic director Dr. Keido Harada denied this claim, but he later admitted that he "cut off the fetus' limbs with scissors and dumped all the parts with the general garbage" and "instructed employees to dismember fetuses aborted at 12 weeks or more to make it easier to dispose them as it was costly to hire medical waste professionals to do the job."[17]

Body-Grinding Technology

The Nazi body disposal squads discovered that the most powerful inferno did not always disintegrate all signs of destroyed humanity. The victims' bones or bone fragments sometimes survived the flames of the crematoriums or pits. Bone-grinding devices and machines were developed to extinguish these final traces of mass extermination. In the euthanasia hospitals, "after cremation the stokers used a mill to grind into a powder the human bones not totally pulverized by the fire."[18] Body eradication expert Paul Blobel devised a similar backup method for getting rid of the remaining incriminating evidence: "The activation of machines to grind the human bones."[19]

After the war, additional information about the operation of the bone-grinding technology was brought to public awareness. The Soviet-Polish Extraordinary Commission, established to investigate crimes committed in the concentration camps, revealed that the body disposers resorted to "grinding small bones in a special 'mill.'"[20]

The bone-crunching devices pioneered in the death camps of the Third Reich are not entirely extinct. Today's counterparts are garbage disposal units installed in the scrub sinks of abortion clinics. On May 31, 1978, plumber Rick Gray found some aborted body parts in a garbage disposer he had removed from the Ladies Center, an abortion clinic located in Omaha, Nebraska. "I saw what looked like a miniature arm. There was a miniature hand. It was very distinctive," he reported to local police authorities. "I saw something that looked like a rib cage. You could see miniature fingernails on the hands." According to deputy attorney general Frank Pane, "There's nothing criminal now about grinding up fetal remains. But it's gross and repugnant and something should be done about it."[21]

In early summer 1992, abortionist Dr. Curtis Stover sent a letter to the Colorado Department of Health (CDH) complaining about abortionist Dr. James Parks's use of a meat grinder "to grind up the fetuses" before dumping them down the sink. In late 1989, Stover had contracted with Parks to purchase his clinic, but Parks canceled the contract because of Stover's refusal to employ this particular method of disposal. Stover thereupon initiated legal action against Parks. In his letter of complaint to the CDH, Dr. Stover submitted an affidavit detailing Dr. Parks's fetal disposal technique:

> At the end of a workday in December 1989, Dr. James J. Parks, the owner of Mayfair Women's Center of Aurora, Colorado, demonstrated to me his method of fetal tissue disposal. We went into a utility room that was used for such things as sterilizing instruments. On a countertop were several white plastic buckets, each containing fetuses from about 15 weeks to 22 weeks size. Dr. Parks reached up to a shelf and brought down several pieces of metal that were parts of a meat grinder and placed them on the counter....
>
> Dr. Parks then began to empty each bucket into the hopper on top of the grinder, and with his left hand pressed the fetal tissue down into the hopper as he turned the handle with his right hand, grinding the tissue. As he did this the tissue oozed out of the end of the grinder like multiple tubes of pink toothpaste....
>
> After all the fetuses were ground up into a large bucket, he dumped the contents into the sink and washed it down the sink with water. Finally, he disassembled the grinder, rinsed it off, and placed it back on the shelf.[22]

Seattle abortion clinic owner and operator Dr. Suzanne Poppema's resolution to the problem posed by "larger pieces of tissue" blocking the disposal pipes was the reduction of "large tissue with a disposal grinder." She lamented not being able to use this "disposal system" because of what she called an "absurd" regulation against reducing "the size of tissue before disposal."[23]

Several key parallels between the body disposal techniques of the Third Reich and those in contemporary society are highlighted in table 4.

TABLE 4. GETTING RID OF THE EXTERMINATED VICTIMS

The Third Reich	Contemporary Society
EXTRACTING THE BODIES	
"They knotted thongs around the wrists … and with these thongs they dragged the slippery bodies to the elevators." (*Dr. Miklos Nyszli on removing befouled bodies out of the Auschwitz gas chambers, 1944–45*)	"I've extracted the whole fetus, and so the risks of having retained fetal parts or tissue is virtually eliminated." (*Dr. Maureen Paul on ensuring the total removal of the aborted body in a partial-birth abortion, 2004*)
"The Germans invented special hook-tipped poles which were thrust deep into the flesh of corpses to pull them out." (*Survivor Olga Lengyel on the removal of entangled corpses from the Auschwitz gas chambers, 1944*)	"And technically it is difficult to grasp the head; it is round, it slips out of the instruments that we generally use." (*Dr. Timothy Johnson on removing a "free-floating head" during a D&E dismemberment abortion, 2004*)
THE BURIAL-BURNING CONTROVERSY	
"But would it not be better to burn the bodies instead of burying them?" (*Dr. Herbert Linden on the disposal of Holocaust corpses, 1942*)	"Only one way to dispose of this material would be by incineration." (*ACLU attorney Elizabeth Schroeder on the disposal of aborted bodies, 1997*)
OBLITERATING THE REMAINS	
"A cool wind carried to us a peculiar … odor, much like that of burning flesh." (*Auschwitz death camp survivor Olga Lengyel, 1944*)	"The most horrible thing was I could smell those babies burning." (*Former abortion clinic employee Luhra Tivris, 1995*)
"The heavy smoke from the crematory building is said to be visible … every day." (*The burning of euthanasia victims in the Hadamar Hospital crematorium, 1939–41*)	"One can observe … the putrid smoke … from the 10,000 square foot abortuary." (*Troy Newman on the burning of aborted bodies in Dr. Tiller's abortion clinic, 2003*)
"Four bodies with hacked-off extremities could be placed in one furnace at a time." (*The body disposal process at the Maidanek concentration camp, 1943*)	"Clinic staff snipped off their arms and legs … to make it easier to throw them out." (*The body disposal process at a Japanese abortion clinic, 2004*)
BODY-GRINDING DISPOSAL TECHNOLOGY	
"Grinding small bones in a 'mill.'" (*Description of a concentration camp body disposal technique by an investigation committee, 1946*)	"Grinding up fetal remains." (*Description of a fetal disposal technique by Nebraska Deputy Attorney General Frank Pane, 1978*)
"After cremation the stokers used a mill to grind into a powder the human bones not totally pulverized." (*Erasing the traces of destruction in euthanasia hospitals, early 1940s*)	"Dr. Parks … pressed the fetal tissue down into the hopper as he turned the handle with his right hand, grinding the tissue." (*Eradicating aborted fetal bodies in a meat grinder at a Colorado abortion clinic, 1989*)
"The activation of machines to grind the human bones." (*Paul Blobel's plan for eradicating any remaining evidence of the Nazi destruction process, 1943*)	The reduction of "large [fetal] tissue with a disposal grinder." (*Dr. Suzanne Poppema's resolution for dealing with fetal body parts blocking garbage disposal pipes, 1996*)

Psychological Responses of Health Care Professionals to Participation in Killing

Direct involvement in destroying human lives even under technically ideal conditions can prove to be profoundly upsetting. All the
more so when periodic hitches develop in the destructive procedures. The perpetrators' reactions run the gamut from intense stress
to emotional indifference to professional pride. In the Third Reich,
not that many medical executioners suffered enough psychological
unease to have any appreciable effect on curtailing the destruction
process. Morale-building speeches, overindulgence in alcohol, and
mutually supportive therapeutic group sessions helped solidify their
commitment to advancing the procedural and technical aspects of
destruction. In contemporary society, confrontation with the harsh
consequences of killing causes some health practitioners of abortion,
assisted suicide, and euthanasia to cease their destructive practices. Many nevertheless continue their involvement, helped along by
supportive statements and policies from medical colleagues, resort
to alcohol, and experience brainwashing under the guise of group
discussions.

Momentary Psychological Turmoil

In his study of Nazi doctors, psychiatrist Robert Jay Lifton found
that those who conducted death selections at Auschwitz were prone

to suffering personal anguish because they had to directly confront those selected for gassing. A typical reaction came from death selector Dr. B.: "When you see a selection for the first time ... you see ... how children and women are selected. Then you are so shocked ... that it just cannot be described."[1]

A particularly excruciating experience for the Nazi perpetrators was to behold nearly dead victims making a last-ditch effort to live. Even Heinrich Himmler became upset by an incident in August 1941, when he saw a mobile firing squad fail to kill outright two out of one hundred individuals. General Erich van dem Bach-Zelewski explained to Himmler how adversely affected the shooting squad members were by this incident: "Look at the eyes of the men in this *Kommando*, how deeply shaken they are! These men are finished for the rest of their lives. What kind of followers are we training here? Either neurotics or savages!" Himmler thereupon made a speech in which he attempted to console them by providing a legal and ideological justification for participation in what was admittedly a "repulsive duty" and a "bloody business." He emphasized that their consciences need not be bothered since they were obeying the highest law and carrying out a necessary operation.[2]

Commanders in the field kept careful track of how their charges were holding up under the strain. The number of speeches and discussions intended to boost morale continued to increase as the killings expanded. Doctors were called in to treat those who broke down or showed signs of cracking under the emotional pressure brought about by involvement in the destruction process. Dr. Ernst Grawitz attributed General Bach-Zeleski's stomach and intestinal ailments to "reliving the shooting of Jews that he himself had conducted."[3]

Contemporary abortion proponents and practitioners are ever alert to the winds of potential revolt among medical and nursing personnel emotionally upset by their participation in killing the unwanted unborn.One of the most revealing accounts came from veteran Colorado abortionist Dr. Warren Hern, who in the late 1970s indicated that his staff members' "reactions to the fetus ranged from purposely not looking at it to shock, dismay, amazement, disgust, fear, and sadness." Some of them described dreams about "vomiting fetuses along with a sense of horror" and felt "a need to protect others from viewing fetal parts."[4]

This severe emotional trauma was attributed mainly to participation in an overt act of destruction in which the physician literally tears apart the unborn with forceps, extracts the mangled body parts piecemeal from the womb, and reassembles all the fragments to ensure the completeness of the procedure. There is nothing ambiguous about this destructive operation. Causality is crystal clear. Dr. Hern does not hesitate to highlight this distinctive feature: "We have reached the point in this particular technology where there is no possibility of denying an act of destruction. It is before one's eyes. The sensations of dismemberment flow through the forceps like an electric current."[5]

Emotional disturbances have continued to plague health care professionals involved in abortions. In workshops sponsored by the National Abortion Federation in 1993, "abortion providers" talked about dreams in which "aborted fetuses stare at them with ancient eyes and perfectly shaped hands and feet, asking 'Why? Why did you do this to me?'" During one of the sessions, an abortion clinic nurse revealed that she didn't know what to say to the women in the recovery room who cried, "I've just killed my baby." The nurse then told the group, "Part of me thinks, 'Maybe they're right.'"[6]

Writing in a 2008 issue of *Reproductive Health Matters*, University of Michigan ob-gyn Dr. Lisa Harris furnished an atypically frank account of what happened when she "was a little over 18 weeks pregnant" while performing a dismemberment dilation and evacuation (D&E) abortion "for a patient who was also a little over 18 weeks pregnant":

> With my first pass of the forceps, I grasped an extremity and began to pull it down. I could see a small foot hanging from the teeth of my forceps. With a quick tug, I separated the leg. Precisely at that moment, I felt a kick—a fluttery "thump, thump" in my own uterus. It was one of the first times I felt fetal movement. There was a leg and foot in my forceps, and a "thump, thump" in my abdomen. Instantly, tears were streaming from my eyes.[7]

Although most of the emotional turmoil over participation in the killing of the unborn takes place during the last two trimesters, when a fetus's human qualities are highly visible, psychological distress sometimes occurs during the earlier stages of pregnancy, when their human attributes are less perceptible. This has even happened during the earliest phases of embryonic development at fertility clinics where "many staff members say they dread destroying embryos when patients request it." Dr. John Garrisi, chief embryologist at the Institute for Reproductive Medicine of St. Barnabas Medical Center in Livingston, New Jersey, acknowledged, "No one wants to be assigned that job." The laboratory director at Chicago's Rush Centers for Advanced Reproductive Care admitted that "he destroyed the embryos himself because so many of his staff members found the task distasteful."[8]

Modern-day assisted suicide and euthanasia practitioners have likewise expressed considerable emotional turmoil in carrying out their destructive procedures. According to an analysis by Oregon Health and Science University emeritus professor Kenneth Stevens, many doctors who have participated in euthanasia and/or physician-assisted suicide report "being profoundly adversely affected, being shocked by the suddenness of the death, being caught up in the patient's drive for assisted suicide, having a sense of powerlessness, and feeling isolated."[9]

For some of the fourteen doctors who wrote prescriptions for lethal medications in 1998, the first year of Oregon's Death with Dignity Act, "the process of participating in physician-assisted suicide exacted a large emotional toll, as reflected by such comments as, 'It was an excruciating thing to do ... ,' 'This was really hard on me, especially being there when he took the pills,' and 'This had a tremendous emotional impact.'"[10] One of the doctors revealed how he felt about prescribing a deadly medication for his patient:

> A big piece is grief.... I have to admit, I am blown away by how different this felt than a natural death.... Just the suddenness of it. It's shocking to have somebody go from telling a family story to being dead. It's a strange, strange, strange transition.[11]

Alcohol Consumption

Extensive drinking aided the SS doctors at Auschwitz in numbing themselves to the killing and their responsibility for its implementation. The reliance upon alcohol precipitated an "altered state of consciousness"—a supportive atmosphere highly receptive to taking on the role of killer, or what psychiatric researcher Robert Jay Lifton referred to as the Auschwitz self:

> Alcohol was central to a pattern of male bonding through which new doctors were socialized into the Auschwitz community.... Drinking enhanced the meeting of the minds between old-timers, who could offer models of an Auschwitz self to the newcomer seeking entry in the realm of Auschwitz killing. The continuing alcohol-enhanced sharing of group feelings and numbing gave further shape to the emerging Auschwitz self.
>
> Over time, as drinking was continued especially in connection with selections, it enabled the Auschwitz self to distance that killing activity and reject responsibility for it.[12]

At some of the extermination sites, drunkenness became so pervasive among the perpetrators that they were not able to do their jobs effectively. The victims were often left bleeding and breathing throughout the entire night. One doctor reported becoming so disturbed by his involvement in the destruction process that "he had to drink a lot of alcohol to stick it out."[13]

Overindulgence in alcohol was a standard component of the 1941 celebration at the Hadamar Hospital that commemorated the cremation of the ten thousandth mental patient. This event called for a staff party at which doctors, nurses, orderlies, and grounds attendants were served wine and beer in the institution's lobby, and they then proceeded to the crematorium in the basement, where the body of the ten thousandth victim—adorned with flowers and small Nazi flags—lay on a gurney in front of the oven. After one of the doctors gave a short inspirational talk about the importance of the task at Hadamar, the body was shoved into the furnace. The rest of the festive occasion included more beer, the music of a local polka band, dancing, and laughter. It concluded with "a drunken march around the sanatorium grounds with lots of singing and shouting."[14]

Some contemporary physician abortionists, like the medical executioners of the Third Reich, resort to alcohol as a means of blotting out any bothersome residues of guilt. "Reports of ... excessive drinking among medical staff at the North Carolina Memorial Hospital" were mentioned as one of the ways they coped with the more repugnant aspects of their abortion work.[15]

Correspondent Norma Rosen uncovered a pattern of guilt, despair, heavy drinking, and nightmares among the abortion doctors she interviewed. Dr. William Rashbaum of the Albert Einstein College of Medicine admitted to being troubled by what he referred to as "a fantasy in the midst of every abortion: He imagined that the fetus was resisting its own aborting, hanging onto the walls of the uterus with its tiny fingernails, fighting to stay inside."[16]

The use of alcohol also serves as a means of lessening the anxiety among today's health care professionals who euthanize the lives of those considered unworthy of existence. In Roger Magnusson's underground euthanasia study, Amanda, a community nurse, revealed how she and a colleague resorted to whiskey after making sure that the administration of a lethal injection had its desired effect: "We opened a big bottle of whiskey and sat down and probably drank the whole bottle within half an hour between us."[17]

Moreover, Magnusson indicated that drinking alcoholic beverages became a part of the celebratory, festive atmosphere accompanying the aftermath of euthanasia deaths. In a scene reminiscent of the celebration commemorating the killing of patients at the Hadamar euthanasia hospital in Nazi Germany, some participants "described a sense of relief, elation, and even celebration after death had been achieved." One nurse reported that "we all just sat there and kissed each other and cried, and laughed and had a drink and all that sort of stuff."[18]

Group Support

Informal and formal group sessions evolved to help the death-selection doctors at Auschwitz ventilate their negative feelings about being required to participate in actions at such radical odds with their healing, life-enhancing professional reason to be. The expression of opposition to or doubts about physicians engaging in killing was permitted as an apt topic for group discussion. After becoming nauseated and extremely agitated at his first selection, Dr. Hans Delmotte was heard saying he "didn't want to be in a slaughterhouse," preferred going to the war front, and that "as a doctor his task was to help people and not kill them."[19]

The purpose of encouraging the expression of such sentiments in the group sessions was not for their reinforcement, but to use the group as a device for veteran medical death selectors to refute them and socialize newcomers into accepting the Auschwitz reality that "mass killing was the unyielding *fact of life* to which everyone was expected to adapt." According to Dr. B., "the essential psychological situation" of Auschwitz doctors was compliance with its killing structure: "I'm here. I cannot get out.... And I have to [make] the best of it."[20] Thus, within the group, it was viewed as understandable to express qualms about and resistance to becoming involved in the destruction process. Through the influence of doctors already socialized in selecting victims for the gas chambers, however, group dynamics were heavily stacked in the direction of pressuring reluctant physicians to drop their objections and incorporate the task of killing as a component of their professional duties.

Similarly, central among the strategies that abortionist Dr. Warren Hern adopted to help staff members cope with the stresses of participating in D&E abortions are such familiar devices as "ample opportunities to talk about the feelings and concerns they have" within "the form of informal meetings" and consciously promoting "the idea of team effort and the need for mutual support."[21] According to the title of his paper, "What about Us? Staff Reactions to D&E," Dr. Hern wants to make sure that peers and colleagues understand and sympathize with the extremely intense psychological responses he and his staff have to endure in carrying out such an undeniably destructive procedure.

Despite acknowledging that "there is violence in abortion, especially in second trimester abortion," medical professor Dr. Lisa Harris continues to perform this act of violence while championing "clinical training for staff who would be directly involved in D&E care" and promoting "focus group intervention with a skilled facilitator to provide staff with formal opportunities to explore their experiences and build team cohesion" with an emphasis on "the burdens of this work" and "the unique rewards it brings as well."[22]

To Drs. Hern, Harris, and their fellow abortionists, tearing apart an unborn child in the second trimester is indeed a violent act that causes emotional distress, but this reaction is but a momentary discomfort that can be readily overcome with the aid of peer group support from networks of colleagues, much like those Nazi doctors at Auschwitz who received solace and affirmation for their destructive actions from fellow medical death selectors within the medium of group sessions and discussions.

The ventilation of feelings within a supportive group atmosphere of like-minded colleagues is also frequently advocated as a means of overcoming the emotional turmoil experienced by today's assisted suicide and euthanasia practitioners. Findings published in a 2004 issue of the *Journal of Palliative Medicine* emphasized "the need for development of supportive forums for discussion" as an approach toward helping alleviate the pronounced "emotional intensity" felt by Oregon physicians who prescribed lethal doses of medications to patients.[23]

Emotional Detachment

One of the most horrifying accomplishments of massive medicalized killing past and present is the propensity of those carrying out the deadly operations to remain psychologically distant from their repugnant tasks. Psychoanalyst Erich Fromm identified the psychodynamics involved in such an extreme state of emotional indifference: "What happens is that the aggressor cuts the other person off emotionally, and 'freezes' him. The other person ceases to be experienced as human, and becomes a 'thing—over there.'"[24] Destruction of the victim is therefore perceived as nothing more significant than operating a mechanical device or implementing a procedure that results in discarding an object or thing. The tunnel vision of the technician, coupled with an abysmal lack of empathy—an inability or unwillingness to identify the victim as a genuine human being—creates the conditions necessary for the suppression of inhibitions against large-scale killing.

Psychiatric researcher Dr. Robert Jay Lifton calls this process of advanced emotional detachment "psychic numbing"—a "diminished capacity and inclination to feel, so that one need not experience oneself as in any way related to cruelties and killings."[25] "The key function of numbing" at Auschwitz, he emphasized, was "the avoidance of feelings of guilt when one is involved in killing." This response provided doctors and their cohorts with the license to "engage in medicalized killing, an ultimate form of numbed violence."[26] While some concentration camp doctors became unnerved during their first forays into exterminative medicine, with further experience, "then it got to be routine—like all other routines in Auschwitz."[27]

Other death technicians likewise remained emotionally dissociated from their destructive tasks. "I had no feelings in carrying out these things," one gassing technician told the Nuremberg tribunal. "That, by the way, was the way I was trained."[28] When in 1939 psychiatric nurse Pauline K. and others were recruited for the euthanasia program, she indicated that no one refused and "none of us had moral reservations." For the next four years, she embarked on a relentless, routinized killing spree directed against patients in psychiatric institutions and other settings. At a postwar trial, she showed "few signs of remorse" and provided evidence in a "matter-of-fact and unreflective" manner.[29]

The posture of emotional numbing is strikingly apparent in the comments of a contemporary doctor who admitted having "harpooned the fetus" like a "fish hooked on a line" in the process of injecting lethal doses of poisonous salt solution into the amniotic sac. "I can feel the fetus move at the end of the needle," he declared. "This gives me an unpleasant, unhappy feeling because I know the fetus is alive and responding to the needle stab.... You know there is something alive in there that you're killing." Nevertheless, he maintained,

"I never had any psychological adverse reaction. Except an occasional feeling that one was destroying life."[30] For him, the placement of the needle in the wrong spot represents only a minor, rare, unpleasant, and awkward component of an otherwise flawless technical procedure. It usually induces only a fleeting moment of discomfort that never reaches his conscience. Neither does it last long enough to put an end to the killing.

Initially, physicians who perform D&E abortions are likely to experience some emotional unease arising from the repulsive nature of a grisly mutilation process in which the doctor is the one who dismembers the victim, extracts the body parts piece by piece, and reassembles the mangled remains to make sure the uterus has been completely emptied. Sarina, an abortion clinic doctor, recalled how she gradually became accustomed to performing D&Es into the sixteenth week of pregnancy, something she previously thought would have been impossible because of how disturbing it was to tear apart an individual with clearly discernible human features:

> I've gotten to the point now that because I've been doing this work five months, four months, I look at it a little differently. I don't see the same things that I did. And, honestly, when I sit down to do one of these now, I am watching to be sure that I'm getting everything I need to get. It's: Do I have two lower extremities? Do I have two upper extremities? Is there a spine? ... And the skull.... It doesn't trigger in me the emotional response [I first felt].... It does become a bit routine after a while.[31]

During an interview with leading ob-gyn abortionist Dr. Thomas Kerenyi, a woman's magazine writer disclosed the extreme emotionally detached, mechanistic mindset he adopted in order to carry out the mutilation process in a D&E abortion:

> He doesn't think about what he's doing while he's doing it, or he'd get up and walk out of the room. He's thinking, *You're taking an airplane apart.* With forceps and the strength of his arms he pulls, removing the fetus piece by piece, ticking them off to himself as he goes, the lungs, the bowels, the limbs. *This is an airplane and you're a mechanic*, his hands tired from squeezing and pulling, now just the big one, the head; he's got it, he expels his breath in one loud sigh, it's almost

over. He takes up the curette, carefully scrapes the uterine wall. He can't leave any fetal tissue behind.[32]

Helped along by the passage of time and further experience, today's assisted suicide and euthanasia practitioners likewise learn to overcome the initial shock associated with deliberately ending human lives. Magnusson's study of the underground euthanasia movement reveals how "a number of interviewees admitted that stress levels do decline as one gains experience in euthanasia." A general practitioner asserted, "It does get easier with time. After doing several ... you get over it quicker." A nurse told Magnusson, "I don't go home and have sleepless nights; I have a very clear conscience about it [administering euthanasia procedures]."[33]

Professional Pride

Some doctors in the Third Reich became so imbued with the National Socialist doctrine of Aryan perfection that their response of emotional detachment toward the plight of the victims was elevated to the level of a wholly positive, gratifying experience. They did not need alcohol or group support to blunt the psychological distress ordinarily associated with killing a human being because they defined what they did, not as a distasteful destructive procedure, but as a good thing in its own right, something to be proud of.

SS doctors and their medical attendants took considerable pride in skillfully implementing proficient methods of killing. This was precisely the mentality of those health professionals who administered lethal phenol injections to patients in Block 20 at Auschwitz. Former prisoner physician Dr. Stanislaw Klodzinki testified at the Auschwitz Trial, "It was a matter of pride that they sometimes killed two or three prisoners in one minute." Another former Auschwitz prisoner physician, a Dr. Fejkiel, revealed, "They all bragged of having acquired a certain degree of skill in injecting the phenol."[34]

Prominent psychologist Bruno Bettelheim offered a profound insight into the compelling role that pride in professional skills and knowledge played in helping SS doctors, their prisoner medical accomplices, and prestigious physicians justify carrying out experimental and other death camp atrocities, as well as the ominous future ramifications of this mentality:

> The Important Issue here is that Dr. Nyiszli, Dr. Mengele and hundreds of other far more prominent physicians, men trained long before the advent of Hitler to power, were participants in these human experiments and in the pseudo-scientific investigations that went with them. It is this pride in professional skill and knowledge, irrespective of moral implications, that is so dangerous. As a feature of modern society oriented toward technological competence it is still with us, though the concentration camps, the crematoria, the extermination of millions because of race, are no longer here. Auschwitz is gone, but as long as this attitude remains with us we shall not be safe from the criminal indifference to life at its core.[35]

While Auschwitz has long since receded into history, the mentality that helped fuel the mass extermination there—pride in the perversion of technology for destructive ends under the guise of medicine—has not gone away but continues to be propagated today by those most directly involved in killing unborn humans. For them, abortion is no longer the lesser of two evils but has been transformed into a life-enhancing experience in its own right. Their justifications reek with prideful statements touting abortion as an intrinsically fascinating, interesting, and personally gratifying procedure that makes essential contributions to women, the field of reproductive medicine, and even society itself by "preventing the birth" of unwanted children.

In her book glorifying physician abortionists before and after *Roe v. Wade*, sociologist Carole Joffe refers to freestanding abortion clinics as "a proud creation of the pro-choice community" and those who work in them as "doctors of conscience." One of the abortionists highlighted in her study, Dr. David Bennett, is described as having found "in abortion work enormous opportunities for creativity and professional growth" and as drawing "the most fundamental source of gratification" from the abortion itself, a form of "artistry" encompassing the "totality of the abortion experience" that "serves as a springboard to a higher degree of self-awareness and esteem."[36]

According to the narratives compiled by social science researcher

Wendy Simonds, the health workers at a feminist abortion center in a southeastern American city "took pride in their nurturing style."[37] Sarina, the center's staff abortionist, expressed immense pride in how adroitly she had mastered the technical challenges of her abortion work:

> I think actually performing an abortion is a very refined technical skill; it's a very delicate skill.... The thing I like about the procedure is that ... when you feel like you are indeed a talented abortionist, you get through the difficult cases.... [T]hen knowing how to do this with such delicate precision that you don't injure the cervix. Those kinds of things help me feel like I have really mastered something that I'm very proud of.... In the past year, I've probably done close to five thousand procedures, which is more than many people do in ten years of work.[38]

Another account extolling a prideful physician abortionist appeared in a 2009 issue of *Newsweek*. Reporter Sarah Kliff asked late-term abortionist Dr. Leroy Carhart about his reason for choosing "a job that attracts death threats and protesters." Carhart said he refused to be forced out of "a legitimate medical specialty" and asserted, "Abortion is not a four-letter word. I'm proud of what I do."[39]

The sense of pride also serves as a prominent rationalization relied upon by Planned Parenthood doctors to justify the destruction of unborn humans and the exploitation of their body parts for sale to researchers. On August 9, 2015, during an interview on a San Francisco television station, Heather Saunders Estes, the president of Planned Parenthood's Northern California chapter, defended these practices soon after they were exposed in the first series of undercover videos released by the Center for Medical Progress. "What we do is legal and ethical and we're proud of it," she stated.[40]

Although some of today's assisted suicide and euthanasia practitioners experience either emotional distress or psychic numbing in ending the lives of patients, others carry out these destructive actions with a great amount of pride and personal gratification. Their rationalizations often echo the justifications invoked by Third Reich health professionals and contemporary abortion practitioners for doing away with their respective victims.

Those in Magnusson's underground euthanasia study expressed a range of highly positive reasons for performing euthanasia procedures. One interviewee said of the euthanasia process, "We felt that ... we had done something really positive" and that "we really helped the person achieve something that was really, really important for him." Gary, a general practitioner, gained enormous satisfaction from describing how we've "refined the techniques" of euthanasia so that "I can do it in three or four minutes." Community nurse Michelle boasted, "I do death well."[41]

In a detailed account of prescribing a deadly medication under the 1998 Oregon physician-assisted suicide law for an elderly patient named Helen, Dr. Peter Reagan expressed immeasurable gratification after some initial misgivings and acknowledged, "there was something a little shocking about Helen's sudden transition from cheerful alertness to death." He joined Helen's family in commemorating "the pride of its accomplishment" and feeling grateful that "we could share that satisfaction." Dr. Reagan concluded by professing how "honoured to have been chosen" to be part of a death experience that "exemplified the elements of determination, courage, pride, compassion, honesty, family devotion, and good humour that embody the best in people."[42]

Table 5 highlights a comparison of Third Reich and contemporary health care professionals' emotional reactions to carrying out their destructive operations.

TABLE 5. PERPETRATORS' EMOTIONAL RESPONSES TO INVOLVEMENT IN MEDICALIZED KILLING

The Third Reich	Contemporary Society	
Nazi Perpetrators	Abortion Doctors	Mercy Killers

MOMENTARY PSYCHOLOGICAL TURMOIL		
"You are so shocked ... that it just cannot be described." (*Auschwitz physician's initial response to viewing death selections, early 1940s*)	"Shock, dismay, amazement, disgust, fear, and sadness." (*Abortion staff members' responses to dismembered fetal bodies, 1978*)	"This was really hard on me ... when he took the pills." (*Oregon doctor who wrote a lethal prescription for a patient, 1998*)
"Look at the eyes of the men ..., how deeply shaken they are! ... What kind of followers are we training here?" (*Gen. Zeleski's view of firing squad members' reactions to killing, 1941*)	"There was a leg and foot in my forceps, and a 'thump, thump' in my own uterus. Instantly, tears were streaming from my eyes." (*Dr. Lisa Harris's response to performing an abortion while pregnant, 2008*)	"It's shocking to have somebody go from telling a family story to being dead. It's a strange, strange, strange transition." (*Physician's response to effects of assisted suicide medication, 1998*)

ANXIETY-ALLEVIATING STRATEGIES		
"A drunken march around the sanatorium grounds." (*Celebration commemorating the ten thousandth patient killed at the Hadamar Hospital, 1941*)	"Excessive drinking among medical staff." (*Doctors who performed abortions at the North Carolina Memorial Hospital, early 1970s*)	"We ... drank the whole bottle within half an hour." (*Nurses' behavior after a lethal injection administered to a patient had its desired effect, late 1990s*)
Groups of colleagues arranged to socialize fellow doctors into performing death selections. (*Auschwitz, early 1940s*)	"Group intervention" and "team cohesion ... for staff ... directly involved in D&E care." (*Dr. Lisa Harris, 2008*)	"Supportive forums for discussion" to aid doctors who carry out assisted suicides. (*Health professionals, 2004*)

EMOTIONAL DETACHMENT		
"I had no feelings in carrying out these things." (*Testimony of gassing technician at the Nuremberg Doctors' Trial, 1947*)	"I never had any adverse reaction." (*Abortionist's reaction to harpooning a fetus with a needle, early 1970s*)	"I have a very clear conscience about it." (*Nurse practitioner's attitude toward performing euthanasia, late 1990s*)
"Then it got to be routine." (*Nazi doctors' reactions to conducting death selections, early 1940s*)	"It does become routine." (*Abortion clinic doctor's response to performing D&E abortions, 1996*)	"It does get easier." (*Physician with experience in euthanizing patients, late 1990s*)

PROFESSIONAL PRIDE		
"It was a matter of pride that they sometimes killed two or three prisoners in one minute." (*Concentration camp survivor Dr. Stanislaw Klozinki, 1947*)	"I have ... mastered something that I'm very proud of.... close to five thousand procedures." (*Physician abortionist's satisfaction with her abortion output, early 1990s*)	"We really helped the person achieve something that was really, really important." (*Euthanasia practitioner's description of euthanasia process, late 1990s*)
"They all bragged of having ... skill in injecting the phenol." (*Testimony of concentration camp survivor Dr. Fejkiel, 1947*)	"Abortion is not a four-letter word. I'm proud of what I do." (*Late-term abortionist Dr. LeRoy Carhart, 2009*)	Commemorating "the pride of its accomplishment." (*Dr. Peter Reagan on a prescribed deadly medication, 1999*)

CHAPTER 6

Experimental Exploitation of
Death and Destruction

Widespread experimental exploitation of human beings does not develop out of a void. It depends on a steady supply of research expendables upon whom every conceivable procedure and indignity can be perpetrated. Only a massive program of killing is up to furnishing the prescribed types of subjects in large enough quantities. Physicians embedded in this kind of milieu are not content with simply killing human beings or pioneering some of the world's most technically advanced methods of killing. They are also intent on draining every possible ounce of scientific data out of their subjects before, during, and after extirpation. During the Nazi era, the experimental population consisted primarily of patients in psychiatric institutions and concentration camp inmates destined for annihilation. Today, an ever expanding number of experimental subjects are being supplied from the ranks of unborn humans slated for abortion in hospitals, abortion centers, and fertility clinics.

Preordained Death as a Pretext for Experimentation

Nazi doctors on trial at Nuremberg repeatedly invoked the condemnation-to-death rationalization to defend their involvement in death camp experiments. Defendant Dr. Gerhard Rose acknowledged a view widely held by medical researchers during the Nazi era—since a person "condemned to death ... has to die anyhow, then it does not make any difference if he dies in a medical experiment or whether he is executed."[1]

Dr. Karl Gebhardt admitted responsibility for experiments testing out sulfanilamide and other drugs on inmates of the Ravensbrueck concentration camp after they had been deliberately wounded and their wounds infected with streptococcus, gas gangrene, and tetanus. Some of the subjects died as the result of the experiments, while others experienced intense pain and suffered serious injuries. Dr. Gebhardt justified the experiments according to the contention that the subjects "were definitely sentenced to death" and "clearly had been condemned to death already."[2]

After World War II, Dr. Fritz Ter Meer, the I. G. Farben German Chemical Corporation's executive officer in charge of synthetic rubber and petrochemical operations at Auschwitz, was questioned by a British officer whether he regretted the experiments performed on concentration camp victims by Farben's pharmaceutical subsidiaries. Ter Meer is reported to have responded that "no harm had been done to these KZ [concentration camp] inmates as they would have been killed anyway."[3]

Contemporary medical researchers, like their medical counterparts in the Third Reich, exploit the plight of a deliberately doomed "superfluous" population—"surplus embryos"—as an occasion to justify conducting experiments that involve their destruction as part of the research process. On November 6, 1998, University of Wisconsin developmental biologist Dr. James Thomson disclosed in the journal *Science* that he and a group of colleagues were the first to successfully harvest embryo stem cells from "spare embryos" supplied by a local fertility clinic. Thomson viewed them as entities "consisting of only a few dozen cells—that were destined for destruction."[4]

Ever since then, other biomedical researchers have likewise invoked the destined-for-destruction declaration as an authorization for destroying and exploiting for research the dismembered remains of human embryos. As a member of the US President's Council on Bioethics in 2002, psychiatrist and columnist Charles Krauthammer identified a broad consensus on allowing embryonic stem cell research because the discarded embryos "were doomed to be destroyed anyway."[5] Writing in a September 2006 issue of the *New England Journal of Medicine*, the justification of the journal's deputy editor, Dr. Robert Schwartz, for enabling the funding of embryonic stem cell lines was based on their portrayal as "fertilized-eggs that are stored in freezers and already tagged for destruction."[6]

Some leading newspapers have likewise jumped on the embryonic stem cell research (ESCR) bandwagon together with its destined-for-destruction rationalization. A *USA Today* editorial reasoned, "The surplus embryos are often destroyed anyway.... If surplus embryos from fertility clinics ... are doomed anyway, why not make the most of them?"[7] According to the *New York Times*, "there is good reason to support work on surplus embryos at fertility clinics that would otherwise be destroyed without any medical or scientific benefit whatsoever."[8]

Harvesting the Parts of Experimental
Victims for Transplantation

In the bone, muscle, and nerve regeneration and bone transplantation experiments conducted at the Ravensbrueck concentration camp between September 1942 and December 1943, the body parts—mainly sections of bones, muscles, and nerves from shoulders, arms, and legs—were amputated from female prisoners for transplantation to wounded members of the German armed forces residing at the Hohenlychen Hospital. Many of the experimental victims were killed after the mutilating procedures were performed or suffered permanent crippling disabilities.

During the course of carrying out her duties as an x-ray technician in Ravensbrueck, physician prisoner Dr. Sofia Maczka provided a revealing account of what happened to the victims and the use of their dismembered body parts for transplantation attempts on Hohenlychen patients. "Almost all of the patients became cripples, and suffered very much as a result of these operations," she wrote in an affidavit submitted at the Nuremberg Doctors' Trial. Regarding the fate of mentally disabled inmates, she indicated that "a few abnormal prisoners (mentally ill) were chosen and brought to the operating table, and amputations of the whole leg (at the hip joint) were carried out, or on others, amputation of the whole arm (with the shoulder blade) were carried out. Afterwards the victims (if they still lived) were killed by means of evipan injections and the leg or arm was taken to Hohenlychen."[9]

Today's counterparts to the destructive, dismembering transplantation experiments imposed on Ravensbrueck prisoners are the destructive, dismembering research procedures conducted on human fetuses and embryos. Fetal and embryonic humans are torn apart, and cells are dissected from their mutilated remains with the long-range goal of transforming these cells into spare parts for transplantation to patients.

As a precursor to their use on behalf of wanted human lives, many of these experiments have involved first determining whether nascent cells and organs cut out of aborted unborn humans can be implanted in pigs, rats, mice, rabbits, sheep, and monkeys. In one such experiment, medical scientists at the Karolinska Institute in Stockholm found that aborted "fetal tissue fragments" grafted to the "cortical cavities of immunosuppressed rats" resulted in a "very good taking and growth of the human fetal tissue" in the "rat host brains."[10]

Several decades of attempts to transplant the body parts of aborted human fetuses for treating and curing illnesses have proven unsuccessful. Many researchers have subsequently abandoned fetal experimentation and have redirected their destructive experimental procedures toward the younger "surplus" embryonic humans at fertility clinics by dismembering their bodies for stem cells to be eventually utilized on behalf of sick patients. The preoccupation of biomedical scientists with such cells—likened to the stem of a plant that spreads out and grows in multiple directions—is based on the premise that at this most rudimentary and least differentiated stage of development, they possess the unlimited capacity and plasticity to be transformed into the two hundred or so specialized cell types in the human body.

Amidst great fanfare in 2006, Harvard University launched an ambitious project designed to clone human embryos and extract their stem cells for research and therapeutic pursuits on behalf of patients with incurable illnesses. An editorial in the *Boston Globe* called it "one of the great scientific quests of the new century."[11] Despite the numerous extravagant claims about pending cures, embryonic stem cell research has never been successful in treating a single human patient. On November 19, 2010, *New York Times* health and medical reporter Nicholas Wade departed from the usual highly positive mainstream media spin placed on embryonic stem cell research with an exposé of its dark underside: "Stem cell researchers have created an illusion of progress by claiming regular advances in the 12 years since human embryonic stem cells were first developed. But a notable fraction of these claims have turned out to be wrong and fraudulent."[12]

Despite the steadfast commitment of some biomedical researchers to killing and exploiting the unwanted unborn for transplantation experiments, there exists a decided movement toward advances derived from adult stem cells and other sources that do not require the destruction of human fetuses and embryos. International expert on stem cell research and cloning Dr. David A. Prentice cites numerous published studies indicating that many people worldwide now receive adult stem cell transplants for treating various cancers, spinal cord injuries, heart damage, multiple sclerosis, sickle cell anemia, and many others.[13]

Testing Survival Technology on the Unwanted for Benefit of the Wanted

A priority item for the German armed forces was the matter of survival in frigid ocean waters. A sudden death response was reported to have occurred among many of those pulled from the water. The possibility that such deaths could rise dramatically in mass catastrophes at sea intensified the need for immediate solutions. Also lamented was the lack of knowledge about the treatment of shipwrecked persons who had been exposed to low water temperatures for prolonged periods. It was not known whether physical, medical, or pharmacological methods of treating chilled individuals were best. Most theories of rewarming frozen individuals favored a slow-warming approach, while rapid-warming advocates challenged this contention.

German medical scientists set about trying to rectify this knowledge gap by simulating the survival conditions at sea and imposing them on Dachau inmates in a series of research projects referred to as the freezing or cooling experiments. The subjects were immersed in enormous basins filled with ice cold water:

> The basin was filled with water and ice was added until the water measured 3° C. The experimental subjects, whether dressed in a flying suit or naked, were placed into the ice water.... It always took a certain time until so-called "freezing narcosis" made the experimental subjects unconscious, and the subjects suffered terribly. The temperature of the victims was measured rectally and through the stomach by galvanometer. They lost consciousness at a body temperature of approximately 33° C. The experiments actually progressed until the experimental persons were chilled down to 25° C. body temperature.[14]

After being forced to remain submerged in water for extended lengths of time, the victims were removed from the basins and exposed to a variety of rewarming techniques. For many it was too late—they had already been chilled beyond revival. Approximately 90 out of 280 subjects died; countless others suffered severe injuries with unknown long-term effects. Despite the indignities, suffering, and deaths imposed on the subjects, the cooling experiments were deemed a success. This was largely attributed to one main finding: the demonstrated effectiveness of rapid rewarming of severely cooled subjects through immersion in a hot bath.[15]

Similarly, contemporary medical scientists have long been involved in trying to develop equipment designed to help prematurely born infants survive a host of afflictions, particularly respiratory distress syndrome, a malady characterized by breathing difficulties due to insufficient lung development. Unborn humans aborted by hysterotomy have been utilized as guinea pigs for testing the operational efficacy of various life support technologies such as artificial placentas and other extracorporeal life support systems. Hysterotomy victims are considered ideal subjects for this type of research because their situations so closely duplicate those of their premature counterparts. Their bodies are aborted from the uterus intact and connected to some type of life-enhancing unit, their lives are momentarily prolonged, and then their reactions are carefully observed to determine how long they can survive. Like the Nazi experiments, the purpose of this research is to exploit unwanted doomed subjects as a means for developing technologies to aid wanted individuals.

One of the most elaborate techniques devised for the ultimate purpose of enhancing the lives of premature infants with respiratory problems was an artificial placenta developed by Dr. Geoffrey Chamberlain while a research fellow at George Washington University in Washington, DC. It was tested on eight human victims, 300 to 980 g (11 oz to 2 lbs, 3 oz) in weight, obtained from hysterotomy abortions. Each fetal subject was encased in a heated and insulated mobile cupboard to allow for constant pressure control and ease of movement. The process of hooking up the eight human fetuses to an extracorporeal circuit followed a similar sequence:

> In 7 cases, the gestational sac was removed intact from the uterus, while in the eighth, the fetus was placed in warmed normal saline at the operating table. The fetus was kept under artificial liquor amnii in the tank.... Cannulation of the umbilical vessels (vein and both arteries if possible) was achieved within 12 minutes in all cases.... In the smaller fetuses blood flow was poor. The most difficult problem was that of establishing a return flow from the fetus to the circuit via the umbilical arteries.... The longest survival in this series came with the largest fetus.[16]

Dr. Chamberlain's experiments were rated a success even though none of the fetal subjects survived for any appreciable length of time. The largest fetus (980 g) survived for five hours and eight minutes and might have lived longer if it had not been for a cannula that "inadvertently slipped and could not be reintroduced."[17]

The availability of intact, well-developed specimens for testing the utility of extrauterine life support systems has subsided owing to the decline in the incidence of hysterotomy abortions. To take up the slack, researchers have turned their attention to exploiting another source of experimental fodder for developing artificial wombs on behalf of the wanted unborn and born: human embryos "left over" at IV fertilization clinics.[18]

Characteristics of Induced Deaths

Although the experimental rescue techniques imposed by Nazi medics were only moderately successful in sustaining life, and then for just a short period of time, a number of them produced what were considered valuable by-products such as detailed descriptions of the subjects as they succumbed to the adverse experimental conditions. The researchers dutifully and methodically went about the task of recording the dying process in an exceedingly exact manner, utilizing the latest scientific measuring devices at their disposal.

The report, "Death after Cooling in Water: Practical and Theoretical Considerations," contains portrayals of breathing difficulties just before death engulfed the experimental expendables in the freezing experiments:

> In two cases breathing ceased simultaneously with the heart activity. These were cases in which it was specifically noted that the neck and the back of the head lay deep in the water. In all remaining cases breathing outlasted the clinical chamber cessation by as much as 20 minutes. In part this was "normal, much decelerated breathing," in part an agonal form of gasping.... Death occurred relatively quickly after removal from the water, which may be compared with rescue. The longest interval involved was 14 minutes.[19]

As was the case with the Nazi cooling experiments, Dr. Geoffrey Chamberlain's report on fetal experiments includes a revealing passage on the dying responses of an aborted fetal human connected to an artificial placenta:

> For the whole 5 hours of life, the fetus did not respire. Irregular gasping movements, twice a minute occurred in the middle of the exper-

iment but there was no proper respiration. Once the perfusion was stopped, however, the gasping respiratory efforts increased to 8 to 10 per minute. The fetus died 21 minutes after leaving the circuit.[20]

At first glance, the designations in the Nazi and contemporary experimental accounts—"agonal form of gasping," "irregular gasping movements," "decelerated breathing"—could well be construed to convey the agonizing, impending deaths of human beings. When incorporated within the framework of scientific reports, however, such phrases lose their power to generate horror and revulsion at what has actually taken place. They are not intended to project images of suffering humanity, but to simply embellish clinical observations with data. When a subject is characterized as gasping or having a hard time breathing, it is not meant to elicit an emotional response, but merely to describe the operation of physiological processes.

Descriptions of Reflex Actions

Another characteristic of the destructive experimental procedures conducted at Dachau was the decided propensity of the scientific perpetrators to concentrate on the reflexive reactions of the victims. A prime example of this is the focus placed on the operation of the reflexes and other biological processes of three Russian prisoners after being shot in the upper left thigh with poisoned bullets in an experiment conducted at the Sachsenhausen concentration camp on September 11, 1944. The purpose of the experiment was to assess how long it would take for the subjects to expire as a means of determining the time needed to prepare an antidote. Reich chief hygienist Dr. Joachim Mrugowsky compiled a meticulous report that is notable for its reduction of the extermination process to the technical, dispassionate level of sheer anatomy: the demise of strictly organic and physiological functions.

> During the first hour of the experiment the pupils did not show any changes. After 78 minutes the pupils of all three showed a medium dilation together with a retarded light reaction.... After 65 minutes the patellar and Achilles tendon reflexes of the poisoned subjects

were negative. The abdominal reflexes of two of them were also negative. The upper abdominal reflexes of the third were still positive, while the lower were negative.... Masseter spasms and urination were observed in one case. Death occurred 121, 123, and 129 minutes after entry of the projectile.

Summary. The projectiles filled with approximately 38 mg. of aconitine nitrate in solid form had, in spite of only insignificant injuries, a deadly effect after two hours. Poisoning showed 20 to 25 minutes after injury. The main reactions were salivation, alteration of the pupils, negative tendon reflexes, motor unrest.[21]

A considerable amount of contemporary fetal research also consists of inducing and observing reflex actions in aborted humans just before their expiration. The bulk of this research was documented in an extensive review of the literature in 1970 by Dr. Tryphena Humphrey, a professor at the University of Alabama Medical School in Birmingham.[22] Equipped with glass rods, clamps, and instruments for measuring tactile sensibilities, the researchers went about the tasks of touching, stroking, probing, and poking every imaginable nook, cranny, orifice, and surface of these expendable subjects. The experimental manipulations imposed are truly staggering: exerting pressure on the amniotic sac housing the victims; causing actions by pulling the subject's umbilical cord; stroking skin surfaces; forcing instruments into the mouth; probing the eye-nose-mouth sector; poking at the fingers, hands, feet, and genitals; and applying oxygen to stimulate fetal movement.

A typical example of the type of experiment conducted is a report on "three stages in a gag reflex elicited from an 18.5-week fetus by inserting a glass rod far back in the mouth." One finding highlighted was a description of the fetal subject's facial response to the stimulator imposed as "characteristic of a gag reflex postnatally." Dr. Humphrey's portrayal of the gag-reflex stages is reinforced by photographic prints from motion picture sequences showing these stages:

Considerable stimulation with a glass rod was required, probably over both the back of the tongue and the posterior wall of the pharynx. No doubt the stimulus included pressure as well as touch. The gag reflex itself was rapid and rather violent, although it was not

accompanied by extremity or trunk activity. Wide mouth opening, laryngeal elevation, spasmodic contraction of the diaphragm,
depression of the floor of the mouth, and partial mouth closure all
occurred.[23]

Another noteworthy fetal reflex experiment featured the analysis
of a 23.5-week aborted human's responses to being resuscitated temporarily with an oxygen mask placed over the face and then removing the mask. After the withdrawal of resuscitation, the subject is described as exhibiting a "characteristic scowl," a "tight eyelid closure," a
"wide mouth opening," and a "pain cry."[24]

Observations on Beating Hearts

Besides manipulating and recording the dying gasps of their experimental subjects, Nazi researchers exhibited a pronounced preoccupation with examining the reactions of the human heart to the destructive conditions imposed. A prime example of such an emphasis
became incorporated in a series of experiments conducted to develop
rescue techniques for German aviators who had to bail out of their
aircrafts at high altitudes. During the spring and summer of 1942, in
what became known as the high-altitude experiments, inmates at the
Dachau concentration camp were locked inside a low-pressure chamber (an airtight ball-like compartment). The pressure in the chamber
was then altered to simulate the atmospheric conditions that an avia-
tor might encounter when falling great distances through space without a parachute and without oxygen. "Approximately 180 to 200 inmates were experimented on, about 70 to 80 being killed as a result."[25]

A report on a victim who failed to survive the high-altitude experiments was accompanied by a meticulous account of his heart's
reactions:

> At 5-minute intervals electrocardiograms from three leads were writ-
> ten. After breathing had stopped, the electrocardiogram was contin-
> uously written until the action of the heart had come to a complete
> standstill. About ½ hour after breathing had stopped, dissection was
> started.[26]

Some contemporary fetal researchers have likewise conducted experiments focusing on the heart rates of aborted humans who have been kept temporarily alive in makeshift extrauterine life support apparatuses. In a series of experiments conducted at the Stanford University School of Medicine during the 1960s, Dr. Robert Goodlin studied the cardiac responses of human fetuses placed in a steel, oxygen-pressured immersion chamber that functioned as a fetal incubator. At intervals of eleven hours, he opened the chamber to see whether any subjects had survived:

> Frequently, the umbilical cord was pulsating or heartbeats were visible; if not, the thorax was opened and the heart was observed directly. When the heart was beating, the fetus was returned to the chamber and the experiment was resumed.... No fetus was living after a third period of immersion of 11 hours.[27]

In the early 1970s, Dr. Bela Resch and fellow researchers from the University Medical School in Szeged, Hungary, compared the "spontaneous contraction rates of in situ and isolated fetal hearts." The in situ hearts remained intact inside the fetal body, while the isolated hearts were cut out and suspended in a nutrient solution:

> The estimated gestational (menstrual) age of the fetuses ranged from 5 to 15 weeks. The hearts were dissected from the fetuses and were mounted in a thermostatically controlled bath.... Under these circumstances the hearts survived for many hours without any significant change in their spontaneous contraction rate.... Electrograms were displayed on a polygraph and served as a basis for determination of the spontaneous heart rate.[28]

Almost ten years later, Drs. Resch and Julius Papp utilized the same procedure—"hearts isolated surgically from healthy human fetuses at legal termination of pregnancy"—for the purpose of studying the effects of caffeine on the fetal heart. After seven hearts, ranging in age from seven to sixteen weeks, "had been beating for 60 minutes in control nutrient solution," various concentrations of caffeine were added to the solution. The strengths of the cardiac responses to the caffeine were found to increase "with advancing age, reaching its maximum in the 16-week-old heart." The researchers therefore concluded, "it seems very likely that moderate to excessive use of caffeine during pregnancy results in stimulation of the developing fetal heart."[29]

Skull Research

Besides cutting out the hearts and other body parts from the condemned subjects, medical researchers in the Third Reich demonstrated a marked partiality for practicing their carving skills on the victims' heads, skulls, and brains. Collecting and analyzing the human skulls of euthanasia patients and concentration camp prisoners became a specialty for several university affiliated medical scientists.

Kaiser Wilhelm Institute world-renowned neuropathology chairman Dr. Julius Hallervorden was an avid practitioner of conducting experiments on the brains of euthanasia victims. During an interrogation in 1945, Dr. Hallervorden admitted to American medical science consultant Dr. Leo Alexander that when those responsible for implementing euthanasia asked him how many brains he required for his research, he replied, "An unlimited number—the more the better." Hallervorden recalled, "I gave them the fixatives, jars and boxes, and instructions for removing and fixing the brains, and then they came bringing them in like the delivery van from the furniture company."[30]

Dr. Hallervorden reaped a vast experimental harvest from the severed heads, serving as the basis for the publication of articles in twelve scientific journals during the postwar years. He was never brought to trial for his involvement in exploiting the euthanasia killings and continued conducting research on the extensive pathological collection until his death in 1966.[31]

An anatomy professor from Reich University of Strasbourg, Dr. August Hirt, exhibited a painstaking attempt to prove the inferiority of the Jewish race through skull measurements. The information for this project was derived from the severed heads of inmates exterminated in the gas chambers. Dr. Hirt provided precise instructions for a special deputy (preferably a junior physician or medical student) commissioned to procure the specimens:

This special deputy ... is to take a prescribed series of photographs and anthropological measurements, and is to ascertain, insofar as is possible, the origin, date of birth, and other personal data of the prisoner. Following the subsequently induced death of the Jew, whose head must not be damaged, he will separate the head from the torso and will forward it to its point of destination in a preserving fluid in a well-sealed tin container especially made for this purpose. On the basis of the photos, the measurements and other data on the head and, finally, the skull itself, comparative anatomical research, research on racial classification, pathological features of the skull formation, form and size of the brain, and many other things can begin.[32]

Like the fixations of Drs. Hallervorden and Hirt on collecting the heads of Nazi euthanasia and concentration camp victims for their research projects, some contemporary biomedical researchers demonstrate a comparable focus on the experimental exploitation of fetal brains. The widespread prevalence of induced abortion has provided an extraordinary opportunity to indulge this passion by severing the heads of fetal bodies and subjecting them to further scientific scrutiny and purported therapeutic usage.

Doctors affiliated with the Montefiori Hospital and Medical Center in New York City and the Harvard Medical School in Boston cut out portions of fetal brains obtained from hysterotomy abortions and homogenized them in glass tubes. They were then compared with the hypothalami dissected from the brains of rats "killed by neck fracture."[33]

Another example of destructive fetal brain research was conducted by Case Western Reserve University pediatrician Dr. Peter Adam and Finnish researchers at the University of Helsinki Children's Hospital who cut off the heads of twelve prenatal humans (twelve to twenty-one weeks' gestation) aborted by hysterotomy and hooked them up to a "system of perfusion" for the purpose of studying fetal brain metabolism through observing and measuring "the utilization and oxidation of both B-OH-butyrate and glucose by isolated perfused human fetal brain[s] early in gestation." After "the head was ... isolated surgically from the other organs," it was "perfused through the internal carotid artery...." The report also features a "schematic drawing of the closed, recirculating system utilized for perfusion of [the] isolated human fetal brain."[34]

Medical Bystanders

Experimental atrocities flourished in the hospitals, psychiatric institutions, and concentration camps of the Third Reich even though only a minority of doctors participated. But the silence, apathy, tolerance, and acceptance by the remainder of the German medical profession played a crucial role in advancing the implementation and expansion of destructive research on people defined as human discards. In his history of Nazi Germany, *The Rise and Fall of the Third Reich*, William Shirer disclosed that although the experiments were known to "thousands of leading physicians of the Reich, not a single one of them, so far as the record shows, ever uttered the slightest public protest."[35]

A lack of critical response was strikingly evident among those who attended the Conference of Consulting Physicians held at the Military Medical Academy in Berlin on May 24-26, 1943, when they heard the detailed presentation of Drs. Karl Gebhardt and Fritz Fischers on the sulfanilamide experiments, which consisted of inflicting serious wounds on Ravensbrueck prisoners for the purpose of testing the effects of sulfanilamide preparations. Part of their report included a chart documenting patient deaths. In an affidavit prepared for submission at the Nuremberg Doctors' Trial, Dr. Fischer acknowledged that "No criticism was raised" by any of the conference attendees.[36] Dr. Fischer also testified during the trial about the discussion following their joint lecture: "I heard no critical utterance during that discussion. I heard no critical objections at all during the course of the entire meeting."[37]

Today, analogous to the situation in the Third Reich, little if any opposition comes from the ranks of the medical establishment against the experimental exploitation of vulnerable unborn human lives slated for extinction. The voices of medical dissent among rank-and-file doctors have been largely silenced as strip mining the bodies of fetal and embryonic humans for research has become an increasingly acceptable medical procedure.

A pervasive medical apathy was in full force at a May 1973 combined meeting of the American Pediatric Society and the Society for Pediatric Research held in San Francisco, during which the attendees heard "at least four reports on work involving human fetal tissue." The most egregious one was Dr. Peter Adam's paper detailing the procedure used in cutting off the heads of hysterotomy abortion victims and hooking them up to a circuit for studying fetal brain metabolism. Dr. Adam admitted that he no longer pursued the decapitation "line of investigation," not because of any ethical qualms, but because the replacement of the hysterotomy method by the prostaglandin abortion technique had reduced the supply of fetuses as suitable research subjects. The *Medical World News* reported that "No one even raised an eyebrow"[38] during Dr. Adam's presentation.

A great tragedy associated with the Nazi research atrocities and the contemporary experimental assaults on the unborn is the researchers' perspectives. They have methodically compiled a host of scientific observations while dispassionately watching their dying charges literally gasp for breath and life and then collapse into extinction. What they have done is lost the big picture—the human being as an irreducible individual whose dignity requires the utmost respect and loving care. Instead, humanity is shorn away and relegated to the level of sheer anatomy. The subjects are perceived as disparate congeries of tissues, organs, and biochemical elements.

Table 6 recapitulates some of the main comparisons linking various aspects of experimental atrocities past and present.

TABLE 6. HARVESTING DOOMED SUBJECTS FOR RESEARCH

The Third Reich	Contemporary Society
PREORDAINED DEATH AS A PRETEXT FOR EXPERIMENTAL EXPLOITATION	
"No harm had been done ... as they would have been killed anyway." *(Justification for experimenting on "surplus populations" at Auschwitz, Dr. Fritz Ter Meer, 1946)*	"The surplus embryos are often destroyed anyway." *(Justification for experimenting on "surplus embryos" at fertility clinics, USA Today, 2001)*
TRANSPLANTATION RESEARCH	
Arms, shoulder blades, and legs were amputated from Ravensbrueck prisoners and transplanted to hospitalized German soldiers in attempts to replace their injured limbs. *(Bone, muscle, and nerve regeneration and bone transplantation experiments, 1942–43)*	Stem cells are being cut out of dismembered human embryos for the ultimate purpose of transplanting them to heal or replace the cells and organs of sick patients. *(Embryonic stem cell research and human cloning attempts, 1998–present)*
TESTING SURVIVAL TECHNOLOGY	
Condemned prisoners functioned as subjects to test rewarming techniques on behalf of German military personnel who became stranded at sea. *(Dachau freezing experiments, 1942-43)*	Aborted unborn humans served as subjects in testing artificial placentas on behalf of wanted unborn and premature newborn infants. *(Artificial placenta experiments, 1968)*
CHARACTERISTICS OF INDUCED DEATHS	
"Much decelerated breathing ... an agonal form of gasping.... Death occurred relatively quickly after removal from the water." *(Responses of a prisoner subjected to the Dachau freezing experiment, Dr. Sigmund Rascher, 1942)*	"Irregular gasping movements ... the gasping respiratory efforts increased.... The fetus died 21 minutes after leaving the circuit." *(Responses of an aborted human subjected to an artificial placenta experiment, Dr. Geoffrey Chamberlain, 1968)*
DESCRIPTIONS OF REFLEX ACTIONS	
"Poisoning showed 20 to 25 minutes after injury. The main reactions were salivation, alteration of the pupils, negative tendon reflexes, motor unrest." *(Dr. Joachim Mrugowsky's report on prisoners killed by poisoned bullets at Sachsenhausen concentration camp, 1944)*	"Wide mouth opening, laryngeal elevation, spasmodic contraction of the diaphragm, depression of the floor of the mouth, and partial closure of the mouth all occurred." *(Dr. Tryphena Humphrey's review of a gag reflex induced in an aborted infant of 18.5 weeks' gestation, 1970)*
OBSERVATIONS ON BEATING HEARTS	
"After breathing had stopped, the electrocardiogram was continuously written until the action of the heart came to a complete standstill." *(Impact on the heart of a prisoner killed in the Dachau high-altitude experiments, 1942*	"The hearts survived for many hours.... Electrograms were displayed on a polygraph ... for determination of the spontaneous heart rates." *(Hearts dissected from aborted humans and mounted in a nutrient solution, 1974)*
SKULL RESEARCH	
"He will separate the head from the torso and forward it ... in a preserving fluid." *(Instructions for the beheading of inmates in Dr. August Hirt's Jewish skull experiment, 1942)*	"The head was ... isolated surgically from the other organs" and then "perfused." *(Medical journal account of severed head from Dr. Peter Adam's fetal brain metabolism experiment, 1975)*
MEDICAL BYSTANDERS	
"No criticism was raised." *(Responses of participants at a conference of German physicians to a presentation on the death-inducing Ravensbrueck sulfanilamide experiments, May 1943)*	"No one even raised an eyebrow." *(Responses of participants at a conference of American pediatricians to Dr. Peter Adam's experiment involving the beheading of aborted humans, May 1973)*

CHAPTER 7

Fronts for the Sanitization
of Medicine's Dirty Work

From Back Alley Butchery to
Main Street Massacre

The destruction of human lives—whether the victims were Jews, Gypsies, patients with disabilities in the Third Reich, or unborn and born humans considered expendable in contemporary society—is a repulsive and dirty business at best. Such a repugnant process requires the most antiseptic fronts to counteract its deeply degrading aspects. During the Nazi era, as numerous laws leading to the final solution and other forms of genocide took hold, mob violence in the streets was replaced by mass extermination in more unobtrusive and often esteemed settings. Ever since the full-fledged legalization of abortion promulgated by the 1973 *Roe v. Wade* decision, the so-called back alley butchers have flocked to convivial health care settings located on contemporary society's main streets, where they destroy the unborn on a massive scale. Owing to an increase in laws sanctioning physician-assisted suicide and euthanasia, a similar movement is occurring today among health professionals who are emerging from the tawdry depths of a euthanasia underground to take the lives of vulnerable patients in respectable locales.

The Nature of Medical Dirty Work

One of the most difficult problems any society encounters is consigning people to perform its "dirty work." There are certain jobs considered so physically repulsive, symbolically degrading, and morally
dubious that they qualify as "dirty work." Low-status jobs requiring
little skill, such as collecting garbage and digging ditches, are often
placed under this classification.

By any yardstick, the killing of human beings constitutes the most
extreme form of dirty work imaginable. The carrying out of society's
dirtiest work is epitomized by the role of the official executioner (the
hangman, the electric chair operator, the gas chamber expert, and the
administrator of lethal injections). Soldiers in combat are delegated to
perform the repugnant job of annihilating the enemy in a gruesome
manner—shooting, blowing up, bayoneting, and so on.

Among the annals of history befouled by endless episodes of destructive dirty work, few if any can match the Nazi Holocaust for its
scope of destruction and utter revulsion. In his seminal article "Good
People and Dirty Work," sociologist Everett Hughes called racial
genocide perpetrated under the Nazi regime "the most colossal and
dramatic piece of social dirty work the world has ever known."[1] An
extremely noisome task consisted of dispatching to the crematory ovens huge numbers of bodies covered with blood, sweat, urine, and ex-
crement. Auschwitz survivor Dr. Miklos Nyiszli supplied vivid details
on the revolting nature of the body disposal process:

> The Sonderkommando squad, outfitted with large rubber boots,
> lined up around the hill of bodies and flooded it with powerful jets
> of water. This was necessary because the final act of those who die
> by drowning or by gas is an involuntary defecation. Each body was
> befouled, and had to be washed.... The "bathing" of the dead was ...
> carried out by a voluntary act of impersonalization and in a state of
> profound distress.[2]

The repellent nature of today's worldwide killing of human lives
inside the womb is periodically acknowledged, even by some abortion
proponents. Professor Carol Joffe draws upon the insights of sociol-

ogist Hughes regarding the monumental dirty work intrinsic to the Nazi Holocaust by underscoring the physically repulsive aspects of abortion—"confrontation with blood, vomit, and, in some instances, discernible fetal parts" and the degradation experienced in "disposing of the products of conception."[3] She thus classifies abortion as "an emerging class of 'dirty work' tasks in the human services."[4]

Sallie Tisdale, a registered nurse who once worked at an abortion clinic, reveals the disgust-inducing side of abortion—"it's dirty work"—in an unusually graphic narrative of the fetal disposal process:

> At the end of the day I clean out the suction jars, pouring blood into the sink, splashing the sides with flecks of tissue. From the sink rises a rich and humid smell, hot, earthy, and moldering; it is the smell of something recently alive beginning to decay. I take care of the plastic tub on the floor, filled with pieces too big to be trusted to the trash.... I slip the tissue gently into a bag and place it in the freezer, to be burned at another time.[5]

On February 18, 2010, a search team consisting of law enforcement and health officials raided Dr. Kermit Gosnell's Philadelphia abortion clinic, where they found unbelievably squalid conditions:

> When the team members entered the clinic, they were appalled, describing it ... as "filthy," "deplorable," "disgusting," "very unsanitary," "very outdated, horrendous," and "by far, the worst" that these experienced investigators had ever encountered.
> There was blood on the floor. A stench of urine filled the air. A flea-infested cat was wandering through the facility, and there was cat feces on the stairs. Semi-conscious women scheduled for abortions were moaning in the waiting room or the recovery room, where they sat on dirty recliners covered with blood-stained blankets.[6]

In the face of these blatant forms of dirty work—genocide in the past and feticide in the present—how was it possible, and how is it still possible, for the perpetrators to sustain their participation? What could be more convenient than a thorough sanitization of such dirty work! The cleansing process involves the transformation of killing into a respectable, unblemished medical endeavor supported by the creation of immaculate settings, the extensive use of antiseptic language, and the presence of comforting and benign surroundings.

Immaculate Medical-Type Settings

Holocaust perpetrators understood the importance of effective environments for carrying out their genocidal program. A considerable number of atrocities—especially mob violence and shootings in the streets—were perpetrated in the most unsavory and transparent circumstances and places. But these actions were viewed as simply stopgap measures, a prelude to the performance of mass extermination in less messy and more unobtrusive settings. Leading Nazi officials expressed concern over the growing incidence of street riots against Jews and their property, the most extensive outburst being the infamous "Night of the Broken Glass" (November 10, 1939), during which many Jews were killed, thousands were arrested, and their shops, homes, and places of worship were demolished. As early as 1935, even the vociferous anti-Semitic propagandist Julius Streicher spoke out against such "excesses," declaring that the Jewish question was being solved "piece by piece" in a legal manner. He further asserted, "We don't smash any windows and we don't smash any Jews. We don't have to do that."[7]

The Nazis were not opposed to killing per se, but the wrong kind of killing (uncontrolled and messy) in inappropriate places (streets) where it was too visible. The systematic annihilation of millions required the admixture of technology, personnel, and settings so that the killing would proceed efficiently, swiftly, and in an unsullied fashion. Eventually, the killing underwent a radical shift from random outbursts of mob violence in German streets to assembly-line annihilation in the antiseptic fronts constructed in state hospitals, euthanasia institutions, and concentration camps.

During the summer of 1940, six killing centers were established to implement the extensive euthanasia program against patients with mental and physical disabilities. Historian Henry Friedlander concluded that "every procedure was designed to conceal the function of the killing center and to simulate a normal hospital. Although the order might differ slightly from place to place, the procedures were generally the same at all killing centers." Patients, often accompanied by male or female nurses, arrived at the institution's reception area, where they undressed. Their clothing and other personal items were sorted, labeled, and assigned a number to convey the impression that their belongings would be "eventually returned to the rightful owner." Next, they were taken into an examination room, where a doctor conducted a brief, superficial examination, comparing the identity of the patients with their medical records. Finally, the patients were herded into gas chambers, which "were disguised to look like shower rooms with tiled floors, wooden benches along the walls, and showerheads along the ceiling."[8]

In the Nazi concentration camps, the presentation of killing as an impeccable medical activity continued to prevail. The architects of Auschwitz, Buchenwald, Dachau, Treblinka, and other camps built upon and perfected a destruction process that began when physicians started exterminating patients in state institutions and euthanasia hospitals.

Upon arrival at Auschwitz, the prisoners were greeted with a reassuring facade of competent medical care. Not only were doctors present, but also their appearance was accentuated as they stood by "in a separate row with their instrument bags."[9] The medical subterfuge was enhanced by the presence of trucks with red crosses emblazoned across their sides. Prisoner survivor Dr. Gisella Pearl recalled that many of those selected for the crematory ovens "were loaded into Red Cross trucks, in a weird mockery of all human decency."[10]

Dachau, a major site for experimental atrocities conducted on human subjects, was a prominent exemplar that combined medical expertise with the most immaculate and up-to-date medical front:

> At first glance Dachau would appear to be a model camp.... The Revier (sick-bay) would seem amazingly clean and tidy. It included rooms for eye and E.N.T. clinics, a physiotherapy room with the most modern apparatus ... two magnificent operating theatres with a sterilization room, an x-ray department, a dental clinic, a well-fitted laboratory, a well-stocked dispensary, and beautiful parquet floors to the wards.[11]

Holocaust survivor Dr. Elie Cohen exposed the horrendous reality concealed behind such an ultraslick veneer: "The Nazis—including the Nazi physicians—pursued but one aim: *extermination*. The whole medical apparatus was nothing but a *décor*, nothing but a lie intended to disguise the massacre."[12]

The passion for cleanliness pervaded every phase of the death selection process. Those chosen for annihilation were told that "they had to take a shower to be clean after the long trip."[13] Great care was taken by the perpetrators to ensure that "everything was spotlessly clean" inside the Auschwitz crematorium:

> Everything was shiny as a mirror in this huge crematorium. Nothing pointed to the fact that only a night before thousands of people were gassed and burnt there. Nothing was left of them, not even a tiny piece of dust on the oven armatures.[14]

Today's physician abortionists, like the Third Reich doctors, stress the importance of antiseptic medical locales for performing their deadly operations. Before *Roe v. Wade*, many abortion proponents maintained that an alarming number of pregnant women were losing their lives at the hands of incompetent, sleazy, nonmedical abortionists under sordid circumstances in the dingy rooms of back alleys and streets. Abortion advocates and those who considered themselves respectable practitioners castigated this brand of feticide as "butchery" and those who perpetrated it as "back alley or back street butchers."

In reality, most of the illegal abortions prior to *Roe* resulted in few maternal deaths because they were performed in large part by physicians. Many of these physician abortionists were commonly portrayed as heroic pioneers for violating what were characterized as harsh, unjust, and antiquated anti-abortion laws. As early as 1933, Dr. Abraham Rongy, a fellow of the American College of Surgeons, described the physician as "the chief agent of abortion" and a "sort of Robin Hood who defies the law to help the needy."[15] By 1960, staunch abortion supporter Dr. Mary Calderone admitted, "90 percent of all illegal abortions are presently being done by physicians.... They must do a pretty good job if the death rate is as low as it is."[16]

After *Roe*, the back alley butchers in effect moved to the friendly

confines of Main Street medical establishments where they continue to commit medical mayhem against unborn human beings under
the cover of law. Modern-day abortion practitioners abhor killing the
unborn only when the destruction process occurs under conditions
where the destructive procedure is more likely to be botched, when
it is carried out by incompetent practitioners in nonmedical, unsanitary settings. The destruction of millions before birth demands an
authorized antiseptic environment in which killing is performed by
credentialed practitioners (doctors) in a speedy, proficient, and non-
transparent manner. Abortion proponents are fully aware that success
in removing the long-standing stigma associated with killing the unborn is greatly contingent upon defining abortion as a "sanitary operation" performed in the "spotless locales" of hospitals and clinics.

In a striking resemblance to those Third Reich killing centers
whose entire facilities were given over to exterminating patients in
immaculate hospital-type surroundings, today's freestanding abortion
clinics assume the lion's share of prenatal killing in establishments
containing all the earmarks of high-quality health care. Some of them
have expanded to engulf not only victims in the first trimester of pregnancy, but also those in the mid to later gestational stages—once the
exclusive domain of contemporary hospitals.

Typically, the trip through the abortion clinic begins when the
pregnant woman, frequently accompanied by a "support person," receives a warm greeting from the receptionist in an attractive waiting
room. From there she is ushered through a series of phases, including
information gathering and laboratory tests. As she is led toward the
procedure room, staff members hover over her every need, and someone is often present to hold her hand while the doctor, with the aid
of nurses and medical attendants, extinguishes the life of her unborn
child. Even a sophisticated, emotionally detached coed from a major
university in the eastern United States expressed gratitude for the opportunity to have her abortion "in a sanitary hospital environment."[17]

Pro-abortion literature is full of references highlighting the immaculate appearance of abortion clinic interiors. A study of abortion
clinics with a variety of settings ranging "from small Middle West

cozy to huge Alphaville labyrinthine" concluded that all of them were "clean, comfortable, well lit," and "tastefully decorated."[18] An architect responsible for the design of a modern New York abortion clinic emphasized that the procedure room should project "a medical environment of manifest cleanliness and surgical correctness."[19]

Cleansing the Destruction Process

The Nazi portrayal of killing as "cleaning up" or "cleansing" was in close harmony with their conceptions of Jews and other unwanted groups as unclean, sinister, inhuman, or foreign elements that threatened to pollute the purity of the German Volk and the Aryan race. What could be more sanitary, it was fervently argued, than the "cleaning out" of elements so harmful to the public health? Such antiseptic terminology aided the killers, symbolically as well as psychologically, to whitewash their activities to themselves and to others. Holocaust scholar Raul Hilberg pointed out that the destruction process came of age as a "cleansing operation" when the lethal product of a German fumigation company was employed to gas a million Jews.[20] German physicians played a leading role in characterizing the extermination of Jews, Gypsies, and "defective" patients as a "cleansing process" against those defined as posing a danger to the health of the German people. In the fall of 1935, Germany's leading medical journal, the *Deutsches Arzteblatt*, announced that the anti-Jewish racial laws would help protect the German people against further intrusion of "foreign racial elements" and would help to "cleanse the body of our Volk."[21]

Sanitized terminology played a central part in obscuring the harsh reality of the Nazi destruction process itself. The execution of more than forty-five hundred mental patients from Polish asylums was classified as "cleanup work."[22] Dr. Hermann Pfannmuller, director of the Eglfing-Haar euthanasia institution, likened the elimination of "unworthy lives" to "a cleansing of the body politic."[23] Heinrich Himmler's order for the annihilation of the Jewish population in the general government was titled "A Total Cleanup."[24]

Modern-day physician abortionists regularly depict their destructive operations as a "cleanup" process. This imagery is considered in close accord with the widespread portrayals of the unwanted unborn as foreign tissue, cell masses, or tumors. Abortion is then readily defined as a legitimate medical procedure consisting of "cleaning out" foreign tissue from the woman's body, just as racial genocide was characterized as a public health measure involving "cleansing" foreign elements from the body of Nazi-occupied Europe.

Antiseptic language has become a standard ingredient in the nomenclature of abortion practitioners, a group continually on the lookout for euphemisms to offset the repellent aspects of destroying human beings before birth. An abortion doctor from Atlanta, Georgia, described his job as "cleaning out the uterus."[25] In dilation and curettage abortion, according to Planned Parenthood of New York City, "the doctor inserts the curette into the uterus and gently scrapes the walls clean," while in "vacuum aspiration" abortion, the "emptying" of the womb is followed by "a final cleanup with a small curette."[26]

The task of reassembling dismembered aborted body parts to ensure the complete evacuation of the uterus is called "sterile-room work" at a feminist abortion clinic in the southeastern part of the United States.[27] Disposal of the "products of conception" in an abortion center located in a northeastern American city is referred to as "the post-abortion cleanup."[28]

Consoling Surroundings

The Nazi death camps consisted of huge compounds with many barrack-type structures, all enclosed by high barbed wire fences. Sand, stone, and wood dominated the environment, while grass, trees, and vegetation were almost nonexistent. Even in the midst of such desolate settings, the camp planners created an atmosphere designed to alleviate anxiety and conceal destruction.

In barracks 29 and 31 at Auschwitz, an elaborate kindergarten functioned as a subterfuge to distract attention from the use of children for Dr. Josef Mengele's experimental atrocities:

Their whitewashed walls were decorated with color paintings featuring scenes from fairy tales. The back yard of barrack 31 was fenced as a playground, complete with sandbox, merry-go-round, swings, and exercise equipment.... The facility was constructed for propaganda purposes, for the benefit of top-ranked SS and civilian officials who often visited the Gypsy camp and the kindergarten, took photos, and filmed the children at play. The truth turned out to be grim: the familiar kindergarten served as a pool of living experimental material for Mengele.[29]

As the internees passed into the camp compound, they observed a hopeful sign: a large inscription over the gate that read, "Arbeit Machi Frei" ("Labor Gives Freedom"). Many believed this meant they would soon be allowed to become productive workers once again. The changing rooms adjoining the gas chambers were designed to look like dressing rooms. Auschwitz survivor Filip Müller revealed that "along the walls stood wooden benches, creating the impression that they were placed there to make people more comfortable while undressing."[30] The elaborate deception continued inside the gas chamber, which was outfitted with all the accoutrements of a public bathhouse, including overhead shower faucets and a "bath director" who was on hand to pass out soap and towels.[31]

Contemporary abortion clinic designers have displayed comparable ingenuity in concealing the unpleasant realities of killing behind a comforting, functional front. A prime example of the lengths to which abortion clinic planners have gone in their efforts to alleviate tensions associated with participation in feticide can be found in architect Herbert McLaughlin's report on the design features of an abortion clinic in New York. The purpose of constructing the patient waiting room as a "large, high-ceilinged, open space with wood bookshelves ... and contemporary furniture of bright, bold colors and solid fabrics" was to communicate "a cheerful and anxiety-free environment." Just outside the procedure rooms were anterooms for the women to change into hospital gowns. "These alcoves are decorated with brightly printed wallpaper and curtains to provide a domestic and specifically reassuring tone."[32]

Others have continued to carry on the legacy of covering up the killing of the unborn within the confines of warm, patient-friendly atmospheres. The locale of Dr. William Waddill's once-thriving abortion practice featured antiques reflecting traditional values in a bygone era. His medical suite was decorated with "oak panels, antique furniture, even antique style examining rooms," and "cotton balls" were "stored in antique jars."[33] The walls of the Lovejoy abortion clinic waiting room in Portland, Oregon, "are covered with textured plaster," and "the chairs arranged around the room have rounded wooden backs and plush purple cushions."[34]

Floral Displays

During the early 1980s, Nazi hunter Simon Wiesenthal told a *USA Today* reporter that many of the perpetrators he tracked down were "good family men" and "gave to the poor." He summed up such an extreme paradox with the statement "They loved flowers. But they killed people."[35] The "love of flowers" served as a compelling guise for covering up the destruction of millions in Nazi hospitals and concentration camps.

A geranium plant comprised a prominent decorative object in the room at the Eglfing-Haar state hospital set aside for the extermination of unwanted children during the Nazi era. In his analysis of human violence, psychiatrist Fredric Wertham highlighted the stark contrast between the well-nourished floral display and the fate of the children dispatched to this room:

> In the children's "special department" there was a small room. It was bare except for a small white-tiled table. At the window was a geranium plant which was always carefully watered. Four or five times a month a psychiatrist and a nurse took a child to this little room. A little while later they came out, alone.[36]

The death selection process at Treblinka was facilitated by the construction of a false railway station and the presence of "flowerbeds ... which gave the area a neat and cheery look." Survivor Jean-Francois Steiner recalled that "the flowers, which were real, made the whole scene resemble a pretty station in a little provincial town."[37]

Other death camps featured a variety of floral arrangements. The Dachau medical front was enhanced by "the charming lay-out of the buildings with flower-beds and an avenue of poplars."[38] Testimony presented at the Nuremberg Doctors' Trial revealed that "a wonderful garden" was constructed for prisoner patients at Buchenwald with "deck chairs in their garden so that recuperating patients could lie in the sun."[39]

Plants and flowers also constitute standard ingredients devised to obscure the destructive reality of contemporary abortion clinic operations. The most distinctive decorations at the Lovejoy abortion facility consist of a six-foot metal sculpture of a sunflower and a vase with fresh flowers.[40] Writing in a January 2013 issue of *Time* magazine, Kate Pickert depicted the botanical-imbued interior of the waiting room at North Dakota's only remaining abortion facility as providing a consoling atmosphere for availing women of "abortion services": "The waiting room is filled with sunlight. Lush houseplants are perched everywhere."[41]

The use of flowers as a backdrop for cosmetizing the destruction of the unborn performs an identical function for facilitating the killing of unwanted human beings after birth. The widespread depiction of Terri Schiavo's enforced starvation and dehydration death on March 31, 2005, in a Florida hospice as a loving and peaceful act focused on the dazzling display of flowers at her bedside. According to a common media account, "A glorious spring bouquet of lilies and roses, red and white, sat on a nightstand by the bed" and "[at] the center of the tableau lay Terri Schiavo in a floral gown."[42]

Father Frank Pavone—who was at Terri's bedside during the final hours of her life except for the five minutes just before her death—provided a sharply contrasting perspective on the significance of the flowers: the presence of well-nourished flowers in a hospice room with a person who was denied the most basic life-sustaining nourishment. In a manner reminiscent of psychiatrist Fredric Wertham's observations about the killing of children in a Nazi psychiatric hospital room containing a carefully watered geranium plant, Father Pavone pointed out the tragic irony and hypocrisy involved in making sure the flowers were amply supplied with water while Terri wasted away from imposed dehydration:

> There was a little night table in the room.... And on that table was a vase of flowers filled with water. And I looked at the flowers. They were fully nourished, living, beautiful. And I said to myself, "This is absurd, totally absurd. These flowers are being treated better than this woman. She has not had a drop of water for almost two weeks. Why are those flowers there? What type of hypocrisy is this?" The flowers were given water. Terri was not. Had I dipped my hand in that water and put it on her tongue, the officers standing around her bed would have led me out under arrest. Something was seriously wrong here.[43]

Musical Accompaniment

When the victims arrived at Auschwitz, they were welcomed by an inmate orchestra, clad in striped pajamas, playing swing tunes. "The gas chamber waited," recounted prisoner physician Dr. Olga Lengyel. "But the victims must be soothed first." As the camp doctors proceeded to select who would be exploited as slave labor and who would be dispatched to the gas chambers, the orchestra played a medley of "languorous tangos, jazz numbers, and popular ballads."[44]

Excerpts from judgments handed down by West German courts in 1965 and 1970 in the trials of Treblinka defendants furnished further details on the role of the orchestra led by a noted conductor in facilitating the killing process:

> During the first weeks of the camp's operations, the orchestra was stationed near the "tube" [the path leading to the gas chambers], where it played lively operetta tunes to drown out the screams of the victims in the gas chambers. Later on ... the orchestra played marches and Polish or Jewish folk tunes mostly during the evening roll call.... These were macabre scenes, for even as these functions were going on, the flames from the cremation grills lit up the sky high above the camp.[45]

Although today's unborn expendables do not have the benefit of an orchestra to greet and accompany them on their journey to extinction, stereophonic music is a standard feature in many abortion centers. Sociologist Donald Ball's analysis of an abortion facility along the California-Mexico border disclosed "the function of the music, piped into every room including the one for the procedure":

> When the patrons first arrive at the clinic the music is quiet, soothing, and relaxing in style; but with the entrance of the first patient into the medical wing, the tempo and timbre increase. The volume of the music then operates to drown out any untoward sounds which might emanate from the medical wing and alarm those patrons still in the waiting room.[46]

Similarly, a woman who had an abortion in the mid-1970s at an American abortion clinic asked about the loud music being played during the abortion procedure. The clinic personnel told her that "the loud music ... was played to camouflage any screams that might come from the procedure room."[47]

The presence of consoling music continues to be a customary ingredient permeating the interiors of most modern abortion clinics. Writing in *Harper's Magazine*, Verlyn Klinkenborg underscored how music contributed a tranquil atmosphere at a Milwaukee abortion clinic: "And in the examination rooms at the Women's Medical Center, small, quiet chambers decorated with birds on the ceiling and filled with aquatic, almost astral music played at low volume" while "abortions were being performed, every half hour or so."[48]

Impact of the Fronts

The extensive planning that went into the design of the Nazi death camps made a profound impression. Few victims actively rebelled; many were fooled or comforted by the subterfuges. Survivor Dr. Olga Lengyel recalled the powerful effect of the medical fronts upon arrival at Auschwitz. It was "rather reassuring" to see the doctors standing by "with their instrument bags" openly displayed. "Four or five ambulances drove up. We were told that these would transport the ailing. Another good sign." Lengyel revealed that she and her fellow prisoners could not have known that "all this was window-dressing to maintain order" and "could not possibly have guessed that the ambulances would cart the sick directly to the gas chambers.... Quieted by such cunning subterfuges, we allowed ourselves to be stripped of our belongings and marched docilely to the slaughter houses."[49]

Disguising gas chambers as bath houses and shower rooms proved to be an exceedingly effective ruse. When the victims entered the Mauthausen camp gas chamber, "some of them were even laughing, and all were expecting to take a shower."[50] Auschwitz prisoner Dr. Miklos Nyiszli recalled how the "Baths and Disinfecting Room" sign allayed the misgivings of even the most suspicious inmates: "They went down the stairs almost gaily."[51]

The victims were not the only ones consoled by the window dressing; the perpetrators also required soothing. In his autobiography, Auschwitz commandant Rudolf Hoess wrote about gaining some respite from the stresses associated with mass destruction by fondly recalling the "paradise of flowers" in his wife's garden and how his "whole family displayed an intense love of agriculture."[52]

In a like manner, Lovejoy abortion clinic director Allene Klass "found her own escape from the pressure" by "redesigning her garden in the spring" and then falling "in love with it—the sculpted stones, the blooms on the rhodies, the ancient trees way in the back she calls her forest." A clinic worker characterized the garden as "Allene's symbolic focus for reestablishing her house as her refuge, imposing order out of increasing chaos."[53]

Contemporary pro-abortion propaganda also highlights stories from women who had abortions about the effectiveness of the clinic surroundings in relieving anxiety. One woman expressed delightful surprise with the setting: "I didn't expect a place as nice as this. I expected a dingy room and all kinds of people like you see at a bus stop.... But nobody in the waiting room seems very upset—they're all sitting there socializing."[54] Still others were made to feel "nice" about themselves "by the physical ambience."[55] Such reassuring environments have greatly facilitated the widespread destruction of unwanted unborn human lives.

Table 7 recaps the components related to whitewashing the destructive medical dirty work performed in the Third Reich and in contemporary society.

TABLE 7. THE SANITIZATION OF MEDICAL DIRTY WORK

The Third Reich	The United States
DESTRUCTIVE DIRTY WORK	
"The most colossal and dramatic piece of social dirty work." (*Professor Everett Hughes's portrayal of Nazi genocide, 1962*)	"An emerging class of 'dirty work' tasks in the human services." (*Professor Carole Joffe's characterization of abortion, 1979*)
IMMACULATE MEDICAL-TYPE SETTINGS	
"Everything was spotlessly clean." (*A description of an Auschwitz crematorium, 1942*)	"A medical environment of cleanliness." (*A description of an abortion procedure room, 1973*)
"Amazingly clean and tidy." (*A description of the Dachau medical front, 1946*)	"A sanitary hospital environment." (*Aborted woman's characterization of an abortion clinic, 1975*)
CLEANSING THE DESTRUCTION PROCESS	
"Cleanup work." (*The execution of Polish mental patients, 1940*)	"Sterile-room work." (*Reassembling dismembered aborted body parts, 1996*)
"Cleansing of the body politic." (*Dr. Hermann Pfannmuller's characterization of euthanasia, 1940*)	"Cleaning out the uterus." (*An abortion doctor's characterization of the abortion process, 1973*)
CONSOLING SURROUNDINGS	
"Their whitewashed walls were decorated with colored paintings." (*The Auschwitz kindergarten front designed to conceal Dr. Josef Mengele's experimental atrocities against children, 1943-44*)	"These alcoves are decorated with brightly printed wallpaper and curtains." (*An abortion clinic changing room, adjacent to the procedure room where unborn children were destroyed, 1973*)
"Along the walls stood wooden benches ... to make the people more comfortable while undressing." (*Changing rooms adjoining the Auschwitz gas chambers, 1942-44*)	"The chairs arranged around the room have rounded wooden backs and plush purple cushions." (*The Lovejoy abortion clinic waiting room, Portland, Oregon, 1995*)
FLORAL DISPLAYS	
"Flowerbeds ... gave the whole area a neat and cheery look." (*The site of death selections at Treblinka, 1942-43*)	"The waiting room is filled with sunlight. Lush plants are perched everywhere." (*Kate Pickert's description of an abortion clinic interior, 2013*)

TABLE 7. THE SANITIZATION OF MEDICAL DIRTY WORK (*cont.*)

The Third Reich	The United States
"At the window was a geranium plant which was always carefully watered." (*Eglfing-Haar state hospital room where children were put to death, 1945*)	"A vase of flowers filled with water" stood on "a little night table." (*Florida hospice room where Terri Schiavo died of imposed dehydration, 2005*)

MUSICAL ACCOMPANIMENT

"The orchestra was stationed … where it played lively tunes to drown out the screams of the victims in the gas chambers." (*A major function of music at Treblinka, early 1940s*)	"The loud music … was played to camouflage any screams that might come from the procedure room." (*A major function of music at an abortion clinic, mid 1970s*)
The orchestra played "languorous tangos, jazz numbers, and popular ballads" while doctors selected gas chamber victims. (*Auschwitz physician prisoner, Dr. Olga Lengyel, 1947*)	"Aquatic, almost astral music played at low volume" while "abortions were being performed, every half hour or so." (*Harper's Magazine writer Verlyn Klinkenborg, 1995*)

IMPACT OF THE FRONTS

"Some of them were even laughing, and all were expecting to take a shower." (*Reactions of victims to gas chamber interior, 1942*)	"I didn't expect a place as nice as this.… They're all sitting there socializing." (*Response of woman patient to abortion clinic setting, 1973*)
He gained some respite by recalling "the paradise of flowers" in his wife's garden. (*Auschwitz commandant Rudolf Hoess's way of managing the pressures of running Auschwitz, 1946*)	She "found her own escape," by "redesigning her garden in the spring." (*Author Peter Korn's description of how abortion clinic director Allene Klass dealt with stress, 1995*)

PART II

RHETORIC IN THE SERVICE
OF MEDICAL MAYHEM

CHAPTER 8

Ideological Foundations of Medicalized Killing

Targeting Lives Not Worth Living

A basic question pertaining to any large-scale destruction of human lives is, How could such a thing happen? What makes it possible for individuals to actually take pride in applying the most advanced technology for doing away with fellow human beings? Even more incomprehensible was the extensive participation of doctors, scientists, and other health professionals in the extermination of Jews, Gypsies, patients with disabilities, unborn humans, and others considered expendable during the Nazi era. Equally incomprehensible are today's medical assaults on the unwanted unborn and the increasing involvement of physicians in assisted suicide and euthanasia. What, then, accounts for the widespread involvement of medical scientists in the successful implementation of such destructive actions as the development of sophisticated technological procedures for the massive extermination of vulnerable human lives and the experimental exploitation of their remains?

The Significance of Ideology

Underlying almost every extensive process of killing, including medical-induced killing, is some kind of ideology—a philosophy, a social theory, a set of interrelated ideas, concepts, beliefs, and values that generate and sustain the application of destructive technology. In his magisterial epic *The Gulag Archipelago*, Aleksandr Solzhenitsyn underscored the centrality of ideology in furnishing the crucial rationale for helping the evildoer define his malevolent actions as benevolent deeds: "To do evil a human being must first of all believe that what he's doing is good, or else that it's a well-considered act in conformity with natural law." As a prelude to his analysis, Solzhenitsyn emphasized that Shakespeare's classic evildoers Macbeth and Iago "stopped short at a dozen corpses. Because they had no *ideology*":

> Ideology—that is what gives evildoing its long-sought justification and gives the evildoer the necessary steadfastness and determination. That is the social theory which helps to make his acts seem good instead of bad in his own and others' eyes, so that he won't hear reproaches and curses but will receive praise and honors....
>
> Thanks to *ideology*, the twentieth century was fated to experience evildoing on a scale calculated in the millions.[1]

The belief in human inequality—the notion that some lives are considered valuable and of great significance while others are deemed of little importance or even valueless—often serves as the dominant ideology for justifying the destruction of those who fail to measure up to the prevailing criteria of worth. Professor Henry Friedlander's *The Origins of Nazi Genocide: From Euthanasia to the Final Solution* emphasizes the importance of "the belief of the Nazi movement in inequality among humans—which provided the ideological underpinning for exclusion and genocide."[2] Physicians and scientists in the Third Reich were especially prone to invoke the hierarchy-of-worth doctrine as a major justification for their participation in the numerous destructive operations directed against individuals before and after birth who were considered too far away from the Aryan standard of acceptability.

Doctors and other prestigious professionals in twentieth-century America also resorted to the dogma of human inequality as a prominent rationalization for their involvement in a proliferating eugenics movement aimed at rooting out the unfit through forced sterilization, euthanasia advocacy and practice, abortion expansion, institutional segregation, and restrictive immigration quotas. An influential editorial published in 1970 under the auspices of the California Medical Association gave a further boost to advancing the quality-of-life ideology with the following statement: "It will become necessary and acceptable to place relative rather than absolute values on such things as human lives."[3]

Today's medical practitioners of abortion, euthanasia, and assisted suicide utilize an identical ideological rationale to explain away their deadly practices. Anyone who falls below the minimum standards of acceptability is placed in imminent jeopardy of being declared superfluous. Unborn children are sacrificed because they are viewed as only potentially human owing to their rudimentary stage of development, or are detected as having defects, or even belong to the wrong gender. Children with disabilities are rendered disposable because they do not possess the requisite physical or mental capacities, while the chronically afflicted elderly have lost theirs. In the practical order, the quality-of-life imperative too often translates to mean the quality of life for some at the expense of life for others.

Extinguishing Life Unworthy of Life Preceding and during the Third Reich

Dr. Leo Alexander, American medical science consultant to the Nuremberg Doctors' Trial, supplied an insightful reflection on how readily millions were defined as expendable in Nazi Germany under the "life not worthy to be lived" ideology:

> Whatever proportions these crimes finally assumed, it became evident to all who investigated them that they had started from small beginnings. The beginnings at first were merely a subtle shift in emphasis in the basic attitude of the physicians. It started with the acceptance of the attitude, basic in the euthanasia movement, that there is such a thing as life not worthy to be lived. This attitude in its early stages concerned itself merely with the severely and chronically sick. Gradually the sphere of those to be included in this category was enlarged to encompass the socially unproductive, the ideologically unwanted, the racially unwanted and finally all non-Germans. But it

is important to realize that the infinitely small wedged-in lever from which this entire trend of mind received its impetus was the attitude toward the nonrehabilitative sick.

It is, therefore, this subtle shift in emphasis of the physicians' attitude that one must thoroughly investigate.[4]

People with Disabilities

Charles Darwin's theory of evolutionary development, which espouses the survival of the fittest through natural selection and the elimination of the unfit in the struggle for existence, has furnished a pseudo-scientific ideology for devaluing the lives of those afflicted with disabilities. In *From Darwin to Hitler*, historian Richard Weikart reveals how the Darwinian emphasis on biological inequality stimulated many late nineteenth- and early twentieth-century German scientists and physicians "to categorize people as 'inferior' or 'superior,' 'more valuable' or 'less valuable.'"[5] In a 1909 speech commemorating the anniversary of Darwin's one hundredth birthday, University of Munich hygiene professor Max von Gruber concluded that, according to Darwin, "the never-ceasing struggle" for existence is "not useless. It constantly clears away the malformed, the weak, and the inferior among generations and secures the future for the fit."[6]

A foremost proponent of Darwinian thought as a foundation for justifying the killing of people with disabilities and other individuals was University of Jena medical professor Ernst Haeckel, who identified a broad array of individuals he considered unworthy of continued existence. Prominent on his list of discards were handicapped newborn children. "What good does it do to humanity," he asked in *The Wonders of Life* (1904), "to maintain artificially and rear the thousands of cripples, deaf-mutes, idiots, etc., who are born every year with an hereditary burden of incurable disease?" According to Haeckel's unworthy lives ideology, even those without genetic difficulties were still inherently flawed: "The new-born infant not only has no reason or consciousness but is also deaf."[7]

Haeckel's pernicious ideology had an enormous impact on the educated sector of society, especially physicians and scientists. Dr. Heinrich Ziegler conjured up ominous images of "a veritable army of the feeble-minded who committed most of the crimes" as fuel for propaganda aimed at their elimination.[8] In their influential 1920 treatise *Permitting the Destruction of Unworthy Life: Its Extent and Form*, Professor Karl Binding and Dr. Alfred Hoche decried the amount of time and resources wasted on "lives no longer worth living." Binding complained about "how much labor power, patience, and capital investment we squander (often totally uselessly) just to preserve lives not worth living," while Hoche lamented the care provided for "human life which has so utterly forfeited its claim to worth."[9]

By summer 1939, an advisory committee—euphemistically called the Reich Committee for the Scientific Registration of Severe Hereditary Ailments—was established to supervise and coordinate the killing of physically and mentally disabled children. Expert medical referees received registration forms filled out by doctors and midwives on newborn children and infants suspected of suffering from such "congenital" diseases as idiocy, Down syndrome, microcephaly, hydrocephalus, physical deformities, and paralysis. Those selected were transferred to special children's wards in some thirty state hospital pediatric clinics throughout the Third Reich, where they were subjected to lethal doses of morphine-scopolamine or luminal and veronal.[10]

The Nazi euthanasia program operated out of a villa located at number 4 Tiergartenstrasse, in the Charlottenburg section of Berlin, and hence became known by the code name "Aktion T-4." Questionnaires and registration forms containing an extensive list of designations for identifying death candidates were sent from T-4 headquarters to state hospitals and nursing homes.[11] Those targeted for extermination included patients suffering from schizophrenia, epilepsy, senile illness, paralysis, syphilitic diseases, feeblemindedness, encephalitis, Huntington's disease, and other terminal neurological conditions; patients institutionalized for criminal insanity; patients institutionalized for five years and longer; patients incapable of any institutional work except strictly mechanical tasks such as weeding; or patients who were neither German nor of German blood. Among the forty T-4 medical experts involved in evaluating the registration forms were nine professors from leading medical schools.[12]

The "life unworthy of life" classification was extended beyond these lists to engulf entire populations of mental hospitals outside of Germany. Those with tuberculosis, arteriosclerosis, cancer, and other disabling diseases were declared "persons who no longer had any value" and were therefore put to death.[13]

Inferior Races

Tracking down the unfit for extermination was not aimed exclusively at those with suspected or actual disabilities; it encompassed individuals from undesired racial groups as well. German racial theorists concentrated on two basic races: a master race of Aryans and an inferior race of non-Aryans populated primarily by Jews who were considered expendable not only because of their imputed impaired status, but also because they were viewed as threatening to taint, corrupt, and destroy the purity and survival of the Aryan race. In 1935, Dr. Edgar Schulz of the Office of Racial Policy declared that "Jewish racial degeneracy" resulted from the hybrid nature of the Jewish race, which contained an "impure" mixture of Black and Asian blood.[14]

These variations on the ideology of Jewish racial degradation helped pave the way for the passage of German racial legislation in the mid-1930s. Moreover, not only did a larger percentage (45%) of doctors than any other profession join the Nazi party, but prominent physicians also participated in the actual construction and implementation of Nazi racial policies, first against Jews and then those who were defined as blights on the Aryan ideal of perfection. The study *Racial Hygiene: Medicine under the Nazis* (1988), by historian Robert Proctor, found "that biomedical scientists played an active, even leading role in the initiation, administration, and execution of Nazi racial programs."[15]

Next on the agenda for annihilation were the Gypsies. They were considered as equivalent to the Jews—a subpar species living a useless existence. All individuals who looked like Gypsies or wandered around in a "gypsy-like" manner were seized and shot. A series of special ordinances aimed at Gypsies culminating in the decree "Combating the Gypsy Plague of December 1938" provided the basis for their deportation to the death camps of the East.[16]

The Dispensable Unborn

The approval of abortion, along with euthanasia and racial genocide, became an established component of the expanding Nazi culture
of death and destruction. In his analysis of the impact of Darwinian
thought on the value of human life in Germany preceding and during
the Nazi era, Richard Weikart disclosed that eugenics functioned as a
powerful engine driving the acceptance of abortion: most of the leading abortion advocates "were avid Darwinian materialists who saw
abortion not only as a means to improve the conditions of women, but
also as a means to improve the human race and contribute to evolutionary progress."[17]

Special hereditary health courts were established to expedite the
killing of unborn humans suspected of being afflicted with some type
of defect or abnormality. In 1934, the Hamburg Eugenics Court cited
a "racial emergency" as the reason for embarking on a program of eugenic abortions. "A pregnancy may be interrupted," it pronounced, "in
case either parent has been legally declared to present hereditary and
transmissible defects." The eugenic rationale for this decision was un-
mistakably clear: "For the sake of the continued existence and health
of the German people, an unborn child that is likely to present hereditary and transmissible defects may be destroyed."[18]

The killing of the unborn was considered a high-priority item
in the overall program of genocide. Abortion—along with gassing,
shooting, imposed starvation, and lethal injections—functioned as a
potent weapon for "reducing the surplus populations" of the East under Nazi occupation. A letter of July 23, 1942, from Hitler's secretary
Martin Bormann to Nazi philosopher Alfred Rosenberg entrusted
Rosenberg with the task of applying population reduction directives
to engulf all populations under the control of the Ministry of the Occupied Territories of the East. Bormann emphasized that "when girls
and women in the Occupied Territories of the East have abortions,
we can only be in favor of it; in any case, German jurists should not
oppose it."[19]

Eugenic ideology also served as a justification for abortions performed on women who were appropriated as slave laborers. Pregnant

eastern workers and expectant fathers were forced to undergo a racial examination in order to assess the quality of their racial characteristics. According to the decree "Concerning Interruption of Pregnancy of Female Eastern Workers," abortions were induced "if on the basis of the racial examination the offspring is expected not to be racially valuable."[20]

In many instances, however, the Nazis did not bother administering racial exams but regularly performed abortions on female eastern laborers because their unborn offspring were considered threats to the dominance of the Germanic Aryan movement. In a letter addressed to the Reich Commissioner for the Strengthening of Germanism, "the designation Race and Settlement II, undesirable population increase,"[21] was used as the rationale for performing abortions on female eastern workers at Auschwitz.

Hunting Down Unfit Lives in the First Half of the Twentieth Century in America

The dogma of human inequality as a justification for sterilizing, euthanizing, aborting, and exterminating lives considered undeveloped, inferior, defective, and seriously impaired was not confined to Germany in the half century preceding and throughout the twelve years of the Third Reich. A similar ideological rationale for doing away with the unwanted unborn and vulnerable born had likewise become implanted in American soil during the early decades of the twentieth century, helped along by a strong commitment to eugenics and acceptance of the biological inequality doctrine stemming from the social Darwinian focus on the survival of the fittest and elimination of the unfit in the struggle for existence.

Expendable Postnatal Defectives

Euthanasia advocacy for individuals deemed defective, useless, and a serious challenge to the survival of the fittest members of society became one of the bedrocks powering the eugenic war against the weak designed to create an American super race. The contention that bad blood—defective germ plasm or genes—was responsible for crime, pauperism, mental illness, alcoholism, and other problems was reinforced by a series of studies done on families with multiple problems. An upsurge of books and reports portrayed such groups as the Smokey Pilgrims of Kansas, the Jackson Whites of New Jersey, the Hill Folk of Massachusetts, the Naim Family of Upstate New York, and nomadic paupers in Indianapolis as "clans of defective, worthless people, and a burden to society and a hereditary scourge."[22]

Influential eugenic family studies published after the turn of the century were conducted by Dr. Henry Goddard, director of the Training School for the Feebleminded at Vineland, New Jersey, and his staff. In *The Kallikak Family: A Study in the Heredity of Feeblemindedness*, he traced the hereditary problems of a "high-grade feebleminded" Vineland resident named Deborah Kallikak back to an illicit affair between her Revolutionary War-era ancestor Martin Kallikak and a feebleminded tavern maid. Goddard maintained that this affair spawned "a race of defective degenerates," including generations of paupers, criminals, and imbeciles.[23]

This and other family studies served as further impetus for the expansion of eugenics programs designed to track down the unfit. A 1913 meeting of the American Breeders Association's (ABA) "Committee to Study and to Report on the Best Practical Means of Cutting Off the Defective Germ Plasm in the American People" declared that the "socially unfit and their supply should if possible be eliminated from the human stock if we would maintain or raise the level of quality essential to the progress of the nation and our race." Social researcher Edwin Black described the ABA eugenicists as "attempting a constantly upward genetic spiral in their insatiable quest for the super race."[24]

Eugenic euthanasia moved from advocacy to practice in the fall of 1915 when Chicago surgeon Harry Haiselden announced he had allowed a child born with physical disabilities to die. Subsequently, he admitted having secretly permitted many other "defective" infants to expire during the previous decade. Over the next several years, he embarked on a public crusade to legitimize these actions, as well as advocate for withholding treatment from and accelerating the deaths of handicapped babies. Dr. Haiselden repeatedly warned, "Our streets are infested with an Army of the Unfit—a dangerous vicious army" and cautioned of the need to protect society from "lives of no value."[25]

After Haiselden's death in 1919, other health professionals carried on his campaign against society's most vulnerable individuals. One of the most adamant was birth control agitator Margaret Sanger, who began her nursing career at the turn of the twentieth century. She expressed an utter contempt for people with physical and mental handicaps in institutions and brashly asserted in *Woman and the New Race* (1920): "The most merciful thing that the large family does to one of its infant members is to kill it."[26] Sanger's commitment to euthanasia was so tenacious that she served on the board of the Euthanasia Society of America (ESA) from 1942 until her death in 1965.[27]

After his election as president of the ESA in 1939, renowned Cornell University neurologist Foster Kennedy promptly revealed, "I believe it would be for the general good that euthanasia be legalized for creatures born defective."[28] Dr. Kennedy's tenure as president lasted less than two months because his position deviated from the official ESA policy that, according to its treasurer Charles E. Nixdorff, "was limited purposely to voluntary euthanasia because public opinion is not ready to accept the broader principle." Nixdorff admitted, nonetheless, "that the society hoped eventually to legalize the putting to death of non-volunteers beyond the help of medical science."[29] Historian Ian Dowbiggen disclosed that "behind closed doors" among the many eugenicists on the ESA's board of directors, a strong sentiment existed in favor of "extending euthanasia to cover unconscious geriatric patients, the incurably insane, and handicapped infants and children."[30] Apparently, Dr. Kennedy spoke prematurely and too forthrightly about ESA's long-range intentions.

Disposable Unborn Victims

The early decades of twentieth-century America were not only a heyday for the promotion of euthanasia, but also an era when eugenics emerged as one of the prime factors prompting the increasing attempts to justify abortion.

The 1933 book *Abortion: Legal or Illegal?* by American surgeon Abraham Rongy includes a host of reasons for promoting abortion, including the eugenic indication "mental defects in the mother." Dr. Rongy exerted considerable effort depicting the opposition to abortion as an outmoded dictate fashioned by "religion and mystical taboos."[31] His two-pronged strategy—the linking of abortion disapproval exclusively with Christianity and the equation of Christianity with superstition—was intended to render abortion opposition impotent by reducing it to a centuries-old irrational and delusional mode of thinking. Such a diatribe is not surprising since one of Christianity's core tenets—the equality and sanctity of all human lives—is the very antithesis of Dr. Rongy's secular, elitist ethic, which places relative values on human lives owing to their rudimentary stage of development or when they are beset with genetic anomalies.

In his influential 1936 book *Abortion Spontaneous and Induced*, Washington University medical professor Frederick Taussig incorporated "eugenic factors" among the broad range of justifications he favored for expanding the acceptance of abortion. "No doubt," he lamented, "too many idiots are being born in the world." He supported directives sponsored by the Eugenics Society of America as guidelines for physicians regarding "the question of a therapeutic abortion" for such "eugenic reasons" as nervous disorders, epilepsy, mental disorders, eye and ear diseases, allergic diseases, cretinism, diabetes, and tuberculosis.[32]

Quality-of-Life Discards in Post–World War II America and Modern Society

The years spanning the last half of the twentieth century and the beginning decades of the twenty-first century have witnessed a resurgence of efforts to expand the indications justifying abortion, particularly situations in which prenatal diagnostic tests detect a growing range of fetal defects. Alongside the movement to abort more and more unborn children because they do not measure up to increasingly elitist quality-of-life criteria, the fate of infants with disabilities and adults beset with afflictions is increasingly dependent upon meeting the ever-demanding standards of worth.

Preborn Human Expendables

In the post-World War II era, abortion advocacy for eugenics and a growing list of other indications experienced a revitalization. At an abortion conference sponsored by the Planned Parenthood Federation of America in 1955, Dr. Sophia Kleegman praised the "eugenic aspect" of abortion as being crucial for protecting and enriching "future generations in regard to our most precious resource—the human race."[33] On June 21, 1967, the American Medical Association's policy-making House of Delegates adopted a resolution approving abortion in cases where "the infant may be born with incapacitating physical deformity or mental deficiency."[34]

Soon after the *Roe v. Wade* decision, the escalation of prenatal genetic tests ushered in the era of eugenic abortions. In the 1970s, amniocentesis—an analysis of samples of amniotic fluid surrounding the unborn child—was the major test employed to detect and subsequently target for abortion those found with chromosomal anomalies during the middle trimester of pregnancy. By the 1990s, the array of tests devised to identify fetal disabilities mushroomed, "including amniocentesis, fetoscopy, ultrasonography, chorionic villus sampling, and fetal blood sampling, along with concomitant laboratory techniques, including cytogenetic and biochemical tests and molecular genetic approaches."[35] Such procedures function, for the most part, as search-and-destroy missions. According to studies of abortion rates, "About 90 percent of women who learn they are carrying a fetus with the extra 21st chromosome that causes Down syndrome choose an abortion."[36]

Prenatal screening tests designed to detect fetal abnormalities have proliferated during the first decade of the twenty-first century. *New York Times* correspondent Amy Harmon revealed that "more than 450 conditions, including deafness, dwarfism and skin disease, can be diagnosed by testing fetal cells." Some doctors told her about being "troubled by what sometimes seems like a slippery slope from prenatal science to eugenics." Other doctors mentioned having seen "couples terminate pregnancies for poor vision, whose effect they had witnessed on a family member, or a cleft palate, which they worried would affect the quality of their child's life."[37] The movement toward designer babies is an expression of an obsessive consumer culture in which vulnerable humans become just another product to be manipulated and assessed for quality control and then discarded if they don't measure up to the prescribed specifications.

The vast majority of abortions, nonetheless, are not performed on individuals detected with disabilities, but simply because they are not wanted. Aborting the unborn is often framed as advancing a global quality of life by preventing the birth of problematic people who would otherwise exacerbate the travail in a world depicted as being already overburdened by overpopulation and environmental depredation. In an interview with the *New York Times* on the nomination of Sonia Sotomayor to America's highest court, Supreme Court Justice Ruth Bader Ginsberg revealed she had originally thought that the 1973 *Roe* decision was enacted to sanction abortion as a prime means of reducing the growth of undesirable populations, thus supporting the Medicaid funding of abortions for poor women:

> Frankly I had thought that at the time *Roe* was decided, there was concern about population growth and particularly growth in populations that we don't want to have too many of. So that *Roe* was going to be then set up for Medicaid funding of abortion.[38]

To the contrary, the 1980 US Supreme Court decision in *Harris v. McRae* upheld the Hyde Amendment, which forbids the use of Medicaid abortion funding. Ginsberg expressed surprise at the ruling and then lamented, "I realized that my perception of it had been altogether wrong."[39]

Vulnerable Postnatal Casualties

Just preceding the *Roe v. Wade* decision, the influential biomedical ethicist and abortion-fetal experimentation-euthanasia proponent Dr. Joseph Fletcher had begun to construct the basic components of an aggressive quality-of-life ideology directed against vulnerable individuals with disabilities. Writing in the *Hastings Center Report* of November 1972, he listed fifteen "indicators of humanhood" viewed as essential for meriting membership in the human community: minimum intelligence, self-awareness, self-control, a sense of time, a sense of futurity, a sense of the past, the capability to relate to others, concern for others, communication, control of existence, curiosity, change and changeability, balance of rationality and feeling, idiosyncrasy, and neocortical functioning.[40]

Drs. Raymond Duff and A. G. M. Campbell relied upon an array of quality-of-life factors to rationalize the withholding of life-saving medical treatment to forty-three seriously ill infants who subsequently expired in the Yale-New Haven special care nursery during the early 1970s. They cited such justifications as their "prognosis for meaningful life was extremely poor or hopeless," individuals with "little or no hope of achieving meaningful 'humanhood,'" and "individuals who have no human potential"[41] in defending their death-inducing decisions.

Pediatric surgeon Anthony Shaw has attempted to enhance the rigor of hospital infanticide with a mathematical formula QL = NE x (H+S) for assessing the infant's quality of life and its implications for medical treatment. According to this equation, "(QL) represents the quality of life and (NE) represents the patient's natural endowment (physical and intellectual)," while "(H) represents the contributions made to the individual by his home and family and (S) represents the contributions made to the individual by society."[42]

It did not take long for someone to put the formula to the test. A multidisciplinary health care committee applied Dr. Shaw's quality-of-life formula to children born with spina bifida at the Oklahoma Children's Memorial Hospital in Oklahoma City from 1977 to 1982.

Those thirty-six infants who passed the quality-of-life examination received vigorous treatment for their afflictions, and "35 are still alive; one child died at 14 months in a motor vehicle accident." The twenty-four children who failed to measure up were dispatched to a shelter where they "died at an average of 37 days" due to the denial of life-sustaining treatment.[43]

Following in the footsteps of Joseph Fletcher and Anthony Shaw, Australian philosopher Peter Singer, the author of *Animal Liberation* and a host of articles and books on ethics, has emerged as an implacable advocate of a biomedical ethics based on quality-of-life concerns. In *Should the Baby Live? The Problem of the Handicapped Infant* (1985), Singer and colleague Helga Kuhse cited Joseph Fletcher's indicators of humanhood as a basis for proposing a series of traits a person needs in order to merit legal protection and survival: "self-awareness, self-control, a sense of the future, a sense of the past, the capacity to relate to others, concern for others, communication, and curiosity." They were particularly enamored of philosopher Michael Tooley's "continuing self" requirement that "only beings with a degree of self-awareness and a sense of the future can have a right to life."[44] Singer elaborated in other books that "infants are sentient beings who are neither rational nor self-conscious,"[45] and "life without consciousness is of no worth at all."[46]

The appointment of Professor Singer to a chair in bioethics at Princeton University's Center for Human Values provided him with a prestigious position from which to promote an elitist ideology with strong eugenic overtones. Singer and other secular philosophers have had a pronounced impact on intensive care units, where a growing number of physicians resort to quality-of-life criteria for determining which children with disabilities are and which are not deserving of life-enhancing medical treatment.

The *New England Journal of Medicine* of March 10, 2005, furnished a platform for Drs. Eduard Verhagen and Pieter Sauer—professors affiliated with the pediatrics department at University Medical Center Groningen in the Netherlands—to promote "the Groningen Protocol" quality-of-life guidelines for justifying the euthanasia of twenty-two

infants born with disabilities. Their account showcases the designations: "a poor quality of life," "a very poor quality of life," and "an
extremely poor quality of life." Among some of the "extremely poor
quality of life" factors Verhagen and Sauer "used to support the decision to end" the lives of the children were "functional disability, pain,
discomfort, poor prognosis, and hopelessness" as well as a "predicted
lack of self-sufficiency," a "predicted inability to communicate," and
an "expected hospital dependency."[47]

Quality-of-life indicators are also increasingly employed in assessing whether vulnerable adults' lives are worth living. In 2009, the Department of the Veterans Administration's National Center for Ethics
in Health resuscitated a fifty-two-page end-of-life planning document,
Your Life, Your Choices, first published in 1997. The primary author of
this publication is Dr. Robert Perlman, chief of ethics evaluation for
the center and a staunch advocate of physician-assisted suicide.[48]

One of the document's main features is a worksheet specifying situations commonly experienced by elderly and disabled patients such
as, "I can no longer walk but get around in a wheelchair," "I live in a
nursing home," and "I cannot seem 'to shake the blues.'" Also inserted
are several guilt-inducing replies: "I can no longer contribute to my
family's well being," "My situation causes severe emotional burden for
my family (such as feeling worried or stressed all the time)," and "I am
a severe financial burden on my family."[49]

The veterans are then asked to check which of these situations
and responses approximate how they feel about their circumstances.
Two of the categories listed for checking under the heading *"Life like
this would be"* include "worth living, but just barely" and *"not* worth
living." The respondents are further instructed to use the following
questions in helping them make sense of and explain their answers to
loved ones and health care providers: "If you checked 'worth living,
but just barely,' for more than one factor, would a combination of these
factors make your life 'not worth living?' If so, which factors?" "If you
checked 'not worth living,' does this mean that you would rather die
than be kept alive?"[50]

Writing in the *Wall Street Journal* on August 19, 2009, Jim Towey, then president of St. Vincent College and director of the White House Office of Faith-Based Initiatives in the George W. Bush administration, exposed this document as a veritable "death book for veterans" with a clear and unconscionable "hurry-up and die message," in which ex-soldiers are led to believe "they're a burden to society." "When the government can steer vulnerable individuals to conclude for themselves that life is not worth living," Towey asserted, "who needs a death panel?" What is more, he disclosed that "a July 2009 VA directive instructs its primary care physicians to raise advance care planning with all VA patients and to refer them to 'Your Life, Your Choices.' Not just those of advanced age and debilitated condition—all patients."[51]

The field of biomedicine has enjoyed an exponential growth over the past several decades, and along with it has emerged a return of eugenics under the respectable guise of scientific genetics. The eugenicists of early twentieth-century America and the racial hygienists of the Third Reich would indeed gasp in awe at the sheer number and utter sophistication of techniques that can be employed against those today whose quality of life fails to meet the prevailing standards of worth.

As recapitulated in table 8, the designations generated by blatant utilitarian ideological perspectives to denigrate historical and contemporary victims possess striking similarities.

TABLE 8. LIVES DEVOID OF QUALITY AND WORTH

Preceding and during the Nazi Era	Early and Contemporary American Society
THE SIGNIFICANCE OF IDEOLOGY	
"The belief of the Nazi movement in inequality ... provided the ideological underpinning for exclusion and genocide." *(Professor Henry Friedlander's analysis of the ideology leading to the Holocaust, 1995)*	"It will become necessary and acceptable to place relative rather than absolute values on such things as human lives." *(California Medical Association on the ideology underlying abortion and euthanasia, 1970)*
DEFECTIVE EXPENDABLES	
"Jewish racial degeneracy." *(Dr. Edgar Schulz's characterization of the Jewish people, 1935)*	"A race of defective degenerates." *(Dr. Henry Goddard's characterization of the Kallikak family clan, 1913)*
"A veritable army of the feebleminded who committed most of the crimes." *(Euthanasia proponent Dr. Heinrich Ziegler, 1904)*	"Our streets are infested with an Army of the Unfit—a dangerous, vicious army." *(Euthanasia practitioner Dr. Harry Haiselden, 1915)*
"The new-born infant not only has no reason or consciousness but is also deaf." *(Euthanasia proponent Dr. Ernst Haeckel, 1904)*	"Infants are sentient beings who are neither rational nor self-conscious." *(Euthanasia proponent Professor Peter Singer, 1999)*
UNWORTHY LIVES	
"Human life which has so utterly forfeited its claim to worth." *(Dr. Alfred Hoche's characterization of individuals with severe mental disabilities, 1920)*	Individuals with "little or no hope of achieving meaningful 'humanhood.'" *(Justification of Drs. Duff and Campbell for denial of life-saving treatment to seriously ill infants, 1973)*
"Persons who no longer had any value." *(Classification of inmates killed in mental institutions under Nazi occupation, 1945)*	"An extremely poor quality of life." *(A designation invoked to justify the killing of infants in Dutch hospitals, 2005)*
"Lives not worth living." *(Professor Karl Binding's characterization of insane and incurably ill patients, 1920)*	"Life like this would be not worth living." *(A phrase from the Veterans Administration's end-of-life planning document, 2009)*
UNWANTED POPULATIONS	
Abortions were performed on eastern slave laborers who failed a racial examination. *(Circular "Concerning Interruptions of Pregnancy of Female Eastern Workers," 1943)*	Life-saving treatment was denied to infants who failed a quality-of-life test. *(Multidisciplinary committee decision, Oklahoma Children's Memorial Hospital, 1977-82)*
"An unborn child that is likely to present hereditary and transmissible defects may be destroyed." *(Hamburg Eugenics Court, 1934)*	"About 90 percent of women who learn they are carrying a fetus with ... Down syndrome choose an abortion." *(Studies of abortion rates, 2007)*
"The designation Race and Settlement II, undesirable population increase." *(The rationale advanced for performing abortions on female eastern workers at Auschwitz, 1944)*	"Concern about growth in populations ... we don't want to have too many of." *(Justice Ruth Bader Ginsberg's view of Roe v. Wade's main reason for legalizing abortion, 2009)*

CHAPTER 9

The Quality-of-Life Ideology
and Semantic Gymnastics

The process of devaluing people for their failure to live up to an increasingly elitist quality-of-life ideology is not only aimed at the destruction of the sanctity-of-life ethic, but also leads inexorably to an extreme corruption of language and thought. An exceedingly forthright and prophetic editorial, "A New Ethic for Medicine and Society," published in the September 1970 issue of *California Medicine*, the journal of the California Medical Association (CMA), contains the rhetorical ingredients essential for the rationalization of killing in the service of healing: a morally relative ideology propagating a relentless outpouring of verbal distortions bolstered by boldface lying and disseminated under the banner of prestigious medical purveyors and their powerful allies:

> The traditional Western ethic has always placed great emphasis on the intrinsic worth and equal value of every human life regardless of its stage or condition. This ethic has had the blessing of the Judeo-Christian heritage and has been the basis for most of our laws and much of our social policy. The reverence for each and every human life has also been a keystone of Western medicine and is the ethic which has caused physicians to try to preserve, protect, repair, prolong and enhance every human life which comes under their surveillance. This traditional ethic is still clearly dominant, but there is much to suggest that it is being eroded at its core and may eventually

even be abandoned. This of course will produce profound changes in Western medicine and in Western society.

There are certain new facts and social realities which are becoming recognized, are widely discussed in Western society and seem certain to undermine and transform this traditional ethic ... and perhaps most important, a quite new emphasis on something which is beginning to be called the quality of life, a something which becomes possible for the first time in human history because of scientific and technologic development....

What is not yet so clearly perceived is that in order to bring this about hard choices will have to be made with respect to what is to be preserved and strengthened and what is not, and that this will of necessity violate and ultimately destroy the traditional Western ethic with all that this portends. It will become necessary and acceptable to place relative rather than absolute values on such things as human lives, the use of scarce resources and the various elements which are to make up the quality of life or of living which is to be sought. This is quite distinctly at variance with the Judeo-Christian ethic....

The process of eroding the old ethic and substituting the new has already begun. It may be seen most clearly in changing attitudes toward human abortion. In defiance of the long held Western ethic of intrinsic and equal value for every human life regardless of its stage, condition or status, abortion is becoming accepted by society as moral, right and even necessary. It is worth noting that this shift in public attitude has affected the churches, the laws and public policy rather than the reverse. Since the old ethic has not yet been fully displaced it has been necessary to separate the idea of abortion from the idea of killing, which continues to be socially abhorrent. The result has been a curious avoidance of the scientific fact, which everyone really knows, that human life begins at conception and is continuous whether intra- or extra-uterine until death. The very considerable semantic gymnastics which are required to rationalize abortion as anything but taking a human life would be ludicrous if they were not often put forth under socially impeccable auspices. It is suggested that this schizophrenic sort of subterfuge is necessary because while a new ethic is being accepted the old one has not yet been rejected.[1]

The Far-Reaching Consequences of the New Ethic

The CMA editorial emphasis on replacing the Judeo-Christian ethic of "intrinsic and equal value for every human life regardless of its stage, condition or status" by a quality-of-life ideology that confers "relative rather than absolute values on such things as human lives" is key to understanding the growing embrace of abortion "as moral, right and even necessary." Even the leaders and followers of some religious denominations and groups fail to grasp the blatant anti-Jewish and anti-Christian nature of the pro-abortion mindset. Paradoxically, they continue to defend a philosophy and movement whose avowed purpose is to ultimately destroy the most fundamental ethic linking both Judaism and Christianity—the sanctity and worth of every human life, whatever its status, condition, or stage of development.

Next, the editorial proposes a policy of extreme linguistic duplicity—fittingly dubbed "the very considerable semantic gymnastics"—as a device for advocating the approval of abortion. It goes a step further by specifying three basic strategies underlying semantic gymnastics: (1) "Avoidance of the scientific fact, which everyone really knows, that human life begins at conception and is continuous whether intra- or extra-uterine until death," (2) "Separate the idea of abortion from the idea of killing, which continues to be socially abhorrent," and (3) present these verbal fabrications as scientific facts when disseminated "under socially impeccable auspices."

Spreading the falsehood that human life does not begin at conception leads readily to denying that human life exists at other stages of prenatal development as well. This deceptive rhetoric has the effect of reducing the unwanted unborn to a subhuman level throughout the entire duration of pregnancy. Separating the idea of abortion from the idea of killing paves the way for burying the harsh reality of intrauterine destruction beneath a comforting blanket of medical metaphors and humanistic designations.

"The very considerable semantic gymnastics" is an apt expression because it signifies the severe twisting and contortion of language "required to rationalize abortion as anything but taking a human life."

Moreover, this level of lying is considered so outlandish that the CMA editorial refers to it as a "schizophrenic sort of subterfuge" but maintains that "this schizophrenic sort of subterfuge is necessary because while a new ethic [the secular humanistic quality-of-life imperative] is being accepted the old one [the Judeo-Christian sanctity-of-life perspective] has not yet been rejected." Comparing this brand of linguistic distortion to a major mental disorder such as schizophrenia is an astonishing acknowledgment and an indication of the radical extremism powering pro-abortion propaganda. Equally astounding is the admission that a tactic of verbal duplicity comparable to a manifestation of pathological lying is actually endorsed as a perfectly legitimate way to promote abortion.

Finally, the editorial provides a revealing insight into how lying bordering on a psychiatric disorder can become so convincing: "The very considerable semantic gymnastics which are required to rationalize abortion as anything but taking a human life would be ludicrous if they were not often put forth under socially impeccable auspices." Thus, under the ordinary standards of honest discourse, it would be deemed ludicrous to deny the scientific fact that abortion destroys an actual human life before birth. In conformity with the tenets of semantic gymnastics, however, when such patent nonsense is circulated under that socially impeccable auspice—organized medicine—it becomes an incontestable truth.

The irony and duplicity underpinning the CMA editorial are mind numbing. Here is a statement formulated under the sponsorship of a reputable medical organization that encouraged its members to work for sanctioning a destructive operation by totally disregarding the undisputed "scientific fact [admittedly, neither a theological dogma nor a philosophical speculation], which everyone really knows, that human life begins at conception" and called abortion something other than killing. Today, more than four decades later, no longer does everyone accept the genuine humanity of prenatal life, nor do they wish to become aware of what abortion does to this life, thanks to the awesome power of big lies in the hands of prestigious perpetrators backed up by an elitist ideology. This pernicious politicization of medicine in the service of a tenacious anti-life agenda has resulted in a monumental hoax—the reduction of undisputed scientific facts to the suspect status of sectarian beliefs.

Although the editorial highlights the endorsement of abortion as a prime example of how the quality-of-life ideology is "eroding the old ethic," the thrust of its verbal duplicity is not confined to encompassing the unwanted unborn but is intended to reach well beyond the womb:

> The part which medicine will play as all this develops is not yet entirely clear. That it will be deeply involved is certain. Medicine's role with respect to changing attitudes toward abortion may well be a prototype of what is to occur.... One may anticipate further development of these roles as the problems of birth control and birth selection are extended inevitably to death selection and death control whether by the individual or by society, and further public and professional determination of when and when not to use scarce resources.[2]

The quality-of-life ideology and its vocabulary of duplicity thus admittedly possess decidedly draconian implications for doing away with vulnerable individuals *after* as well as before birth. Since semantic gymnastics are invoked to deny the humanity of the unwanted unborn, they are also being conjured up to question the humanity of the expendable born. Since semantic gymnastics are relied upon to call abortion something other than killing, they are also summoned to gloss over the killing of the unwanted after birth. Helped along by the enormous inroads made by big lies in the promotion of abortion, today's medical practitioners of euthanasia and assisted suicide increasingly resort to similar linguistic subterfuges to justify their deadly practices.

The goal of the foreboding CMA statement is not to lament the far-reaching consequences of a quality-of-life ideology for determining who will live and who will be declared superfluous. It clearly exhorts members of the medical profession to embrace this ethic and lead the way for its global expansion. In a manner reminiscent of Aldous Huxley's *Brave New World*, physicians are urged "to examine this new ethic, recognize it for what it is and will mean for human society, and prepare to apply it in a rational development for the fulfillment and betterment of mankind in what is almost certain to be a biologically oriented world society."[3]

To the contrary, the reliance of physicians on quality-of-life factors to justify extinguishing the lives of vulnerable individuals before and after birth transforms the doctor into an incomparably lethal force for the debasement rather than betterment of humankind. Today's medical proponents of placing a hierarchy of worth on human lives would do well to heed the warning of Dr. Christoph Hufeland, who more than a century and a half ago warned, "If the physician presumes to take into consideration in his work whether a life has value or not, the consequences are boundless and the physician becomes the most dangerous man in the state."[4]

A Long-Standing Legacy of Name Calling

A quality-of-life ideology that imposes relative values on human lives considered expendable, and even goes so far as to deny their humanity outright, inevitably spawns a series of derogatory terms for further reinforcement. Such demeaning labels as "subhuman," "nonhuman," "nonperson," "lower animal," "parasite," "vegetative existence," "research material," "waste product," "garbage," "disease," "germ," and "appendix" then become readily incorporated into the lexicon of dehumanization. The other basic semantic distortion emanating from this ideological perspective—what is done to the victims is called something other than killing—is a highly influential source for the creation of sugarcoated terminology designed to cover up the destructive deeds performed. The euphemisms generated—many with a decided medical spin—are intended to shore up this component of the duplicitous vocabulary constructed: "choice," "selection," "evacuation," "removal," "reduction," "treatment," "procedure," "operation," "humane service" "release," "deliverance," and "cleanup."

Despite numerous references in the CMA editorial to the quality of life as a new ethic, there is hardly anything new about this ethic. It is simply another incarnation of an extreme moral relativism responsible for all kinds of atrocities down through history. Dressing up this ideology of human inequality in a garb of medical jargon and respectability is not new, either. In many respects, it bears a close resemblance to the situation in the Third Reich when doctors and scientists played a central role in subverting language to justify participation in a wide range of destructive actions. Moreover, the big lies circulated throughout the Third Reich were the products of influential elites, including a number of prominent physicians. This phenomenon is likewise prevalent in contemporary society, where some medical scientists from the most prestigious universities and institutions lead the way in propagating outlandish falsehoods to further entrench the medicalization of destruction as a legitimate component of mainstream medical practice.

Regarding the actual content of the big lies, the denial of the victims' humanity in the Third Reich was reinforced through the imposition of demeaning expressions. Subhuman labels and a plethora of degrading synonyms were directed primarily against Jews, but also aimed at people with disabilities, the unborn, Gypsies, Poles, Russians, and any individual or group viewed as departing too far from the Aryan ideal of perfectionism. Today, the unwanted unborn are the major targets of these same epithets. Increasing numbers of undesired and vulnerable individuals in the postnatal phases are also being subjected to an ever expanding vocabulary of denigration.

Similarly, what was done to the Nazi victims, like the fate of contemporary victims, was called something other than killing. The Nazi doctors had a strong aversion to calling their deadly practices by their proper names and instead resorted to inoffensive and clinical sounding phraseology. Contemporary medical proponents of abortion, assisted suicide, euthanasia, and destructive experiments on humans deemed expendable avoid the word "kill" just as vehemently as did their predecessors in the Third Reich. Modern-day practitioners of medicalized killing rely on identical medical appearing terminology to mask the harsh nature of their lethal procedures.

Furthermore, the same litany of verbal fabrications was disseminated by medical elites and their confederates in other professions during the early decades of twentieth-century America, when the eugenics movement became a pervasive cultural force. The corruption of language was directed at that time mainly against people with disabilities, the rural poor, immigrants from southern Europe, and unborn children.

Table 9 highlights the dehumanizing and euphemistic designations generated by the ideology of human inequality and implemented under the guise of socially impeccable medical auspices. The remaining chapters in part II focus on documenting the enormous number of striking similarities between the linguistic distortions of the past and those of the present.

TABLE 9. IDEOLOGY AND VERBAL DUPLICITY

QUALITY-OF-LIFE IDEOLOGICAL GOALS

A. Destruction of the Judeo-Christian ethic of intrinsic and equal value for every human life regardless of stage, condition, or status.

B. Replacement of the Judeo-Christian ethic with an elitist quality-of-life ethic that imposes relative values on human lives.

IMPLEMENTATION OF GOALS VIA SEMANTIC GYMNASTICS

(1) Dehumanization of the Victims
The victims are called something other than human—avoid the scientific fact that human life begins at conception and is continuous, whether intra- or extrauterine, until death

Subhuman	Nonhuman	Nonperson
Lower Animal	Parasite	Vegetative Existence
Waste Product	Garbage	Research Material
Disease	Germ	Appendix

(2) Euphemisms in the Service of Killing
What is done to the victims is called something other than killing—separate the realities of abortion, physician-assisted suicide, euthanasia, racial genocide, and destructive experimental exploitation from the idea of killing

Choice	Selection	Evacuation
Removal	Reduction	Treatment
Procedure	Operation	Humane Service
Release	Deliverance	Cleanup

(3) Dissemination of These Schizophrenic Subterfuges under Socially Impeccable Auspices
The transformation of fabrications into the truth when put forth by prestigious medical purveyors and their influential accomplices

Physicians	Scientists	Bioethicists
Nurses	Professors	Legislators
Philosophers	Attorneys	Jurists

CHAPTER 10

The Imposition of Dehumanizing Labels

The language of denigration generated by the quality-of-life ideology is relentless. It varies from sowing doubts about the human status of vulnerable individuals to outright denials of their humanity altogether. The result is a proliferation of deeply degrading expressions, some of its major purveyors being physicians in league with other professionals. Holocaust scholar Raul Hilberg identified the main functions of the demeaning stereotypes constructed in the war against the Jews: "They are used as justifications for destructive thinking; they are employed as excuses for destructive action."[1] Disparaging stereotypes serve identical purposes in today's destructive actions against the unwanted unborn and the escalating assaults on the vulnerable born—to justify destructive thinking and excuse destructive action.

Subhuman

The word *untermensch* (subhuman) and such associated terms as "nonhuman" and "not a human being" comprised a lexicon of derogatory expressions deployed during the Nazi era to demonize Jews and others considered alien to the Aryan standard of worth. In *Accounting for Genocide*, Helen Fein concluded that extermination of the Jews could not have occurred "had not the victims been previously defined as basically of a different species, outside of the common conscience, and beyond the universe of obligation; this was the precondition."[2]

A widely circulated pamphlet, *The Subhuman*, published in 1942 by the RuSHA (Race and Settlement Main Office), contained numerous degrading stereotypes—both printed and pictorial—directed against the Jewish people:

> The sub-human, that biologically seemingly complete creation of nature with hands, feet and a kind of brain, with eyes and mouth, is nevertheless a completely different, dreadful creature. He is only a rough copy of a human being, with human-like facial traits but nonetheless morally and mentally lower than any animal.... Sub-human, otherwise nothing. For all that bear a human face are not equal.[3]

Medical practitioners of extermination employed identical terminology to rationalize their lethal procedures. Dr. Friedrich Mennecke called concentration camp prisoners he selected for the gas chambers "only silhouettes in human form" and a "shabby heap of humanity."[4] Dr. Hans Heinze expressed hope that after the war this "fight against or extermination of subhumanity ... will take its honored place as a further great deed beside those already accomplished."[5]

Resort to dehumanizing labels was especially prevalent among doctors who exploited concentration camp inmates for experimental atrocities. Anatomy professor Dr. August Hirt's rationale for demonstrating the inferiority of the Jewish race through measurements on skulls collected from gas chamber victims appeared in a report submitted on February 9, 1942: "By procuring the skulls of the Jewish-Bolshevik Commissars, who personify a repulsive, yet characteristic subhumanity, we have the opportunity of obtaining tangible scientific evidence."[6]

The lexicon of subhumanity devised to denigrate the unwanted unborn in modern times closely mirrors the vocabulary used against the victims of the Nazi Holocaust. A 1968 issue of the *Journal of Marriage and the Family* provided a forum for University of California, Santa Barbara, biology professor and abortion advocate Dr. Garrett Hardin to put forth an influential version of anti-fetal linguistics containing an admixture of blatant arbitrariness and subjectivism: "Whether the fetus is or is not a human being is a matter of definition, not fact; and we can define in any way we wish.... It would be unwise to define the fetus as human (hence tactically unwise ever to refer to the fetus as an 'unborn child')."[7]

Writing in the journal *Society* (March/April 1976), Columbia University sociologist Amitai Etzioni proposed developing "procedures and criteria for determining who and what shall live or die and which fetuses are tissue and which are human." He characterized the early phase of prenatal life as "the subhuman stage" and maintained that most scientists and much of the public view the "previable" fetus as "not alive, not human, and basically a piece of tissue." Etzioni therefore concluded, "For the first four and one-half months the fetus is subhuman and relatively close to a piece of tissue."[8]

Health workers at a feminist abortion center in the early 1990s appropriated subhuman terminology to offset the shock of encountering what they instinctively defined as a "baby" in late-term abortions. When a worker acknowledged getting upset by the sight of blood and fetal parts, her initial reaction was, "By the second trimester ... it's a baby, and by eighteen weeks it's definitely a baby." She nonetheless overrode this reality with the rhetoric that abortion involves "ending something ... that is alive that I don't believe is really a human being yet."[9]

Subhuman designations also comprise a significant component in contemporary euthanasia advocacy and practice, particularly when directed against individuals afflicted with genetic anomalies and those dependent for survival on respirators, feeding tubes, and other life-sustaining devices. Theologian-biomedical ethicist Joseph Fletcher characterized a child born with Down syndrome as "a sadly non- or un- or subhuman creature."[10] Nobel Prize-winning scientist Dr. Francis H. Crick once proposed that "no newborn infant should be declared human until it has passed certain tests regarding its genetic endowment and that if it fails these tests it forfeits the right to live."[11]

Nonperson

The word "nonperson" has joined the parade of disparaging expressions designed to justify doing away with vulnerable individuals and groups. For many perpetrators, it serves as just another synonym for "subhuman" and "nonhuman." Other perpetrators, while acknowledging the humanity of their victims, find nonperson to be a convenient term for consigning them to the human race's outermost margins, where they can be manipulated, mutilated, and annihilated with impunity.

Defining Jews as "non-Aryans" (the Nazi equivalent of nonperson) functioned as a key semantic device for removing Jews from the protected status of legal personhood. This classification furnished a basis for the enactment of more than four hundred laws, ordinances, and decrees against Jews leading to "the final solution." Its significance is attested to by Holocaust scholar Raul Hilberg: "When in the early days of 1933 the first civil servant wrote the first definition of 'non-Aryan' into a civil service ordinance, the fate of European Jewry was sealed."[12]

Another milestone on the path to the legalization of racial genocide occurred in 1936 when the highest court of Germany, the Reichsgericht, equated Jews with sickness and death. According to German legal scholar Ernst Fraenkel's assessment, "The *Reichsgericht* itself refused to recognize Jews living in Germany as 'persons' in the legal sense."[13] A further step toward the full-fledged denial of legal personhood to Jews occurred on March 28, 1938, with the passage of a law depriving Jewish religious congregations of legal protection. Historian George Mosse concluded that from then on, Jews were no longer considered "legal personalities."[14]

Jews were not the only victims subjected to the nonperson epithet; it also was a central term of denigration bolstering the Nazi euthanasia program against disabled and mentally ill individuals. During a 1964 interview in *Der Spiegel*, former Nazi euthanasia selector Dr. Werner Catel defended infanticide, calling disabled children "creatures ... beyond help" that "will never become a person" and "were not people, but simply beings produced by people."[15]

Political scientist Hannah Arendt and theologian Richard Rubenstein captured the essence of nonpersonhood in totalitarian societies as involving the consignment of victims labeled nonpersons to a condition of statelessness: a veritable nonentity under the law. Arendt found that the hallmark of a tyrannical regime like Nazi Germany was the exclusion of people declared stateless from the protected ranks of "legal persons."[16] In his reflections on Auschwitz, Rubenstein stated, "One of the most difficult conclusions to which we have come is that the Nazis committed no crime at Auschwitz since no law or political order protected those who were first condemned to statelessness and then to the camps."[17]

On January 22, 1973, the US Supreme Court's decision in *Roe v. Wade* ushered in the modern era of legal nonpersonhood in the United States by declaring, "The unborn have never been recognized in the law as persons in the whole sense" and ruling that "the word 'person,' as used in the Fourteenth Amendment, does not include the unborn."[18] This decision in effect constitutes a continuation of the nonperson legacy of the Third Reich underscored by Arendt and Rubenstein: the unwanted unborn in contemporary American society—like the Jews and other unwanted victims in Nazi Germany—have been reduced to the statelessness of nonpersons outside the protection of the law. Furthermore, like the Nazi perpetrators, physician abortionists commit no crime in the abortion clinics since neither today's law nor the political order protects the unborn, who have been first condemned to the statelessness of nonpersonhood and then to the clinics.

Ever since 1973, abortion proponents have unremittingly utilized professional journals, the judicial system, and prestigious conferences as platforms for reinforcing the legal nonpersonhood doctrine upholding the abortion liberty. Keeping the unborn in the rightless status of nonpersonhood perpetuates as well as expands their destructive procedures and related forms of exploitation. Inevitably, the nonpersonhood doctrine ensnares in its arbitrary and ever expansive orbit a wide array of victims after birth who lack the prescribed physical, cognitive, social, and psychological capacities considered essential for membership in the moral community of bona fide persons. Although people with disabilities and other vulnerable individuals have not yet been officially defined as nonpersons under the law, philosophers, physicians, bioethicists, and like-minded ideologues are working toward achieving this goal.

An essay in a 1976 issue of the *New England Journal of Medicine* by Vanderbilt bioethicist John Lachs maintained that infants afflicted with hydrocephalus could not become persons because they lack the most fundamental attribute of personhood—a functioning brain. Lachs pointed out what he believed was a basic mistake made by their caretakers: "The child itself (and to make the point more forcefully, I should not even call it a 'child') is not a person, and the fundamental error of our ways consists in thinking that it is one."[19]

In *Abortion and Infanticide* (1983), philosopher Michael Tooley built an elaborate case for justifying the killing of infants as well as unborn humans according to the premise that they do not possess the most essential qualities of persons—especially self-consciousness: "New-born humans are neither persons nor even quasi-persons, and their destruction is in no way intrinsically wrong."[20] The concepts "nonperson" and its pseudo-derivative "quasi-person" are exceedingly slippery constructions with ambiguous boundaries containing wide latitude for targeting a huge variety of victims at all phases of the human life span.

Drs. Alberto Giubilini and Francesca Minerva have joined the group of prominent philosophers and bioethicists who rely upon the nonperson designation to condone the killing of human lives *after* as well as before birth. Writing in the *Journal of Medical Ethics*, they asserted, "The moral status of an infant is equivalent to that of a fetus, that is, neither can be considered a 'person' in a morally relevant sense" and "neither is a 'person' in the sense of 'subject of a moral right to life'" because of their inability to pursue aims due to the lack of even a "minimal level of self-awareness." This encroaching definition of nonperson leads Giubilini and Minerva to conclude, "What we call 'after-birth abortion' [killing a newborn] should be permissible in all the cases where abortion is, including cases where the newborn is not disabled."[21]

The nonperson epithet is fast becoming a leading designation for denigrating unborn and born humans considered not worthy of life.

It has inaugurated a new litmus test for survival—no longer is one's humanity a sufficient basis for meriting the right to life; one must also be a person. The definition of personhood required for existence is an increasingly restrictive one whereby expanding numbers of people are declared expendable and relegated to the rightless category of "legal nonpersons."

Lower Animal

Consignment of vulnerable human beings deemed superfluous to a form of animal life has long been another linguistic stratagem for rationalizing their victimization. Before and during the Nazi era, animal analogies were invoked to dehumanize the unborn and degrade a broad spectrum of postnatal victims. In 1904, human evolutionary proponent and National Socialism forerunner Dr. Ernst Haeckel based his support for abortion and infanticide on the evolutionary theory that the human organism first passes through the evolutionary stages of its nonhuman ancestors, traversing the protozoon, amphibian, and primitive mammalian stages before reaching the fully human stage sometime after birth. Haeckel stated that "the developing embryo, just as the newborn child ... is a pure reflex machine, just like a lower vertebrate."[22] Placement of unborn and newborn infants in an evolutionary phase comparable to "our animal ancestors" led him to conclude that killing them could not be equated with murder since it was nothing more significant than killing another animal.

One of Dr. Alfred Hoche's main contributions to the 1920 treatise *Permitting the Destruction of Unworthy Life* included the use of animalistic terminology to malign people with serious brain injuries. These "mentally dead" individuals, he stressed, stand "far down in the animal kingdom; even their emotional movements do not rise above the level of elementary processes bound to animal life."[23] Hoche's portrayal established a standard of discourse that paved the way for the extermination of physically and mentally handicapped patients in the Third Reich.

Descriptions of the experiments conducted on concentration camp prisoners were saturated with references to the victims as experimental animals. The opening statement of the prosecution at the Nuremberg Doctors' Trial on December 9, 1946, emphasized how the treatment of the inmates closely reflected the animalistic images foisted on them: "To their murderers these wretched people were not individuals at all. They came in wholesale lots and were treated worse than animals."[24] University of Strasbourg medical researcher Dr. August Hirt reprimanded a colleague for expressing qualms about continuing poisonous gas experiments on test subjects. "You must not forget," he insisted, "that the prisoners here are animals before all else."[25]

The unwanted unborn in contemporary society have been likewise subjected to a host of demeaning animal references. In 1970, nurses at a New York hospital became distraught when they encountered an aborted baby who moved. The attending physician told them they were simply witnessing "a reflexive response of a spinal animal."[26]

According to philosophy professor Mary Anne Warren, "Even a fully developed fetus" in the final months of pregnancy is "considerably less person-like than is the average mature mammal" or "the average fish." Therefore, she maintained, it "cannot be said to have any more right to life than, let us say, a newborn guppy."[27] Cornell University neurology professor Hart Peterson resorted to a similar characterization in an attempt to neutralize the horror of the abortion depicted in the film *The Silent Scream*. "What we're seeing here is a primitive response, much like that of a primitive animal that's poked with a stick."[28]

Astronomer Carl Sagan and his wife, scientist Ann Druyan, resurrected a pseudo-evolutionary perspective paralleling Dr. Ernst Haeckel by comparing the unborn human at different phases of development to forms of animal life. Sagan and Druyan specified that the human embryo resembled "a segmented worm" by the third week and "a newt or tadpole" during the fourth week. They called the embryonic face "reptilian" by the sixth week and "mammalian but somewhat piglike" at the end of the seventh week.[29]

Some individuals after birth in contemporary society are also increasingly at risk of being reduced to animals. "Until a living being can take conscious management of life and its direction," declared biblical studies professor George Ball, "it remains an animal."[30] He included under this classification unborn humans, newborn infants, and comatose adults.

Animal liberation philosopher Peter Singer favors consigning infants with serious disabilities to a status even below that of some animals: "If we compare a severely defective human infant with a nonhuman animal, a dog or a pig, for example, we will find the nonhuman to have superior capacities, both actual and potential, for rationality, self-consciousness, communication, and anything else that can plausibly be considered morally significant."[31]

Parasite

The parasite is one of the most despicable creatures in nature. It invades another organism, attaches itself to the organism, and voraciously consumes the host's tissues, blood, and food supply. This relationship invariably results in the debilitation and death of the organism. Many parasites are also disease carriers that infect their host with deadly illnesses and germs. Throughout the annals of infamy, such a repulsive image has been imposed on a variety of human victims to justify their extermination under the guise of a public health program against a dangerous, repulsive, disease-ridden alien bent on exploiting, afflicting, and destroying defenseless human lives.

In America as far back as the early twentieth century, the words "parasite," "parasitic," and "parasitism" emerged as common expressions of disparagement imposed on poverty-stricken rural families, mentally and emotionally disturbed individuals, those with serious physical ailments, and immigrants from southern and eastern Europe. The parasitism attributed to these groups was presented to the public as an irreversible condition resulting from the hereditary transmission of defective germ plasm from one generation to another.

Physicians played a key role in invoking the parasite epithet as a basis for promoting medicalized violence against unwanted human lives. In a paper, "Race Suicide for Social Parasites," presented before a joint meeting of the Physicians' Club and the Law Club of Chicago on December 13, 1907, Dr. W. T. Belfield railed against "the hordes of social parasites who crowd our costly and ever multiplying public infirmaries."[32]

Bolstered by the involvement of doctors, parasitic rhetoric flourished in influential segments of American life. At a national meeting held in Cincinnati in 1899, Charles Henderson, president of the National Conference of Charities and Corrections, told the superintendents of institutions for the care of feebleminded patients, "We wish the parasitic strain ... to die out."[33] A popular 1914 high school textbook, *A Civic Biology: Presented in Problems*, warned about "hundreds of families ... spreading disease, immorality, and crime to all parts of this country.... Largely for them, the poorhouse and the asylum exist. They take from society but they give nothing in return. They are pure parasites."[34]

The castigation of non-Aryans—overwhelmingly Jews but also Gypsies and Germans with handicaps—as grasping, unscrupulous, and dangerous "parasites" intent on exploiting and annihilating the people and institutions of Germany emanated from reputable intellectual circles long before the Nazis came to power. German philosopher Friedrich Nietzsche employed a medical ethical foundation for placing a parasitic label on people with disabilities. In *Twilight of the Idols and the Anti Christ* (1888), Nietzsche began his moral code for physicians with the statement "The invalid is a parasite on society" and advised doctors to engage in the "ruthless suppression" of this "cowardly" type of "degenerating life."[35]

Portrayals of Jews as "parasites" had their most telling impact during the twelve years of the Third Reich. A booklet issued by Nazi officials—*The Jew as Global Parasite*—served as an influential source for motivating those entrusted with carrying out the Holocaust. Its hatred-inducing pages are saturated with references to the Jew as a dangerous, contagious, all-encompassing parasitic creature: "The Jew is the parasite among men. He can infect the individual as a single parasite, entire nations as a social parasite and mankind as a global parasite." These fearsome images furnished an urgent justification for National Socialism's "resolute struggle against the Jewish Global Parasite."[36]

European Gypsies were viewed as identical to Jews—a rootless, alien species living a parasitic existence. A 1937 study on the "antisocial properties" of 136 individuals from two large Gypsy clans by Dr. Otto Finger of the Institute for Hereditary Health and Race Preservation resulted in dispatching these "racially alien parasites" to Nazi concentration camps.[37] A 1938 memorandum proposed "a National Socialist solution for the Gypsy question" to counter the presence of "parasites within the body of our people, causing immense damage and imperiling the purity of the borderland peasant's blood and way of life."[38]

The parasite analogy has become a mainstay in contemporary pro-abortion semantics. Implacable abortionist Dr. Warren Hern likened the development of the "fetoplacental unit" to the "local invasion" of "a parasite" and portrayed abortion as an effective "medical treatment" for "the blocking of the deleterious effects of the parasite or its destruction."[39]

The presentation of abortion as a medical procedure designed to eradicate the preborn human defined as a ravenous, disease-spreading parasitic intruder has been wholeheartedly embraced by some feminist ideologues. Rosalind Pollack Petchesky claims, "On the level of 'biology alone,' the dependence is one-way—the fetus is a parasite ... it contributes nothing to her sustenance. It only draws from her: nutrients, immunological defenses, hormonal secretions, blood, digestive functions, energy."[40] Rachel Conrad Wahlberg maintains that pregnancy reduces the woman's body to "an incubator growing a parasite" and calls the unborn human a "parasitical," "cannibalistic" creature feeding "on the mother's body without any consideration for her needs" by draining energy, nourishment, and strength from an unwilling host.[41]

The parasite epithet also shows signs of engulfing today's vulnerable individuals after birth, especially aged individuals, owing to their greater utilization of medical and hospital services. Increasing numbers of cost-conscious biomedical ethicists devote considerable energy to building a case for denying life-sustaining treatment to the aged and others dependent upon various technologies (pacemakers, respirators, feeding tubes, antibiotics, dialysis). Daniel Callahan, founder of the prestigious ethics think tank the Hastings Center, once warned that "a denial of nutrition may in the long run become the only effective way to make certain that a large number of biologically tenacious patients actually die."[42] This form of disparagement conveys the image of a relentlessly grasping group clinging as tenaciously to life support as would a parasite to its host.

Vegetative Existence

Throughout history and up to the present, the reduction of victims to the level of unwanted plants such as weeds or vegetative existences has long operated as a prime designation to justify mass destruction. Such an analogy has the effect of transforming killing into the agricultural task of clearing out "weeds" and "extraneous vegetation" to ensure the survival of worthwhile plants in a garden, or getting rid of unwanted individuals reduced to a "vegetative existence" devoid of value.

Nazi propagandists frequently characterized euthanasia as equivalent to "weeding out" a garden overflowing with hostile, worthless vegetation. Hitler's notorious SS director Heinrich Himmler carried the plant analogy to its most extreme lengths by comparing the role of the Holocaust perpetrator to "the plant breeding specialist who, when he wants to breed a pure new strain from a well-tried species that has been exhausted by too much cross-breeding, first goes over the field to cull the unwanted plants."[43]

In an affidavit introduced at the Nuremberg Doctors' Trial on May 14, 1947, Irmgard Grube, a secretary in the Chancellery of the Führer, stated how firmly entrenched the word "vegetate" had become in the mindset of euthanasia administrator Viktor Brack: "The decisive factor was always Brack's frequently expressed views that these people were merely vegetating and their existence was of no value."[44] On April 3, 1940, at a secret conference of mayors in Berlin, Brack said about patients in city mental institutions, "They vegetate like animals, and are antisocial people unworthy of living."[45]

"Vegetate" and "vegetating" became standard components in Nazi books and films promoting euthanasia. *Mission and Conscience* (1936), a novel written by ophthalmologist Helmut Unger, highlights the plight of a young woman suffering from multiple sclerosis who asks her physician husband to relieve her misery with a poisonous substance. He administers the fatal injection while a friend (also a doctor) plays soothing music on the piano. Afterward he is brought to trial for murder and is acquitted on the grounds that what he did was "an act of mercy." In his defense, the accused posed the question to the jury, "Would you, if you were a cripple, want to vegetate forever?"[46]

A contemporary dependence on the plant analogy involves the portrayal of seriously disabled children and adults as "vegetables," "vegetating," or existing in a "persistent vegetative state." In November 1973, pediatrician Raymond Duff invoked the phrase "vegetated individuals who have no human potential"[47] in referring to infants born with serious handicaps who were denied life-sustaining medical treatment at the Yale University-New Haven Hospital intensive care nursery.

Among philosopher John Lachs's extensive roster of dehumanizing expressions are references to "the 'gardens' that flourish in our major hospitals—of the thousands of human vegetables we sustain on life-preserving machines without any hope for their recovery." His prescription for them involves "a formalized system of easing death" because, according to him, "I cannot make myself believe that the unconscious vegetables in our hospitals are in any real sense human."[48]

On March 15, 1986, the American Medical Association's Council of Ethical and Judicial Affairs classified food and water as forms of medical treatment that could be withdrawn or withheld. This change in policy opened the floodgates to an increasing number of decisions authorizing the removal of life-sustaining feeding tubes from patients. Many of these cases are invariably accompanied by the contention that such patients are in a "persistent vegetative state."[49]

The 2005 imposed starvation-dehydration death of Terri Schiavo in a Florida hospice is a prime case of what happens to a cognitively impaired patient repeatedly subjected to the persistent vegetative state (PVS) label. Physician-assisted suicide advocate Dr. Timothy Quill affirmed the decision to remove her feeding tube, contending that "her neurological examinations have been indicative of a persistent vegetative state, which includes ... no signs of emotion, willful activity, or cognition."[50] He stood by the "diagnosis of a persistent vegetative state" despite testimony challenging the PVS designation plus the desire of Terri's parents to care for their daughter and obtain the therapy and rehabilitation denied to her by husband Michael Schiavo.

Waste Matter

For some perpetrators and their defenders, reducing undesired individuals to subhuman, nonhuman, nonperson, animal, and vegetative levels is not degrading enough. Instead, the victims are relegated to the bottom of the subhuman scrap pile. The result is an outpouring of demeaning designations comparing them to waste products, trash, rubbish, garbage, refuse, and debris. This repulsive lexicon was prevalent in late nineteenth- and early twentieth-century America, dominated the Third Reich, and persists today. It has been used to malign and continues to denigrate individuals at all phases of the human life cycle.

Criminology professor Nicole Hahn Rafter's analysis of the eugenic family studies conducted on the rural poor before and soon after the turn of the twentieth century in the United States found the "central, confirmational image" projected to be "that of the degenerate hillbilly family, dwelling in filthy shacks and spawning endless generations of paupers, criminals, and imbeciles." The inhabitants in such families were commonly classified as "white trash."[51]

Dr. E. E. Southard, director of the Psychopathic Hospital in Boston, presented a paper in 1915 at the National Conference of Charities and Corrections that referred to "the feeble-minded" as "waste materials" and expressed concern about "what to do with these waste materials."[52]

Margaret Sanger was fond of reducing "the feebleminded" and others to the level of "a dead weight of human waste." She castigated the state of New York for squandering money on the upkeep of "this dead weight of human waste" institutionalized "in alms-houses, reformatories, schools for the blind, deaf and mute, in insane asylums, in homes for the feeble-minded and epileptic." Sanger also maligned maternity homes for helping "slum mothers," since the "cruelty" of such organized charities "encourages the healthier and more normal sections of the world to shoulder the burden of unthinking and indiscriminate fecundity of others; which brings with it ... a dead weight of human waste."[53] Dr. Alfred Hoche invoked similar expressions to characterize the lives of "wholly worthless" people. He thereupon justified their destruction as equivalent to the disposal of "dead weight existences" and "empty human shells."[54]

According to Leon Poliakov's *Harvest of Hate: The Nazi Program for the Destruction of the Jews of Europe*, "even in their subconscious minds the Germans had been trained to consider the Jews as pariahs, the refuse of humanity." Nazi rhetoricians dubbed Poland—the major locale for the extermination and disposal of millions—the "trashcan of Europe."[55] After inspecting the Warsaw ghetto in 1939, Nazi propaganda minister Joseph Goebbels reported to Hitler, "The Jew is a waste product."[56]

Furthermore, burning victims in the crematorium came to be viewed as the disposal of "waste material." According to one of the medical perpetrators at Auschwitz, "the problem of the crematorium and its capacity ... was equal to the ordinary problem of sewerage."[57]

Waste analogies are likewise cited by contemporary health care officials to neutralize the unsavory aspects associated with the disposal of aborted humans. In February 1982, when more than sixteen thousand aborted human bodies were found in a huge metal storage container outside Los Angeles, assistant coroner Dr. Richard Wilson stated that this unnerving discovery did not constitute "evidence of foul play" but only the possibility of minor "health code" violations "concerning the disposal of medical waste."[58] The following year, Wichita, Kansas, public health director Mary Ellen Conlee referred to the pictures taken of aborted human bodies about to be burned in the city owned incineration along with dead cats and dogs as "pathological waste."[59]

Waste-product terminology has been further appropriated to rationalize harvesting fetal organs for transplantation purposes. At a 1987 forum on genetic engineering, *Harper's Magazine* editor Lewis Lapham supported the exploitation of fetal brain implants for Alzheimer's patients with the statement, "We're talking about a waste product here: thousands of fetuses are discarded every day."[60]

Relegating aborted humans to the status of waste matter continues to persist in the twenty-first century. On March 24, 2014, a report came to public attention regarding the incineration of aborted and miscarried children as "clinical waste" in twenty-seven British hospitals over the past several years. The remains were burned in "waste to energy" facilities as a means of generating power for heating the hospitals.[61] Similarly, a month later, a former worker at the Covanta Marion power plant in Brooks, Oregon, revealed that this waste-to-energy facility was burning the remains of aborted bodies shipped from British Columbia under the medical waste designation.[62]

The contemporary reliance on such degrading expressions also encompasses vulnerable individuals in the postnatal stages of development. Health care professionals at a major Southern American university medical center utilized the word "garbage" to portray "troublesome" patients.[63] Listed among the glossary of slang expressions used by Harvard University Medical School house physicians is the entry "*Garbageman*, a baby born with serious defects."[64]

A sociological study of medical staff working in the accident and emergency departments of three British hospitals revealed that the term "rubbish" was commonly resorted to in castigating "undesirable" patients: "If there's anything interesting we'll stop, but there's a lot of rubbish this morning.... We have the usual rubbish, but also a subdural hemorrhage.... It's a thankless task, seeing all the rubbish, as we call it, coming through.... We get our share of rubbish."[65]

Research Material and Specimens

Generally, the most degrading waste metaphors are utilized when the victims of mass extermination are viewed as having no worth whatsoever, and their only legitimate destination is burial, incineration, or disposal in the sewage system. Conversely, the victims' bodies and body parts are often endowed with convenient value by medical researchers who are intent on draining every possible ounce of information, blood, and tissue out of their ravaged remains.

From his exalted position as chairman of neuropathology at the Kaiser Wilhelm Institute in Berlin-Buch, Dr. Julius Hallervorden utilized for his research more than six hundred brains severed from psychiatric patients. In a report to the German Association for Scientific Research on December 8, 1942, he wrote, "This material is constantly being added to by the post-mortem department of the mental hospital in Görden."[66]

Dr. Josef Mengele looked upon Auschwitz as an incomparable scientific laboratory containing a huge captive population of "scientific material" and "specimens" for unlimited experimental utilization. Besides studying, performing experiments on, and having victims killed, he "collected human specimen material from the Auschwitz inmates and this material was forwarded to the Kaiser Wilhelm Institute in Berlin-Dahlem.... These specimens included human eyes, human heads, and blood samples."[67] Chief Auschwitz physician Eduard Wirths characterized Mengele's research as a "valuable contribution to anthropological science by making use of the scientific materials available to him."[68] Dr. Mengele was especially fascinated by the study of heterochromia, a condition in which the two eyes of an individual are of different colors. Six Gypsy twins with this condition were killed by phenol injection, and their eyes were dissected and sent to Mengele's former professor Helmut Verschuer, who considered them "enormously interesting specimens."[69]

University of Munster anatomy professor Johann Paul Kremer viewed debilitated Auschwitz inmates who were killed by phenol injections as "suitable specimens" and "fresh human material" for experiments on the subject of starvation.[70] After the war, he hoped to establish a small laboratory consisting of "materials from Auschwitz which absolutely must be worked on."[71]

Just as the words "material" and "specimens" functioned to justify the experimental exploitation of Jews and other expendable victims in the Third Reich, these same designations had become incorporated in the vocabulary of American biomedical researchers by the mid-1980s. In anatomical studies carried out at the Good Samaritan Medical Center and the Oregon Health Sciences University in Portland, a method was devised for identifying the remains of induced abortions. Among the most common designations created to describe the dismembered body parts were "suctioned or curetted material," "cellular material," "abortion material," and "material removed from the uterus."[72]

At a parliamentary hearing on the use of human embryos for therapeutic, scientific, industrial, and commercial purposes convened by the Council of Europe in 1985, the conference chairman asked Swedish fetal researcher Dr. Arne Andersson about his reaction to "the Finnish use for scientific purposes of fetuses of 21-weeks age where they cut off the heads." Andersson defended the experiments, stressing that "the research people" have nothing to do with "the choice of abortion technique. They just take advantage of the fact that they have had the opportunity to use this material."[73]

American fetal researchers often depend upon special technicians to scavenge the remains of aborted humans for potentially valuable "experimental material" at today's abortion centers. In his book on the Lovejoy abortion facility in Portland, Oregon, Peter Korn furnishes revealing information on a medical assistant from a biological supply company who searches the remains of aborted babies according to "regular faxes detailing what body parts are needed by which researchers around the country." She places "the body parts into glass jars with preserving fluid" and "then packs the jars in Styrofoam boxes full of ice and calls Federal Express." This process is referred to as "allowing the extracted material to be used for medical research."[74]

The series of undercover videos released in summer 2015 by the Center for Medical Progress that exposed the experimental utilization of aborted body parts by Planned Parenthood physicians bear a striking resemblance to the methods and terminology employed by Dr. Josef Mengele to rationalize dissecting the bodies of Auschwitz victims for experimental exploitation. In the first video, Dr. Deborah Nucatola provides a number of graphic details about obtaining intact aborted specimens: "We've been very good at getting heart, lung, liver, because we know that, so I'm not gonna crush that part, I'm gonna to basically crush below, I'm gonna crush above, and I'm gonna see if I can get it all intact. And ... if you do it starting from the breech presentation ... you can evacuate an entire calvarium [the head]."[75] In the second video, one of the actors posing as a buyer from a human biologics company asks Dr. Mary Gatter whether her facility could supply "intact specimens" aborted at ten to twelve weeks. She replied, "I wouldn't object to asking Ian, who's our surgeon who does the cases, to use an IPAS [manual vacuum aspirator] at that gestational age in order to increase the odds that he's going to get an intact specimen" and "to see how he feels about using a 'less crunchy' technique to get more whole specimens."[76] Another video reveals Planned Parenthood Gulf Coast Research Director Melissa Farrell admitting how adept doctors have become at harvesting intact fetal specimens for research purposes: "Because some of our doctors have projects and they're collecting the specimens so that they do it in a way they can get the best specimens."[77]

Table 10 underscores the stunning resemblances between the dehumanizing designations imposed on victims in Nazi Germany and the degrading expressions fabricated to dehumanize vulnerable individuals in past and contemporary America and elsewhere.

TABLE 10. PORTRAYALS OF EXPENDABLE POPULATIONS

Before and during the Third Reich	Past and Contemporary Society
SUBHUMAN	
"Sub-human, otherwise nothing." *(Description of Jews in anti-Semitic pamphlet, 1942)*	"A sadly non- or un- or subhuman creature." *(Portrayal of Down Syndrome child, 1968)*
"The Jewish-Bolshevik Commissars, who personify a repulsive subhumanity." *(Dr. August Hirt, 1942)*	"For the first four and a half months the fetus is subhuman and . . . close to a piece of tissue." *(Sociology professor Amitai Etzioni, 1976)*
NONPERSON	
"The Reichsgericht itself refused to recognize Jews as 'persons' in the legal sense." *(Ernst Fraenkel on a 1936 German Supreme Court decision)*	"The unborn have never been recognized in the law as persons in the whole sense." *(Roe v. Wade US Supreme Court decision, 1973)*
"Creatures . . . beyond help" that "will never become a person." *(Former Nazi death selector Dr. Werner Catel's defense of infanticide during a 1964 interview)*	"Neither [infant nor fetus] is a 'person' in the sense of 'subject of a moral right to life.'" *(Drs. Alberto Giubilini and Francesca Minervas espouse "after-birth abortion," 2012)*
LOWER ANIMAL	
"A pure reflex . . . like a lower vertebrate." *(Dr. Ernst Haeckel's view of the embryo and the newborn, 1904)*	"A reflexive response of a spinal animal." *(Physician's view of an aborted child who moved, 1970)*
"Mentally dead" individuals stand "far down in the animal kingdom." *(Dr. Alfred Hoche's description of brain-injured people, 1920)*	"A primitive response, much like that of a primitive animal that's poked with a stick." *(Dr. Hart Peterson on the fetal reaction to being aborted, 1985)*
PARASITE	
"The invalid is a parasite on society." *(Friedrich Nietzsche's moral code for physicians, 1888)*	"They are pure parasites." *(American textbook view of poor and disabled people, 1914)*
"The Jew is the parasite among men." *(Nazi anti-Semitic booklet titled The Jew as Global Parasite, 1938)*	"The fetus is a parasite." *(Feminist professor Rosalind Pollock Petchesky, 1984)*
VEGETATIVE EXISTENCE	
"These people were merely vegetating and their existence was of no value." *(Irmgard Grube's description of euthanasia administrator Viktor Brack's attitude toward mentally ill patients, 1947)*	"Vegetated individuals who have no human potential." *(Dr. Raymond Duff's portrayal of disabled infants born in the Yale-New Haven Hospital intensive care nursery, 1973)*
"Would you, if you were a cripple, want to vegetate forever?" *(Dr. Helmut Unger's pro-euthanasia propaganda novel titled Mission and Conscience, 1936)*	"Her neurological examinations have been indicative of a persistent vegetative state." *(Dr. Timothy Quill's depiction of imposed starvation-dehydration victim Terri Schiavo, 2005)*

TABLE 10. PORTRAYALS OF EXPENDABLE POPULATIONSM *(cont.)*

Before and during the Third Reich	Past and Contemporary Society
WASTE MATTER	
"Dead weight existences." (*Dr. Alfred Hoche's characterization of the lives of "wholly worthless" people, 1920*)	"A dead weight of human waste." (*Margaret Sanger's description of institutionalized disabled people, 1922*)
"The Jew is a waste product." (*Nazi propaganda minister Joseph Goebbels, 1939*)	"We're talking about a waste product here." (*Editor Lewis Lapham on "discarded fetuses," 1987*)
RESEARCH MATERIAL AND SPECIMENS	
"This material." (*Dr. Julius Hallervorden's characterization of the brains severed from euthanasia victims used in his experiments, 1945*)	"This material." (*Dr. Arne Andersson's description of the heads severed from aborted victims used in Dr. Peter Adam's fetal brain experiment, 1985*)
"These specimens." (*Harvesting for research the heads, eyes, and blood samples from inmates killed at Auschwitz by Dr. Josef Mengele, 1944*)	"The best specimens." (*Harvesting for research the heads, hearts, lungs, and livers from babies aborted by Planned Parenthood doctors, 2015*)

CHAPTER 11

Treatment for Disease

The Lexicon of Medicalized Killing

Doctors intent on carrying out destructive procedures under the cover
of medicine have appropriated disease metaphors as a major semantic
device to justify the most extreme perversion of medicine—killing as
a form of medical treatment for victims reduced to the level of disease
entities. What better way for physicians to rationalize participation
in destructive operations than by defining their victims as essential
segments of the universe of pathology? Past and present victims before
and after birth have been lowered to the level of diseases, defective
components, degenerates, contagions, menaces, plagues, epidemics,
germs, infections, malignant cells, and gangrenous body parts. These
degrading designations have set the stage for portraying the annihilation of those subjected to them as legitimate forms of medical treatments, procedures, and operations.

Disease Entities in Early Twentieth-Century America

The movement toward building a super-race by reducing vulnerable populations to expendable, defective entities is most often associated with what happened in the Third Reich. But the early decades
of twentieth-century America also constituted a veritable heyday of
eugenics, a pseudo-science obsessed with developing a superior Nor-
dic race through the selective breeding of people from the best racial

stocks and the elimination of defective hereditary strains. The Eugenics Section of the American Breeders Association was founded in 1906 to "investigate and report on heredity in the human race, and emphasize the value of superior blood and the menace to society of inferior blood."[1]

This organization set the pace for what followed as other organizations, groups, people, and projects—all oriented toward an "insatiable quest for the super race"—became part of "an alliance between biological racism and mighty American power, position and wealth." Some of the most influential forces were the American Eugenics Society, the Race Betterment Foundation, the Galton Society, the Eugenics Record Office, the Carnegie Institute, the Rockefeller Foundation, the Fitter Families Contests held at state fairs, and integration of eugenics doctrine in the high school curriculum and in the biology, zoology, social science, psychology, and anthropology departments at the nation's leading universities.[2] Such a wide-ranging movement provided fertile ground for the expansion of disparaging disease labels against society's weakest and most marginalized individuals because they were considered to be an obstacle to the relentless goal of purifying the American people.

The terms "defective," "infection," "contamination," and "defective germ plasm" were some of the degrading characterizations imposed on vulnerable individuals (mainly the poor and those with physical and mental disabilities) during the late 1800s and early 1900s. This terminology permeated a series of eugenic family studies purporting to demonstrate that the disproportionate incidence of crime, insanity, feeblemindedness, epilepsy, and other maladies among white families living in Appalachia and other impoverished rural areas was due not to a subpar environment but to a deficient hereditary endowment commonly portrayed as "defective germ plasm or protoplasm" (the seriously flawed hereditary substance transmitted across generations).

Influential American physicians resorted to demeaning disease analogies in sounding the alarm about the threat posed by mentally and physically handicapped patients. In 1900, Dr. John Fitzgerald, superintendent of the Rome State Custodial Asylum, spoke before the

New York Conference of Charities and Corrections about the "idiotic child" as "a source of moral contagion to the other children which is far reaching in its results."[3] Dr. Martin Barr, director of the Pennsylvania Training School for Feeble-Minded Children, referred to "imbeciles" as "festering sores in the life of society."[4]

The early decades of twentieth-century America—an era marked by the massive social and cultural transformations of unprecedented immigration and industrial and urban growth—turned out to be an auspicious time for expansion of the disparaging disease expressions to engulf the new waves of immigrants from eastern and southern Europe. In *The Rising Tide of Color against White World-Supremacy* (1922), American eugenicist Lothrop Stoddard likened "inferior stocks" to "bacteria" and "bacterial invasions." Writing on the indispensability of "immigration restriction," he declared, "Just as we isolate bacterial invasions, and starve out the bacteria by limiting the area and amount of their food supply, so we can compel an inferior race to remain in its native habitat."[5]

Disease Metaphors Preceding and during the Nazi Era

The decades leading up to the Third Reich witnessed an outpouring of disease-laden expressions against German "defectives" that were strikingly similar to those employed against the "unfit" and marginalized people in early twentieth-century America. During the last quarter of the nineteenth century, prominent physician and biology professor Ernst Haeckel warned about the hundreds of thousands of "incurables" who posed a danger to the survival of the German people.[6] In 1918, Dr. Heinrich Ziegler, one of Haeckel's most avid disciples, declared that most murderers came from the ranks of the "feeble-minded or epileptic."[7]

Adolf Hitler's anti-Semitic tirade *Mein Kampf* (1924) is saturated with such disease-ridden images of Jews as "infections," "this world plague," and "the alien virus ... in the national body." He was obsessed with drawing associations between Jews and the venereal disease syphilis, and placed the lion's share of blame on "this Jewish disease" for the "spreading contamination of our sexual life" and "the resulting syphilization of our people." The Führer referred to the moral degeneracy accompanying venereal disease as the "Jewification of our spiritual life."[8]

The German doctors' appropriation of disease analogies endowed them with a compelling aura of medical authority. In what became known as the "medicalization of anti-Semitism," Jews were relegated to the status of disease entities. Dr. Gerhard Wagner, an influential proponent of this terminology and a leader of the German medical profession, called Jews "a diseased race" and Judaism a "disease incarnate."[9] Dr. Kurt Klare, cofounder of the Nazi Physicians' League, portrayed Jewry as a kind of sickness—the "decomposing influence of Jewry" within the German organism.[10]

During the height of the killing season at Auschwitz, Nazi physician Fritz Klein utilized the phrase "gangrenous appendix" in defending the extermination of Jews in the crematorium. As the black smoke spewed continuously from the huge chimneys, prisoner physician Ella Lingens-Reiner pointed to the chimneys and asked Dr. Klein: "How can you reconcile that with your oath as a doctor?" He replied, "Of course I am a doctor and I want to preserve life. And out of respect for life, I would remove a gangrenous appendix from a diseased body. The Jew is the gangrenous appendix in the body of mankind."[11]

Gypsies likewise became a prime target of the disease-saturated expressions. They were accused of spreading malignant epidemics or were equated with death-inducing illnesses. Nazi medical authorities called Gypsies a "health risk" to the German people, while Dr. Otmar von Verschuer characterized most Gypsies as members of an "asocial and genetically inferior" race.[12] The Nazi-controlled press reported that the "plague" of Gypsies threatened the provinces of Brabant and Limburg.[13]

The Disease of Unwanted Pregnancy

Reduction of undesired pregnancy, and along with it the unwanted unborn, to the status of a disease has taken a toehold in the discourse of contemporary mainstream medicine. Like early twentieth-century American doctors and the Nazi physicians who depicted their respective victims as "germs," "diseases," "infections," and "epidemics" that endangered the health and life of the wanted members of the populace, today's physician abortionists and their defenders call upon identical terminology in portraying pregnancy as an illness that threatens the life and health of women.

An early version of the pregnancy-as-disease mentality can be found in a 1967 issue of *Time* magazine under the heading "Disease of Unwanted Pregnancy." In this article, Dr. Kenneth Ryan, then associated with Case Western Reserve School of Medicine, is quoted as saying, "The 'disease' of an unwanted pregnancy is not usually fatal, but living with it is so onerous that many women risk death via criminal abortion rather than suffer its far-reaching effects."[14] In 1970, psychiatrist Natalie Shainess compared unwanted pregnancy to "the alien germ ... deep within the body," a malady that "insists on expression through one symptom or another."[15]

An especially mind-boggling version of the unwanted-pregnancy-as-a-disease orthodoxy was put forth by influential medical ethics professor Joseph Fletcher, who once wrote, "*Pregnancy when not wanted is a disease—in fact, a venereal disease.*"[16]

Another variation of this disease-ridden imagery appeared in an address by Dr. Willard Cates and colleagues from the Centers for Disease Control and Prevention before the 1976 annual meeting of the Association of Planned Parenthood Physicians. Cates and his associates identified gonorrhea as the number one venereal disease, with unwanted pregnancy holding down the second slot, and asserted that "although rarely classified as a venereal disease, unwanted pregnancy is transmitted sexually, is socially and emotionally pathologic, and has many other characteristics of the conventional venereal diseases."[17]

Echoes of the dehumanizing appendix analogy invoked by Dr. Fritz Klein at Auschwitz have also reverberated in the rhetoric of pro-abortion doctors. A 1968 meeting on abortion convened by the Association for the Study of Abortion featured leading abortion proponent Dr. Alan Guttmacher, who invoked the diseased appendix metaphor in portraying abortion as a legitimate way of "aiding nature" when nature fails to spontaneously eject its defectives: "Since he [the doctor] aids nature in every other way, for example, by operating on an appendix or removing gangrenous bowel, he would aid her further if he did abortions in these cases."[18]

Dr. Bernard Smith—a veteran abortionist known for driving six hundred miles per week to perform abortions in three midwestern states (Illinois, Michigan, and Wisconsin)—likewise relied upon the diseased appendix analogy to justify his destructive practices. In 1993, Dr. Smith told a *New York Times* reporter that after having performed thousands of abortions, "he looked upon the embryo much as another doctor might view an appendix he had just removed."[19]

Medical Treatments

Consignment of past and contemporary individuals to the status of diseases, pathological conditions, epidemics, and infections has prepared the way for defining their extermination as a legitimate component of medical practice. The word "treatment" dominates a vocabulary of medical euphemisms designed to bolster the most radical perversion of medicine—the transformation of killing into healing.

The expression "the treatment" figured prominently in decrees that pertain to the destruction of the unborn offspring of female workers in Nazi-occupied territories. One such decree, issued on April 5, 1943, by Reich Health Leader Dr. Leonardo Conti, states:

> Application has to be made to the Advisory Committee for Interruption of Pregnancy.... The advisory committee will make a decision and charge a surgeon with the treatment. The sick bays established for Eastern laborers, particularly those in which the confinements of female Eastern workers take place, may also be considered as suitable establishments for the treatment.[20]

Before the Nuremberg Doctors' Trial in 1947, Dr. Hermann Pfannmuller, former director of the Eglfing-Haar state hospital, testified about the lethal injection of luminal as a method of killing children at his institution. Yet he avoided the word "kill" altogether and instead repeatedly resorted to the designation "the treatment" as a means of endowing this destructive procedure with the highly positive imprint of a curative medical endeavor:

> A decision was made in Berlin and an authorization was sent back to the institute [at Eglfing-Haar] saying that within the framework of the directives of the Reich Committee the child should be accorded the treatment.... [T]hen finally I received notice when the treatment began and relatives were informed—not about the treatment, but that they should visit the child.[21]

Treatment semantics also came in handy as a tool for implementing euthanasia against German adults. At the Hadamar Euthanasia Trial in 1947, Hadamar defendant nurse Heinrich Ruoff was asked, "What would you say to these people as you came into the bedrooms and prepared to inject them with this deadly drug?" Ruoff replied, "We told them that it was for treatment of their lung disease."[22]

Killing in the name of healing came of age on a monumental scale in the Nazi death camps. One Nazi doctor dubbed the medically supervised process of death selection Auschwitz's "system of treatment."[23] A secret order issued in 1941 instructing that Gypsies "should be treated in the same way as Jews" was fulfilled in the spring of 1943 when thousands of Gypsies were gassed at Auschwitz as "suspected typhoid cases."[24]

The Nazis even employed treatment polemics when portraying the places where the victims were exterminated. According to the logic underpinning this use of semantics, what could be more fitting than having killing redefined as a form of treatment that takes place in a "treatment room"?

Inside a small room in Block 20 at Auschwitz, the "treatment" for thousands of ill and debilitated prisoners consisted of phenol injections directly into the heart. Testimony presented during the Auschwitz Trial in 1964 revealed that "at least 119 children were murdered with phenol injection in the closing days of February 1943." The site where these barbaric actions took place was called "the treatment room."[25]

Contemporary abortion doctors also depend extensively on treatment semantics to endow their destructive actions with professional respectability. Dr. Willard Cates and associates' paper comparing unwanted pregnancy to a venereal disease—"Abortion as a Treatment for Unwanted Pregnancy: The Number Two Sexually-Transmitted Condition"—promotes abortion as "the preferred medical treatment" for the "sexually-transmitted condition" of unwanted pregnancy. Citing a series of statistical estimates, they maintain that "abortion is ten times more effective for treating unwanted pregnancy than penicillin is for treating gonorrhea." Their polemic ends in a predictable manner: "Therefore, we conclude that unwanted pregnancy should be considered a sexually-transmitted condition of epidemic proportion; moreover, legal abortion is an effective, safe, curative treatment for that condition."[26]

Abortion doctors in the obstetrics and gynecology department at the University of Pisa in Italy relied upon extensive doses of treatment semantics to medicalize the killing of 147 unborn humans with the prostaglandin derivative sulprostone under a variety of conditions. Their depictions of sulprostone abortions include the phrases "medical treatments," "iv treatment," "sulprostone treatment," "the treatment," "each treatment," "drug treatment," and "different treatment schedules."[27]

Abortion practitioner Dr. Suzanne Poppema views pregnancy as "a condition of their own bodies" and abortions as belonging under the classification "health-care treatments." She is extremely proud of having had her "clinic" chosen as a site for testing the efficacy of the abortion drug mifepristone and repeatedly referred to this method of destroying unborn humans as "Mifepristone treatment," "this treatment," and "the drug treatment."[28]

Furthermore, the transformation of killing patients into a component of mainline medical practice is becoming increasingly prevalent in contemporary American society. Attorney Rita Marker, executive director of the Patients Rights Council, provides a perceptive insight into how radically the meaning of "treatment" has been perverted to justify euthanasia and physician-assisted suicide: "Current attempts to categorize intentionally prescribed fatal overdoses and lethal injections as 'treatment' are the culmination of a carefully constructed bridge built from the traditional understanding of the term (i.e. an attempt to cure or ameliorate a medical condition) to a new, deadly, and very final 'treatment' (i.e. killing)."[29]

In a critique of the US House of Representatives' passage on March 20, 2005, of emergency legislation intended to halt the enforced starvation-dehydration of Terri Schiavo, health ethics attorney George Annas described the removal of her feeding tube as being in line with "treatment decisions … based on the patient's best interests."[30]

"Treatment room" rhetoric did not cease with the fall of the Third Reich. It is also invoked to describe locales for putting to death today's unwanted prenatal and postnatal children.

From January 1979 through December 1980, Harvard University obstetrics professors taught medical residents how to perform dilation and evacuation dismemberment abortions on 1,392 preborn victims at Boston's Brigham and Women's Hospital. These destructive procedures were carried out in "the treatment room" of the "pregnancy termination unit."[31]

In September 1990, a baby boy was born alive in a Las Vegas hospital after surviving two abortion attempts. The doctor who performed the botched abortions ordered the child be taken off oxygen and placed in "the treatment room," where it took him over an hour to expire.[32]

Operations, Procedures, and Medical Matters

In his study of Nazi doctors, psychiatrist Robert Jay Lifton concluded that "the killing came to be projected as a medical operation."[33] A survivor who witnessed the destruction process told Lifton, "Auschwitz was like a medical operation" and "the killing program was led by doctors from the beginning."[34] Auschwitz commandant Rudolf Hoess viewed gassing as a "procedure" superior to shooting because of its efficiency and bloodless effect. After watching his first gassing, he stated being "impressed" by how well "the whole procedure" worked and proclaimed, "Now we had the gas, and we had established a procedure."[35]

At the 1961 trial of Adolf Eichmann in Jerusalem, defense attorney Robert Servatius expressed the fully entrenched perception of killing by lethal gases as a legitimate medical procedure when he referred to "the collection of skeletons, sterilizations, killings by gas, and *similar medical matters.*" At this point, Judge Benjamin Halevi interrupted, stating, "Dr. Servatius, I assume you made a slip of the tongue when you said that killing by gas was a medical matter." Servatius replied, "It was indeed a medical matter, since it was prepared by physicians; *it was a matter of killing, and killing, too, is a medical matter.*"[36]

Today, abortion doctors draw extensively upon similar expressions to endow their destructive actions with professional respectability. This utilization of terminology was well underway by 1969 when the American Psychiatric Association issued a policy statement placing the killing of the unborn within the realm of mainstream medicine: "A decision to perform an abortion should be regarded as strictly a medical decision and a medical responsibility."[37] Dr. Zigmund Lebensohn concurred, declaring that "we must regard ... abortion as comparable to any other surgical operation."[38]

The word "kill" is nowhere to be found in a medical journal article describing the plunging of a needle into the heart of an unborn twin with Down syndrome. The word "procedure," on the other hand, is mentioned fifteen different times to describe what was done.[39] By 1989, such language had become so deeply embedded in prominent medical circles that an attorney representing the position of the American Medical Association reported, "Abortion is the most widely performed surgical procedure for women in this country,"[40] a boast repeated ad infinitum up to the present time.

Throughout his death-inducing career, Dr. Jack Kevorkian persistently referred to his actions as "medical procedures" and "medical services." Kevorkian's attorney, Geoffrey Fieger, was in complete accord with such portrayals. In August 1996, Dr. Kevorkian assisted in administering death to a forty-two-year-old registered nurse who was overweight and "suffered from chronic fatigue syndrome" but had no life threatening condition. Feiger called this "a medical procedure" carried out by "a caring doctor."[41]

Table 11 focuses on a comparative summary of the medical semantics constructed to facilitate the destruction of human lives past and present.

TABLE 11. MEDICAL RHETORIC AND ITS DESTRUCTIVE EFFECTS

Preceding and during the Third Reich	Twentieth-Century America and Contemporary Society
DISEASE ENTITIES	
A "genetically inferior" race responsible for "spreading infectious diseases." (*Vilification of Gypsies by Dr. Otmar von Verschuer and medical authorities in Bulgaria, 1944*)	"Bacterial invasions" of "inferior stocks" from other countries. (*Castigation of immigrants from southern and eastern Europe by eugenicist Lothrop Stoddard, 1913*)
The effects of "this Jewish disease" on "the resulting syphilization of our people." (*Adolf Hitler's equation of Jews to syphilis, 1925*)	"Pregnancy when not wanted is a disease—in fact, a venereal disease." (*Biomedical ethics professor Joseph Fletcher, 1958*)
"The alien virus . . . in the national body." (*Adolf Hitler's caricature of Jews, 1925*)	"The alien germ . . . deep in the body." (*Dr. N. Shainess on unwanted pregnancy, 1970*)
"I would remove a gangrenous appendix from a diseased body. The Jew is the gangrenous appendix in the body." (*Auschwitz physician Fritz Klein's medicalized justification for the destruction of Jews, mid-1940s*)	"He looked upon the embryo much as another doctor might view an appendix he had just removed." (*A reporter's description of Dr. Bernard Smith's medicalized justification for killing the unborn, 1993*)
MEDICAL TREATMENTS	
"The treatment." (*A decree authorizing abortions performed on female eastern slave laborers, 1943*)	"The preferred medical treatment." (*Dr. Willard Cates's justification of abortion for the disease of pregnancy, 1978*)
"The treatment room." (*Block 20 at Auschwitz, where phenol was injected into the hearts of prisoners, 1943*)	"The treatment room." (*A Las Vegas hospital where a baby aborted alive was forced to expire, 1990*)
"The treatment." (*Dr. Hermann Pfannmueller's account of deadly luminal injections administered to children at the Eglfing-Haar Hospital, 1947*)	"The treatment." (*Lethal injections of prostaglandins administered to unborn humans at the University of Pisa ob-gyn department, 1988*)
"We told them it was treatment for their lung disease." (*Nurse Heinrich Ruoff's description of lethal drug overdoses at Hadamar Hospital, 1947*)	"Treatment decisions . . . based on the patient's best interests." (*Attorney George Annas's depiction of Terri Schiavo's enforced starvation death, 2005*)
OPERATIONS, PROCEDURES, AND MEDICAL MATTERS	
"The killing came to be projected as a medical operation." (*Dr. Robert Jay Lifton's analysis of medical-imposed death selections at Auschwitz, 1986*)	Abortion is "comparable to any other surgical operation." (*Dr. Zigmund Lebensohn's promotion of abortion as a positive health factor, 1973*)
"We had established a procedure." (*Auschwitz commandant Rudolph Hoess's portrayal of the gas chamber extermination process, 1947*)	"A medical procedure." (*Attorney Geoffrey Fieger's portrayal of Dr. Jack Kevorkian's assisted-suicide method, 1996*)
"It was indeed a medical matter, since it was prepared by physicians." (*Defense attorney Robert Servatius's characterization of gas chamber killing at Adolf Eichmann trial, 1961*)	"A decision to perform an abortion should be regarded as strictly a medical decision." (*American Psychiatric Association's placement of abortion within mainstream medicine, 1969*)

CHAPTER 12

Choice and Selection

Slogans for the Reduction of Vulnerable Populations

The rhetoric of choice and selection is a strongly modern phenomenon that contains numerous historical precedents. Today, pro-choice designations are relied upon extensively as justifications for facilitating the huge number of abortions performed throughout the world and are becoming an integral part of the discourse employed in the contemporary movement to legitimize physician-assisted suicide and euthanasia. The last time doctors were so fully implicated in choosing large numbers of individuals for annihilation occurred during the Nazi era, when the words "selection," "select," and "selected"—close equivalents to today's "choice," "choose," and "chosen"—were used as expressions for concealing the extermination of victims in the Holocaust. The word "selection" has likewise emerged on the contemporary scene to obscure the killing of the unwanted unborn and infants born with disabilities. The significance of these concepts derives in large part from their naturally close association with such cherished ideas as rights, freedom, and autonomy. This thrust is intended to bypass the horrendous reality of what specifically is chosen or selected—the destruction of human beings on a vast scale.

Choices in the Womb

In contemporary society, the slogans "choice," "pro-choice," "choose," and "right to choose" are rallying cries for pro-abortion militants and even many individuals outside the abortion establishment. The use of these highly positive designations has had the effect of endowing the most extreme pro-abortion position—the right to choose to kill the unborn as an absolute, fundamental right (literally, abortion on demand)—with all the trappings of moderation, reason, and respectability. Advocates of legalized abortion often brand those who oppose the abortion regime as "anti-choice zealots" or "anti-choice extremists" who are intent upon undermining the woman's freedom of choice or conscience.

Pro-choice rhetoric possesses a highly seductive quality, especially in a democratic society where great importance is placed on personal autonomy. The "right to choose" has been linked with many of the options opened up for women in the long-standing drive to gain true equality. Its appeal is compelling, given the current preoccupations with lifestyles devoted to self-indulgence and interminable identity seeking. Within such a climate, "choice" has attained an unparalleled position of dominance; it is overwhelmingly defined as the key option without which all other possibilities for personal growth and development could not be obtained. "The existence of a choice," asserted Dr. Malkah T. Notman, "supports the validity of other priorities" and "confirms a woman's self-image as someone who is valued not only for her child-bearing role."[1]

After being convicted of manslaughter in 1975 for performing a late-term abortion, Boston City Hospital obstetrician Kenneth Edelin resorted to pro-choice rhetoric to justify what he had done:

> Women since they've been on this earth have been making that choice, whether they want to carry that baby or not.... The only humane thing we can do is make sure that when they make that choice they have the opportunity to make it under the best conditions possible.[2]

Such noble-sounding sentiments make it easy to lose sight of a stark reality—the choice not to carry the baby is an expression designed to cover up the choice to kill the baby.

Another typical display of right-to-choose semantics can be found in an interview conducted with a female physician abortionist published in *Mademoiselle* (February 1988). This particular abortionist called "choice" a form of "reproductive freedom." The most basic issue in abortion, she declared, is "that women should be able to choose" and presented herself as "the facilitator" of "that choice."[3]

Many doctors are so wedded to "pro-choice" sloganeering that they have created an organization called Physicians for Choice. According to one of their promotional pieces, "choice" is defined as "a most basic human right: the right to decide whether or not to bear a child."[4] An associated organization, Medical Students for Choice, circulated a petition demanding, ironically, mandatory abortion training in obstetrics/gynecology residency programs.[5] The American Psychiatric Association reaffirmed "its position that abortion is a medical procedure in which physicians should respect the patient's right to freedom of choice."[6] More recently, the word "choice" has assumed an even more prominent spot in the persevering efforts to institutionalize the pro-abortion mindset. During the first week of January 2003, in conjunction with the thirtieth anniversary of the *Roe v. Wade* decision, the National Abortion and Reproductive Rights Action League announced expunging the word "abortion" from its lexicon and renaming itself NARAL Pro-Choice America, along with a nationwide campaign intended to further entrench the "pro-choice" mentality in the public square. A press release announcing the change is saturated with eighteen references to "choice" or "choose." The only reason it mentions the word abortion just twice is to make sure everyone understands that "NARAL Pro-Choice America is now the legal name of the organization formerly known as the National Abortion and Reproductive Rights Action League."[7]

The unabated reliance on pro-choice rhetoric to gloss over the deluge of destructive procedures directed against the unwanted unborn is not confined to physician abortionists and pro-abortion organizations. One of its most radical and all-encompassing manifestations is the Freedom of Choice Act (FOCA), a legislative proposal introduced in the US Congress over the past several decades (from 1989 to its most recent version in 2007) aimed at enshrining abortion on demand in American law and wiping out even the most minimal state and federal restrictions on abortion permitted under *Roe*. Beneath the guise of a democratic-appearing, autonomy-endowed title, this draconian bill would invalidate such measures as partial-birth abortion bans, prohibitions on taxpayer funding of abortion, informed consent laws, parental consent and notification laws, waiting period requirements, and conscience rights for health care providers who refuse to participate in abortions. Adamant pro-abortion proponent Senator Barbara Boxer defended the broad reach of FOCA, asserting that it "supercedes any law, regulation or local ordinance that impinges on a woman's right to choose."[8]

Postnatal Choices

For years, euthanasia advocacy groups have observed with more than passing interest how deeply embedded the word "choice" has become in the pro-abortion vocabulary and mindset. The Hemlock Society, one of North America's most aggressive proponents of physician-assisted suicide, has struggled with the highly negative imagery projected by a name based on a poisonous plant. For well over a decade, Hemlock founder Derek Humphry has been replicating a style of discourse basic to abortion advocacy in asserting that "unless we have a right to choose when and how to die, we are not truly free people."[9] Inspired by the success of abortion supporters in selling abortion on demand as a positive, democratic, and private choice, the Hemlock Society's official incorporation of choice sloganeering occurred in July 2003 with the announcement that it had changed its name to End-of-Life Choices.[10]

But it soon became evident that choice alone was not enough to shore up the assisted suicide/euthanasia movement; it still required a more extensive verbal makeover. Another leading pro-death organization—Compassion in Dying—seemed to contain the missing ingredient: an emphasis on the caring nature of choice. Thus in January 2005, End-of-Life Choices joined with Compassion in Dying to form an organization with the newly minted moniker Compassion and Choices (C&C). This merger is considered a public relations coup because it combines the best of two worlds: both the compassionate and autonomous aspects attributed to assisted suicide and euthanasia. The most soothing rhetoric has evolved with choice leading the way. C&C describes itself as a "comprehensive choice-in-dying organization" that works "to improve care and expand choice," advances the "patient's choice to shorten a dying process," and "uses the power of choice and comfort to restore hope to individuals and their loved ones at the end of life."[11]

Armed with a terminological change of expansive proportions, C&C has proven to be extraordinarily active in furthering the acceptance of assisted suicide. One of its most successful accomplishments was spearheading the November 4, 2008, voter-approved passage of Initiative 1000 (the Washington Death with Dignity Act), which legalized physician-assisted suicide in Washington State. Compassion and Choices is also involved in orchestrating voter initiatives, filing lawsuits, and promoting legislative bills in other states viewed as vulnerable to its assisted suicide goals.[12]

Compassion and Choices' implacable pro-choice spin has become increasingly embedded in the semantics of the health care reform movement: "Compassion & Choices is leading the charge to make end-of-life choice a centerpiece of any program that emerges. We are working hard to reach our goal to make end-of-life choice a centerpiece of national health insurance reform."[13]

Selection of the Unfit in Nazi Germany

In the Third Reich, the catchword "selection"—the Nazi counterpart to today's "choice"—served as a key construct to expedite getting rid of huge numbers of victims defined as "defective" according to the Aryan standard of worth. Its historical roots can be traced back to the influential physician, biologist, and philosopher Dr. Ernst Haeckel, who drew upon Charles Darwin's "theory of selection" as a basis for attributing the survival of the fittest in the struggle for existence to the process of "natural selection" whereby weak, defective, and degenerate individuals would inevitably perish. Haeckel proposed various forms of "artificial selection" (exposure, lethal drugs, and capital punishment) to take up the slack in instances where "natural selection" failed to do away with a sufficient number of lives considered below par and expendable.[14]

The "selection" of physically and mentally handicapped patients for euthanasia in the Third Reich was made by committees of medical experts—many of them professors from leading universities—on the basis of questionnaires mailed throughout Germany to target patients residing in hospitals, nursing homes, children's institutions, sanitariums, and psychiatric facilities.

A noticeable expansion of euthanasia took place in the fall of 1941 as commissions of physicians visited concentration camps "to select" for extermination rebellious prisoners and those no longer able to work. This large-scale "patient selection" engulfed a broad range of victims in its lethal orbit. These visits were dubbed "selection tours."[15] By the summer of 1942, the commissions of physicians discontinued their trips to Nazi concentration camps in search of death selection candidates because a number of camps were in the process of being transformed into extermination centers with their own contingent of destructive machinery and death selection specialists (overwhelmingly physicians).

From October 1942 until autumn of 1943, "the selection process" at the Maidanek concentration camp consisted of gassing Jews who were deemed incapable of working. SS-Hauptscharfuhrer Erich Muhsfeld, in charge of the camp's gas chambers and crematoria, testified on August 4, 1947, while a prisoner in Poland that "the arriving convoys were always submitted to a selection process. . . . Those unfit for work were asphyxiated in the gas chamber."[16]

In his study of Nazi doctors, psychiatrist Robert Jay Lifton revealed how the extensive participation of physicians in the destruction process at Auschwitz was perpetrated under the cover of "medical-block selections":

> Nazi doctors were best observed—and perhaps most revealingly— when selecting on the medical blocks. In those selections, the SS doctor performed his healing-killing reversal within a medical context. They were therefore a key to medicalized killing and a special truth of Auschwitz. Selections on a medical block were a murderous caricature of triage: the doctor sorted out the sick and the weak to be fed to the killing machinery.[17]

The word "selection" took on a pronounced medical character when defined as a method of countering the numerous epidemics that raged throughout the camps. Because selections for the gas chambers actually resulted in the eradication of epidemics by eradicating those afflicted with typhus, typhoid, scarlet fever, and other infectious diseases, doctors who performed them consoled themselves that they were involved in an essential public health measure. Professor Fejkiel recalled "the big typhus selection on August 29, 1942. The hospital was surrounded and trucks pulled up to take the people selected to the gas chambers."[18]

Selection of the Vulnerable in Contemporary Society

In league with the contemporary development of prenatal screening tests, selection has emerged as a widespread expression to characterize the substantial increase in abortions done on victims detected as possessing some type of genetic defect. Doctors from the Mount Sinai Medical Center in New York City invoked the phrases "selective termination" and "selective birth" in announcing, on June 17, 1981, what was considered a scientific breakthrough: piercing the heart of a twin with Down syndrome at twenty weeks' gestation while allowing the normal twin to survive. A combination of ultrasound guidance and fetal blood samples helped verify that "the correct selection [bloodletting of the twin with Down Syndrome]" had taken place.[19]

Acutely aware of the significance of language for conferring credibility upon destructive procedures inside the womb, Dr. Mark Evans and colleagues have devoted long-standing attention to evaluating "the use of words" as "a moral choice, especially to describe actions that result in death." They concluded that "selective termination" is the preferable way to describe the destruction of abnormal fetuses in multiple pregnancies, "aware of its potential to mask the directness of killing one or more fetuses."[20]

Selection is increasingly invoked as a code word for aborting unborn girls, especially in China, India, Korea, and other Asian countries where there is a pronounced preference for boys. In *Unnatural Selection: Choosing Boys over Girls, and the Consequences of a World Full of Men* (2011), science journalist Mara Havistendahl estimates that during the past three decades, the number of "missing women" in Asia alone has risen to more than 160 million, a great preponderance of them due to abortions resulting from the extensive use of ultrasound technology for prenatal sex detection. Her book overflows with examples of how selection in association with "sex" and other designations serves to promote aborting unborn babies of the undesired (overwhelmingly female) gender. The text contains an abundance of such characterizations as "sex selection's ubiquity," "sex selection is widespread," "sex selection is a medical act," "gender selection," "prenatal sex selection," and "America's elite pushed sex selection on the developing world."[21]

Despite exposing how the rhetoric of selection sheds light on the harsh reality of 160 million missing women, Havistendahl insists that "this is not a book about death and killing. I do not talk about feticide or gendercide or genocide." Instead, she reduces life before birth to the insignificant status of an "unanswerable question; not an actual life, but only a potential life at best." This distortion provides her with the justification for concluding, "In the end this book is not about life and death but about the *potential* for life—and denying that potential to the very group responsible for perpetuating our beleaguered species."[22]

Although alarmed at the extreme gender discrimination fueling the 160 million missing women, Havistendahl's rigid compliance with one of the pro-abortion movement's most sacrosanct pieces of dog-

ma—avoidance of the scientific fact that human life begins at conception—prevents her from fully owning up to the enormity of such
a calamity. Writing in the *New York Times*, op-ed correspondent Ross
Douthat rightly asserted, "The tragedy of the world's 160 million missing girls isn't that they're 'missing.' The tragedy is that they're dead."[23]

Some of today's leading pediatricians are continuing the legacy of
death selection established by Nazi doctors and contemporary abortion doctors. The intensive care nursery of modern medical centers
has become another prime locale for imposing the label "selection"
and its devastating consequences. A pioneer in the withholding of
life-saving treatment from infants with spina bifida according to the
rhetoric of selection is British pediatrician John Lorber. A typical example of his "policy of selection" appeared in a 1973 issue of the *British
Medical Journal*: out of thirty-seven newborn children with spina bifida referred to the Department of Child Health at Sheffield University,
twenty-five were "selected for nontreatment" by a "paediatric team." In
a triumphant statement intended to vindicate "the proposed criteria
for selection," Lorber concluded that "death occurred in all 25" infants
who were "selectively untreated." He claimed credit for inaugurating
"the second revolution in the management of myelomeningocele—
namely, an almost universal acceptance of selection" as a legitimate
medical practice.[24]

The key features involved in putting to death society's "unfit"
members after birth were fully incorporated in "a program of early selection and treatment of the infant with myelomeningocele" published
in *Pediatrics* (October 1983). This report reveals how a multidisciplinary team of health care professionals headed by Dr. Richard Gross
at the Oklahoma Children's Memorial Hospital in Oklahoma City
used a quality-of-life formula to select thirty-six infants born with spina bifida for "vigorous treatment," while twenty-four were selected to
receive "supportive care." Vigorous treatment consisted of surgery to
close the opening in the spinal column, insertion of a shunt, and antibiotics to prevent infection. Those selected for supportive care were
sent to a children's shelter where they were denied corrective surgery,
shunt therapy, and antibiotics. The death selection team considered

their selection process a resounding success: "all 24 babies who have not been treated at all have died at an average of 37 days."[25]

In reading through Dr. Gross's report, one is struck by how often the word "selection" is used to shore up the actions denying life-sustaining therapy to these children. He and his associates emphasize the importance of utilizing a team of health care experts for implementing "this approach of early selection" and note the significance of "selection criteria" in decision making. They point with pride to the effectiveness of "our selection process"—there were no survivors among those "selected only for supportive treatment."[26]

Selection of Surplus Populations for Reduction

The rhetoric of selection was also employed in the past and holds sway in the present as a basis for doing away with individuals, not necessarily because of any defect on their part, but because they constituted and continue to constitute an unacceptably large number of unwanted individuals crowded into limited spaces. During the Nazi era, huge numbers of Jews, Gypsies, Poles, and other groups were herded into jam-packed ghettoes and concentration camps. Today, owing to the overuse of infertility drug treatments, women's wombs often become crammed with multiple unwelcome preborn humans. The expressions "reduction," "reduce," and "reduced" have been frequently combined with "selection" to further gloss over the actual fate of past and current groups defined as superfluous.

Selections dominated the ecology of Auschwitz as an endless stream of victims came from many parts of Nazi-occupied Europe. Although a large majority of death camp victims ended up in the gas chambers and crematoria, others were selected for lethal injections of phenol into the heart when the Auschwitz hospital became overcrowded. Dr. Stanislaw Klodzinski, a Polish prisoner survivor, furnished details on the fate of individuals who lined up for sick call. "Those were not sick calls meant to save the lives of prisoners, but only inspections, to see whether the hospital wasn't overcrowded. If there was overcrowding, then he [Josef Klehr, the nurse-medical corpsman on duty] would select patients for killing. Those were the so-called small selections."[27]

The words "selection" and "reduction" comprised key components in the nomenclature constructed to hasten the extermination of the "surplus populations" of the East under Nazi domination. Just before launching the attack on the Soviet Union, Heinrich Himmler told a group of SS generals that "one of the goals of the campaign was to reduce the Slav population by 30,000,000."[28] In the summer and fall of 1942, "a giant selection" resulted in dispatching the inhabitants of the Warsaw ghetto to the Treblinka death camp: "300,000 people had been deported" and "the size of the ghetto had also been reduced."[29]

According to German and Russian reports, asphyxiation in gas vans constituted one of the methods used in 1942 for "the daily reduction of hospitals, asylums, and orphanages" in the territories under German control.[30] In testimony before the Nuremberg War Crimes Tribunal, the chief physician of the Main Race and Settlement Office, Dr. Helmut Poppendick, admitted that a major goal of Nazi racial policy involved the extermination of non-Aryans, which was categorized under the phrase "measures to reduce the non-Aryan population."[31]

The semantics of reduction, however, was not confined to covering up the fate of victims outside Germany. An economic analysis of the Rummelsburg Workhouse in Berlin conducted by Ludwig Trieb, administrative inspector of the Reich Association for Institutions, stated that since its Working Group 1 contained a number of individuals "supposedly incapable of work," then it "could be reduced accordingly," while "the remainder [of non-reduced members]" would have to "achieve increased performance." Conversely, Working Group 2 would only have to be "reduced to a limited extent" because it had higher-skilled workers who did "valuable work."[32]

Similarly, along with the designation "selection," the word "reduction" serves as a basic ingredient in the evasive vocabulary invoked to resolve what some contemporary abortion doctors call the predicament of being "too pregnant." The Sloane Hospital for Women affiliated with the Columbia University Medical Center served as the site for a "pregnancy reduction" process involving the injection of potassium chloride "into the area of the beating heart" of "148 multifetal pregnancies."[33]

Doctors affiliated with the Chaim Sheba Medical Center in Israel made use of the expressions "selective reduction," "selective fetal reduction," and "fetuses selected for reduction" to portray the implementation of "needle-guided procedures" in ten "multiple gestations."[34] In another study conducted at this same institution, "multifetal pregnancy reduction" was the expression chosen to depict the fate of "ninety-five high-order pregnancies following assisted conception": "46 triplet pregnancies [were] reduced to twins at 11-12 weeks' gestation," while "49 triplet pregnancies were reduced to twins at 13-14 weeks' gestation." The practitioners of these destructive procedures further revealed that "all fetal reductions ... were performed by transabdominal intrathoracic injection of potassium chloride."[35]

"Selective reduction" is one of the main code expressions utilized by Dr. Mark Evans to justify plunging a needle filled with potassium chloride into the heart of one or more unwanted children targeted in a multiple pregnancy. In 2009, he wrote an essay published in *Newsweek* describing himself as a member of "a small cadre of experienced high-risk obstetricians who now offer selective reduction for higher-order multiples."[36]

Back in 1998, after an assessment of "the ethical and technical problems associated with multifetal pregnancy reduction," Dr. Evans and some associates agreed "that reduction of multifetal pregnancies to twins is probably the more appropriate number in the majority of instances."[37] By 2004, he reconsidered his position and announced in the journal *Obstetrics and Gynecology* that "reducing twin pregnancies to singletons" was also an acceptable ethical option. One of the reasons given for this change was that Evans and his fellow "reduction practitioners" had become more proficient at performing this procedure without any complications for the woman, resulting in the likelihood that "taking home a baby is higher after reduction than remaining with twins."[38]

In the *New York Times Magazine* of August 14, 2011, journalist Ruth Padawer relied upon an abundant use of reductionistic semantics to describe doing away with one of the unborn victims in a twin pregnancy, not because of any defect in the aborted twin, but simply because the pregnant woman wanted only one child and not two. Padawer characterizes this choice as a "twin reduction," which consists of "selecting one fetus over another, when either one is equally wanted." She even furnishes an unusually frank portrayal of what actually happens during the reduction process: "The procedure ... involves a fatal injection of potassium in the fetal chest. The dead fetus shrivels over time and remains in the womb until delivery." But this reality gets lost in the shuffle, as the rest of Padawer's account of the lethal operation is largely dominated by a persistent resort to the euphemistic expressions "reductions," "pregnancy reduction," "reduction to a singleton," "twin reduction," "an elective two-to-one reduction," and "reducing twins." Furthermore, she conferred the designations "early practitioner of pregnancy reduction" and "reduction pioneer" upon those doctors who led the way in destroying the unwanted unborn twin, and called women who underwent these procedures "two-to-one patients."[39]

The Real Meaning of Choice and Selection

Beneath the democratic-appearing words "choice" and "selection" lurks an especially insidious form of oppression—the right to choose or select victims for extinction. Just as the Nazi doctors claimed the *right to select* who would expire in gas chambers, today's physicians in conjunction with others insist upon the *right to choose* or *select* who will perish inside the uterus and in the intensive care nursery of contemporary hospitals.

The parlance of "choice" and "selection" comprises a perversion of the first order—it exploits the language of rights as a pretext for taking away the most fundamental right of all, life itself. It is an essentially arrogant, elitist assumption of the awesome power to destroy those unable to defend themselves, an extreme manifestation of the powerful victimizing the powerless. It is the same kind of power so extensively exercised against inmates and prisoners by Nazi doctors who, under the guise of selection, also had the "right to choose" at the time which of their expendables would be dispatched to annihilation.

Moreover, the catchwords "choice" and "selection" constitute a flagrant sham because the individuals most drastically affected—the victims—are the very ones who are denied the right to choose or select survival. It is death at someone else's choice or selection. This is not reproductive or any other type of freedom, but the worse kind of tyranny. It needs to be repeatedly reasserted that a major reason Nazi Germany came to be is that some physicians and others took it upon themselves to choose who would live and who would be extinguished. And, under the cover of similar and even sometimes identical terminology, this is precisely what some contemporary doctors are doing to the unwanted unborn and vulnerable born.

At an international abortion conference in 1967, Nobel Prize-winning author Pearl S. Buck, the mother of a child with disabilities, gave compelling testimony against allowing the choice of death over life before and after birth:

> I fear the power of choice over life or death at human hands. I see no human being whom I could ever trust with such power—not myself, not any other. Human wisdom, human integrity are not great enough.[40]

In table 12, the focus is on examples derived from the terminology of choice and selection designed to conceal the destruction of human lives in contemporary society and in the Third Reich.

TABLE 12. THE RHETORIC OF CHOICE AND SELECTION

THE OMNIPRESENCE OF CHOICES

PRENATAL CHOICES

"Women since they've been on this earth have been making that choice."
(*Dr. Kenneth Edelin's justification for performing a late-term abortion, 1975*)
"Women should be able to choose."
(*A physician abortionist who characterized herself as "a facilitator of choice," 1988*)
"Physicians should respect the patient's right to freedom of choice."
(*American Psychiatric Association statement on reproductive rights, 1992*)
"NARAL Pro-Choice America."
(*A press release announcing the new name for the organization formerly known as the National Abortion and Reproductive Rights Action League, January 2003*)
"Freedom of Choice Act."
(*A federal legislative proposal aimed at enshrining abortion on demand in American law, 1989-2007*)

POSTNATAL CHOICES

"Unless we have a right to choose when and how to die, we are not truly free people."
(*Hemlock Society founder Derek Humphry, 1988*)
"Compassion & Choices."
(*Announcement of a new name to replace the names of the former pro-death organizations the Hemlock Society, End-of-Life Choices, and Compassion in Dying, January 2005*)
"We are working hard to reach our goal to make end-of-life choice a centerpiece of national health insurance reform."
(*Compassion and Choices' promotion of assisted suicide under the banner of choice, August 12, 2009*)

The Third Reich	Contemporary Society
THE PERVASIVENESS OF SELECTIONS	
"Medical-block selections"	"The correct selection."
(*Asphyxiation of patients in the Auschwitz gas chambers, early 1940s*)	(*Piercing the heart of an unborn twin with Down syndrome, 1981*)
"Typhus selection."	"Policy of selection."
(*Extermination of concentration camp inmates afflicted with typhus, 1942*)	(*Dr. John Lorber's description of the killing of infants with spina bifida, 1973*)
"A selection process."	"Our selection process."
(*Gassing Jews deemed unfit for work at the Maidanek concentration camp, 1942-43*)	(*Denial of life-saving treatment to impaired infants at an Oklahoma children's hospital, 1977-82*)
"Selection tours."	"Sex selection."
(*Dispatching concentration camp victims to their deaths in euthanasia institutions, early 1940s*)	(*Abortions performed on unborn humans of the female gender throughout Asia, 2011*)
SELECTION OF SURPLUS POPULATIONS FOR REDUCTION	
"The ghetto had also been reduced."	"Triplet pregnancies were reduced."
(*Dispatching Warsaw ghetto inhabitants to the Treblinka death camp, summer-fall, 1942*)	(*The killing of surplus fetuses with potassium chloride injections, 2001*)
"The reduction."	"Selective reduction."
(*The selection of Jews living in a crowded Polish ghetto for asphyxiation in gas vans, 1944*)	(*A method of killing one or more children in a multiple pregnancy, 2009*)
"The daily reduction."	"An elective two-to-one reduction."
(*Gas-van extermination of patients in hospitals, asylums, hospitals, and orphanages, 1942*)	(*The destruction of the unwanted unborn twin in a twin pregnancy, 2011*)

CHAPTER 13

Distortions of the Evacuation Designation

Among the most common definitions of the word "evacuation" are
(1) the removal of persons or things from an endangered area and
(2) the action of emptying (a receptacle) or removing (the contents of
anything). Nazi perpetrators considered "evacuation" to be a highly
convenient designation of deception, especially during wartime, when
many legitimate evacuations from battle zones and other unsafe re-
gions took place. The purpose of the Nazi evacuations was just the
opposite—the subjection of huge numbers of victims to the induced
disasters of lethal injections, shooting, gassing, and burning. In addition, the Holocaust practitioners seized upon the second definition of
evacuation as a means of concealing their destructive actions under
the guise of "emptying" or "removing" people from ghettos. Contemporary physician abortionists have appropriated the second definition
of evacuation to convey the impression of abortion as simply a minor
medical procedure in which contents, products, or tissue are "emptied" out of or "removed" from the uterus. Such abstract, emotionally
detached language is intended to obscure the concrete, repulsive task
of pulling apart and extracting the often identifiable remains of tiny
human beings dismembered in the process of "evacuation."

Evacuation to the East

Evacuation rhetoric served as an essential weapon in facilitating
every aspect of the Nazi Holocaust. It was invoked relentlessly to dis-

guise the euthanasia of people with mental and physical disabilities, as well as the program of racial genocide waged against Jews, Gypsies, Poles, "asocials" and others reduced to the status of subhuman expendables or considered dangerous threats to Aryan supremacy. Along with other Nazi elites, German physicians were among the foremost purveyors of this widespread euphemistic terminology.

Mentally ill and physically disabled patients of the Third Reich became prime targets for annihilation under the guise of "evacuations." At a secret meeting held in Berlin before the mayors of German cities on April 3, 1940, leading euthanasia administrator Viktor Brack unveiled a plan to eliminate "incurably ill patients of all kinds who are completely useless to humanity." He announced that "in order to carry out this operation, a *commission of physicians has been appointed* to sift through all asylums involved" to identify which patients fit under this category. Those "sifted through" would then be "evacuated to other institutions"—that is, *"packed into very primitive special asylums"* where "nothing must be done to maintain these seriously ill patients; on the contrary, everything must be done in order to have them die as quickly as possible."[1]

Another example of how the evacuation fabrication operated to conceal the euthanasia program can be seen in the case of eight-year-old Anny Wild and fellow patients who were killed at the Eglfing-Haar institution. On December 14, 1940, Anny's mother wrote to Eglfing-Haar director Dr. Hermann Pfannmuller concerning her daughter's condition and whereabouts. He wrote back, stating in part, "I have been assured that you will be informed about the condition of your daughter Anny Wild in a short time by the receiving institution. The transfer of the patient occurred within the frame of a planned evacuation of the institution for the purpose of making room for evacuees."[2]

By 1942, evacuation served as a pretext for exterminating psychiatric patients on a massive scale. In one of many such incidents, German SS troops dispatched more than 2,450 "mentally defective" patients from Polish hospitals to the outskirts of Riga, where they were shot to death. A doctor in one of the hospitals involved testified he was instructed to write on the sick lists simply—"Evacuated by SS."[3]

During the Nuremberg Doctors' Trial, a legal brief submitted on behalf of Dr. Karl Brandt, codirector of the Nazi euthanasia program, contained multiple euphemistic references to evacuation that were intended to demonstrate how extremely protective the Nazi regime was of its psychiatric patients. The brief stated that wartime conditions such as "evacuation of districts endangered by air raids, evacuation on account of proximity to the front and evacuation under consideration of inner displacements" necessitated the "evacuation" of patients from mental hospitals. "The evacuation from Warstein to Hadamar," it stated, "was made for reasons of air raid precaution," and "this evacuation was carried out by the Cooperative Ambulance Company."[4] In actuality, evacuation served as a code word to conceal the fact that Warstein was one of the collecting sites through which the victims were dispatched on the way to their deaths in the infamous euthanasia institution of Hadamar. The Cooperative Ambulance Company was a front organization responsible for transporting the patients to the euthanasia hospitals.

The establishment of evacuation as a major designation for covering up the extermination of Jews was set forth during the "Final Solution Conference" at Berlin-Wannsee on January 20, 1942. Reinhardt Heydrich announced to an audience composed of high-ranking Nazi officials that the Führer had given approval for "the evacuation of Jews to the East." He displayed a chart that identified "the Jewish communities to be evacuated."[5]

At the Auschwitz death camp, the word "evacuation" was often used to conceal the medicalized killing of individuals defined as being debilitated or in ill health. As reported by a Polish officer who escaped from Auschwitz, "during these actions [so-called delousings] everybody was examined, and those who appeared unhealthy or in weakened bodily condition were, according to the camp doctor's mood, destined for gassing. They were simply led to the 'infirmary,' from where 40 to 50 percent of them were 'evacuated.'"[6]

Accounts of the massive killings of Jews in the Polish ghettos and the eastern territories under Nazi occupation were repeatedly obscured by the omnipresent term "evacuation." The dispatching of Jews from the Lodz ghetto to the extermination centers was carried out under the ruse of "a total evacuation."[7] During the spring of 1943, in a report on *The Final Solution of the European Jewish Question*, statistician Dr. Richard Korherr furnished a numerical perspective on the impact of "the evacuation measures" up through 1942: "Two and a half million Jews had disappeared from the Reich and from Poland."[8]

Evacuation of the Uterus

The destruction of unborn humans with sharp curettes and vacuum devices in the first three months of pregnancy is saturated with the rhetoric of evacuation. Dr. Philip Green, a professor of obstetrics and gynecology at the Rutgers Medical School, maintained that "uterine evacuation" carried out in doctors' offices is "the ideal site" for a "speedy evacuation" and "a complete evacuation."[9] The designations "suction evacuation," "the evacuation procedure," "the evacuation," "evacuation of the uterine contents," "reevacuation," "uterine evacuation" and "the evacuation method"[10] were used to describe 16,410 first-trimester abortions performed over a thirty-month period at Reproductive Health Services, a St. Louis abortion center.

By the 1980s, dismemberment of the unborn in the second trimester with suction machines, curettes, and forceps gained a position of prominence and along with it an extensive rhetoric of evacuation featuring the phrase "dilatation and evacuation," or D&E for short. Among the array of designations deployed by Dr. Phillip Stubblefield in conducting second-trimester abortion techniques are "instrumental evacuation," "the uterus was then evacuated," "evacuation of the uterine content," "uterine evacuation," and "evacuation of a pregnancy."[11] Dr. Warren Hern dubbed the "sharp dissection of presenting fetal parts" as a "forceps evacuation of the uterus ... under direct intraoperative ultrasound visualization."[12]

Evacuation semantics pervaded the testimony of Planned Parenthood medical officer Dr. Maureen Paul during a 2004 California federal court trial convened to contest laws banning partial-birth abortion. The questions asked by a Planned Parenthood attorney and

Dr. Paul's responses typify how the clinical, emotionally detached language of evacuation is exploited to mitigate the disturbing aspects associated with performing later-term abortions:

Q: What is the first thing you do to evacuate the uterus?
A: I break the bag of water....
Q: And when you begin the evacuation, is the fetus ever alive?
A: Yes.
Q: How do you know that?
A: Because I do many of my procedures at 16 weeks under an ultrasound guidance, so I will see a heartbeat....
Q: So, after you've broken the bag of water and the fluid is either drained or you've suctioned out the fluid, what do you do next?
A: I evacuate the fetus....
Q: And can you describe how you do that?
A: Yes. I do it using an instrument called [a] forceps. So I insert the forceps and grasp the fetus and pull ... and sometimes the fetus comes out in pieces, and I make instrument passes until the entire fetus is evacuated.[13]

Moreover, evacuation occupies a key spot in postgraduate medical programs for training physicians to become expert abortionists. On September 14, 2009, Joe Ortwerth, director of the Missouri Family Policy Council, brought to public attention that the Washington University Medical School's Family Planning Fellowship Program joined forces with Planned Parenthood of St. Louis and Barnes-Jewish Hospital to furnish clinical training sites where "fellows will learn" and "ultimately teach and supervise residents" in performing "first and second trimester surgical abortion and medical abortion." Ortwerth also found that one of the program's abortion services listed is that ubiquitous designation, "uterine evacuation procedures."[14]

The Emptying and Removal Processes

The expression "empty" and its various forms were often invoked in conjunction with the dispatching of Jews and myriad victims from the Nazi-occupied ghettos of the eastern territories to the death camps. The year 1942 was when "the ghettos began to be emptied out."[15] On February 13, 1943, German officer Max Merten told Chief Rabbi Zvi Koretz that the Baron de Hirsch ghetto in Salonika, Greece, "would have to be emptied" because of the dangers posed by Communists.[16] From 1942 through August 1944, more than 150,000 Jews in the Lodz ghetto were shipped to extermination centers. Upon completion of this enormous process of annihilation, the Gestapo announced, "The ghetto was empty."[17]

During the fall of 1945, a project of massive destruction took place in Hungary. It resulted in "emptying the hospitals and institutions" of the sick, newborn infants, the blind and deaf, mentally ill patients, and prisoners.[18]

Nazi medical scientists played a significant role in furthering mass destruction under the cover of "removal." Dr. Walter Gross, head of the Office of Racial Policy, spoke on the possible solutions to the Jewish question at a meeting of the Institute for Research on the Jewish Question on March 27-28, 1941, in Frankfurt, Germany. The final solution, he maintained, could occur only with the complete "removal of Jews from Europe."[19] A health conference held in Poland during the summer of 1943 served as a prime occasion for Hans Frank, the governor general of Nazi-occupied Poland, to announce that the "removal" of the "Jewish element" from Poland made an important contribution to better health in Europe.[20]

Medical bureaucrats resorted to "remove" as a pertinent term for accelerating the destruction of Germany's psychiatric patients. A letter dated May 12, 1941—typical of many fabricated during this period—was sent from Berlin to the director of the hospital of the District Association of Swabia, Kaufeuren/Bavaria. It states in part: "By order of the Reich Defense Commissioner I must remove mental cases from your institution ... to another institution."[21]

One of the most memorable uses of removal rhetoric occurred in Nazi-occupied France. The victims consisted of forty-one children who were hiding out in a home located in the village of Izieu, fifty miles east of Lyon. On the morning of April 6, 1944, SS Obersturmführer Klaus Barbie, the infamous butcher of Lyon, and a contingent of Gestapo troops invaded the home, ransacked the premises, terrorized the children, and forced them at gunpoint into several trucks. When one small boy ran away in confusion, he was beaten with rifle butts and thrown, bleeding, into one of the trucks. Another young child was so paralyzed with fear that he had to be carried into the truck. The children were taken to the cellar of a local prison and then transported to the gas chambers of Auschwitz in cattle cars. Barbie's benign version of this atrocity appears in a telegram dispatched to Gestapo headquarters in Paris that stated in part, "A total of 41 children from 3-13 in age were removed."[22]

Many physician abortionists of today are comparably fond of portraying abortion as an inconsequential procedure that merely "empties" or "removes" nondescript material out of the uterus. According to Dr. Warren Hern, "the purpose of an abortion is to empty the pregnant uterus of its contents."[23] At his abortion clinic in Boulder, Colorado, women undergoing late outpatient abortions are "taken into the procedure room where membranes were ruptured and the uterus was emptied."[24] Dr. T. P. Dutt and colleagues in London utilized ultrasound to assess "uterine emptying" in first-trimester abortions induced by prostaglandins. They found this method effective for "the emptying of products of conception" during the first seven weeks of gestation.[25] Besides repeatedly relying upon the word "evacuation" to mitigate her deadly assaults against the unborn, Dr. Maureen Paul concluded, "My objective is to empty the uterus in the safest way possible."[26]

The word "emptying" can also be found in a description of the aborted body disposal procedure at a contemporary abortion clinic. A letter of complaint to the Colorado Department of Health disclosed that Dr. James Parks, owner of the Mayfair Women's Center in Aurora, used a meat grinder to obliterate fetal remains into a large bucket, which were then dumped into the sink and washed down the drain. This process became known as "emptying the buckets."[27]

The designations "removed" and "removal" are deployed today to obscure the horrendous details of dismembering human lives inside the womb. According to an influential version of such sugarcoated semantics put forth on WebMD.com, no one is sucked to smithereens in the vacuum aspiration abortion procedure, but instead "the tissue is gently removed from the uterus."[28]

Among American abortionists, Dr. Warren Hern ranks as one of the most steadfast proponents of removal terminology in pioneering an extensive array of destructive surgical techniques for the "thorough removal of devitalized tissue." He utilizes special backup forceps during "the fetal removal stage" from eighteen to nineteen weeks' gestation "since fetal parts are significantly larger and more difficult to morcellate [break into small pieces]." Dr. Hern advises that "care must be taken in removal," especially of the skull, "because ossification [hardening] is occurring and the edges are sharp." He furthermore advocates "intraoperative ultrasound visualization" as an invaluable tool "to facilitate removal of the tissue."[29]

Dr. Carolyn Westhoff, a Columbia University obstetrics and gynecology professor and late-term abortion practitioner, testified in a 2004 New York abortion case soon after presiding Judge Richard Casey had already heard a steady diet of evacuation rhetoric from a procession of veteran abortion doctors. His impatience with this mode of discourse was manifestly noticeable as he continually pressed Dr. Westhoff to divulge what she really tells her patients about the destructive abortion dismemberment operations she performs. Most of the time, she tried to avoid answering the questions posed by Judge Casey or replied with euphemistic removal phraseology:

> THE COURT: And when you discuss the D&E, do you discuss dismemberment?
> THE WITNESS: I tell them that my responsibility is to remove the fetus and the other—
> THE COURT: Doctor, that isn't my question. Do you discuss dismemberment? Do you tell them about ripping or tearing a limb off the fetus?
> THE WITNESS: I may very often discuss that I remove the fetus in pieces but that is not necessarily a uniform part of the discussion.[30]

Table 13 contains a comparison of the typical variants of evacuation semantics that prevailed in the Third Reich and continue to be invoked in contemporary society.

TABLE 13. EVACUATION RHETORIC IN THE SERVICE OF EXTERMINATION

The Third Reich	Contemporary Society
EVACUATION	
"A planned evacuation of the institution." (*Dr. Hermann Pfannmuller on what happened to patients killed at Eglfing-Haar, 1940*)	"Evacuation of the uterine contents." (*A portrayal of the 16,410 abortions carried out in a St. Louis clinic, 1980*)
"A total evacuation." (*Dispatching Jews from the Lodz ghetto to the extermination centers, 1944*)	"A complete evacuation." (*Dr. Philip Green's promotion of abortions performed in doctors' offices, 1980*)
"Evacuated by SS." (*A medical report on the shooting of mentally disabled patients, 1942*)	"The uterus was then evacuated." (*Dr. Phillip Stubblefield's description of a second-trimester abortion technique, 1986*)
"Evacuation of the Jews to the east." (*Notes compiled by Adolf Eichmann at conference on the plans to exterminate the European Jews, 1942*)	"Forceps evacuation of the uterus." (*Dr. Warren Hern's characterization of dissecting fetal parts in late-term abortions, 2001*)
"40 to 50 percent of them were 'evacuated.'" (*Auschwitz infirmary patients who were exterminated in the gas chambers, 1943*)	"The entire fetus is evacuated." (*Dr. Maureen Paul's use of forceps in extracting all of the aborted dismembered fetal parts, 2004*)
EMPTY	
"The ghettos began to be emptied out." (*Transporting victims to the Nazi concentration camps, 1942*)	"The uterus was emptied." (*Dr. Warren Hern's description of late-term outpatient abortions, 1984*)
"The ghetto was empty." (*Gestapo account of the destruction of the Jews residing in the Lodz ghetto, 1942-44*)	"My objective is to empty the uterus." (*Dr. Maureen Paul's characterization of the abortion procedure, 2004*)
"Emptying the hospitals and institutions." (*Annihilation of disabled and vulnerable patients in Hungary, 1945*)	"Emptying the buckets." (*Dumping obliterated fetal remains into an abortion clinic sink, 1991*)
REMOVAL	
"Removal of Jews." (*Dr. Walter Gross on the fate of Jews destined for extermination, 1941*)	"Removal of the tissue." (*Dr. Warren Hern on grasping the fetal skull during the abortion process, 1984*)
"I must remove mental cases." (*An order for accelerating the destruction of German psychiatric patients, 1941*)	"My responsibility is to remove the fetus." (*Dr. Carolyn Westhoff on the process of performing dismemberment abortions, 2004*)
"41 children from 3-13 . . . were removed." (*Klaus Barbie's description of what happened to children dispatched to the gas chambers, 1944*)	"The tissue is gently removed." (*WebMD version of what happens when the unborn is obliterated during a suction abortion procedure, 2013*)

CHAPTER 14

Decent Perpetrators and Their
Humane Services

Throughout history, the predominant role of the physician has been
to save, preserve, and heal human lives. It is this humanitarian orientation that has attracted so many idealistic and gifted individuals
to the profession of medicine and is responsible for the incomparable
esteem in which physicians have been held. The image of the selfless
doctor totally committed to the welfare of the patient and humanity is
a pervasive one that transcends numerous cultures.

Medical participation in the deliberate destruction of human
lives—as was the case in the Third Reich and is the situation in contemporary society—represents a radical departure from the legacy
of healing intrinsic to medicine since the time of Hippocrates. Those
implicated in medicalized killing face the monumental challenge of
reconciling two opposing forces—retaining their perceptions of themselves as decent, humane professionals while carrying out destructive
operations on vulnerable human lives. Their strategy for overcoming
this formidable obstacle is to not only define themselves as altruistic
healers performing legitimate medical procedures, but also invariably to clothe their destructive actions in the finery of benevolence.
The doctors of the Third Reich laid as much claim to humane motives
for their involvement in killing as do today's abortion, assisted suicide, and euthanasia practitioners. The medical perpetrators of Nazi
Germany repeatedly maintained that their destructive procedures

were based on purely altruistic considerations, either for the sake of humanity in general or for the victims in particular. Contemporary health professionals invoke identical motivations to rationalize doing away with the unwanted unborn and vulnerable born.

Profiles of Decent, Idealistic Medical Executioners

The overriding view of the Nazi Holocaust has long been that of an unimaginable orgy of violence committed by brutal and crazed sadists. Doctors who participated in the barbarities are commonly portrayed as the most repulsive and demented members of the medical profession. The extermination centers, according to this interpretation, operated as opportune settings for them to act out their sadistic impulses at the expense of defenseless human victims. Some of the doctors of infamy most often singled out include Erwin Ding, August Hirt, Josef Mengele, and Sigmund Rascher. Rascher forced Dachau inmates to undergo agonizing deaths in the freezing and high-altitude experiments. Ding kept a diary of the murderous experiments in which the subjects were injected with typhus. Hirt collected the skeletons of gas chamber victims. Mengele conducted death selections and experimental atrocities at Auschwitz.

In one of his morale-building speeches, Heinrich Himmler attempted to counter the perception of Holocaust perpetrators as sadists by praising those entrusted with implementing "the final solution" as individuals of strength and decency:

> Many of you must know what it means when 100 corpses are lying side by side, or 500, or 1,000. To have stuck it out and at the same time, apart from exceptions caused by human weakness, to have remained decent fellows, that is what has made us hard. This is a page of glory in our history.[1]

The doctors and scientists who planned and implemented the Nazi euthanasia program were far from hacks on the fringes of mainstream medicine but saw themselves as competent, decent, and humane professionals possessing all the hallmarks of civic and scientific respectability. American psychiatrist Fredric Wertham found in his research that "among them were more than twelve full professors at universities" who had "made valuable contributions to scientific psychiatry" and were "still quoted in international psychiatric literature."[2]

The Federation of German Chemists protested the sentences handed down by the Nuremberg tribunal against the directors of the I. G. Farben Chemical Corporation for their complicity in the enslavement, mistreatment, terrorization, torture, and murder of concentration camp inmates. In a letter addressed to the tribunal, the chemists said of the defendants, "We know them to be decent men.... Knowing these men, we cannot believe that any dishonorable convictions or actions have actually been proven."[3]

Dr. Josef Mengele—widely regarded as the "Angel of Death"—participated in a series of repulsive crimes against humanity at Auschwitz, including death selections, gassing, lethal injections, shootings, brutal beatings, and experimental atrocities. The monstrous images so often associated with Mengele tend to obscure his respectable professional origins and the effort he expended in projecting himself as a humane medical healer and researcher. In 1935, Mengele earned a PhD from the University of Munich, where he studied anthropology and medicine. Three years later, he was awarded an MD from the University of Frankfurt. Fellow physician Dr. B. (a pseudonym) said of Dr. Mengele, "He was the most decent colleague I met there [at Auschwitz]," and it was "humanitarian reasons" that prompted him to make sure that the practical aspects of gassing were being carried out properly.[4]

It is noteworthy that Mengele's career in exterminative medicine under the banner of healing did not end with the dissolution of the Third Reich. In 1949, helped along by the possession of a Red Cross passport, Mengele found a safe haven in Argentina, where, according to Argentine archives finally opened in 1992, he practiced medicine in Buenos Aires during the 1950s and had established "a reputation as a specialist in abortions."[5]

Dr. Karl Brandt, Hitler's personal physician and a leader in the Nazi euthanasia program, was the prototype of the "decent Nazi"—"such a doctor was usually from an aristocratic or professional, often medical family whose general cultivation and pre-Nazi ethical concerns seemed strikingly at odds with the depth of his Nazi commitment." Brandt portrayed himself as an idealist and identified the great humanitarian physician Albert Schweitzer as his ultimate role model. He claimed he had once even aspired to join Schweitzer in his medical missionary work in Africa. One close medical colleague called Brandt "a highly ethical person ... one of the most idealistic physicians I have ever met."[6]

For an extended period of American history, abortion doctors were considered the scum of the medical profession. Doctors who flouted the laws strongly protective of unborn human life were viewed as a despicable minority of unscrupulous and deviant hacks who exploited desperate women by subjecting them to dangerous, unsanitary, and often fatal operations for the sake of a fast buck or for giving vent to sadistic and perverted instincts. In their sociological study of illegal abortions, Jerome Bates and Edward Zawadzki underscored case studies intended to be reflective of typical illegal medical abortionists: "Almost without exception, the physician abortionist is a deviate in some manner."[7]

As early as the 1930s, the image of American physicians who performed illegal abortions began to undergo a radical makeover. A profound reversal took place whereby the laws designed to protect the lives of human beings in the womb were labeled "harsh," "unjust," "unenforceable," and "antiquated," while doctors who violated them were elevated from the status of unsavory pariahs to bold, altruistic doctors in the forefront of progressive change. According to Rickie Solinger's book glorifying illegal abortionists, "decent, competent practitioners performed the lion's share of abortions in the criminal era."[8]

With the wholesale legalization of abortion by the US Supreme Court in 1973, the "backstreet butchers"—most of whom had long been in reality respectable licensed physicians—moved to Main Street. Ever since then, the image of abortion doctors as decent, upstanding, compassionate members of mainline medicine has been increasingly promoted. Upon receiving a humanitarian award from the National Abortion Federation in 1985, Harvard abortionist Dr. Phillip Stubblefield was eulogized as "a human being who is upright and honorable and decent" for having "done countless abortions for women who wanted them, did them with compassion and respect and skill, still does them, and does some of the hard ones—early, and late."[9] During the summer of 2009, environmentalist Tim Murray declared Canada's notorious abortionist Dr. Henry Morgentaler to be "a decent man of professional competence."[10]

Vociferous Colorado abortionist Dr. Warren Hern portrays himself as a renaissance man who possesses a strong humanitarian motivation for whatever he does. Like Dr. Karl Brandt, who viewed his leadership in Nazi euthanasia as the natural extension of idealism derived from Albert Schweitzer's humanitarian medical ethic, Dr. Hern exploits Schweitzer's idealistic legacy as a basis for pursuing his abortion specialty. It all began, he recalled, with his first abortion on a high school student:

> I had helped her change her life ... and realize her dreams. I felt I had found a new definition of the idea of medicine as an act of compassion and love for one's fellow human beings, an idea that I gained from learning about Albert Schweitzer. I had followed that ideal by working as a medical student at a Schweitzer-inspired hospital in the Peruvian Amazon in 1964 and later as a Peace Corps physician in Brazil.[11]

The story about being motivated by Albert Schweitzer appeared once again in a highly positive piece on Hern authored by John Richardson for the September 2009 issue of *Esquire* magazine. According to this version, Hern told Richardson that after reading "a book about Albert Schweitzer healing the sick in Africa," he announced to his mother, "I'm going to go to Africa before I go to medical school."[12]

During a death-dealing career in which he boasted about having helped more than 130 individuals commit suicide, retired pathologist Dr. Jack Kevorkian characterized himself as a true humanitarian following in the footsteps of famous human rights pioneers. An editorial in the *British Medical Journal* supported this claim by declaring him "a hero" for living "by a personal code of honour" and acting "to end what he perceived as suffering." The journal editors considered his campaign of "heroism" comparable to the actions of prominent historical personages who courageously opposed the errors and practices of their times.[13]

The Humaneness of the Destruction Process

In order to solidify their self-imposed perceptions as decent professionals, doctors involved in mass killing invariably go one step further—not only do they deny the destructive nature of their actions, but they also elevate them to the unimpeachable level of sheer altruism. Thus, when performed by self-proclaimed idealistic physicians, killing is no longer killing, nor is it merely an unpleasant or even emotionally neutral task, but a highly desirable form of charity. Consequently, everything about the killing process is steeped in a language of benevolence, including the killing method itself, the way it is administered, and its impact.

A widespread rhetoric of compassionate destruction functioned as a major factor in doing away with the mentally and physically disabled populations of Nazi Germany. Early in 1940, an experiment conducted on mental patients at the Brandenburg state hospital revealed that carbon monoxide gas did a more effective job of killing than lethal injections. Dr. Karl Brandt later reported to Hitler that gassing would also be "the most humane form of death."[14]

Dr. Albert Trzebinski likewise justified administering lethal injections to children at an abandoned school in Hamburg on April 21, 1945. "I *cannot* reproach myself for giving the children a merciful injection of morphine before their execution," he wrote in preparation for his trial. "On the contrary, this was a humane act."[15]

Similarly, during a 1969 interview conducted in his prison cell, a public health physician condemned to multiple life sentences for active participation in the murders of twenty-six mentally deficient adults in 1945 reiterated a humane rationale for choosing poison over shooting as the preferred method of extermination. "If I had not intervened the whole thing would have been a bloody mess," he explained. "So of course I had to urge a more humane way—poison."[16]

The vocabulary of benevolence in the service of euthanasia was in full swing at the Nuremberg Doctors' Trial. According to the defense put forth to justify medical participation in child euthanasia, "from a medical standpoint, it is a humane motive to shorten the lives of children not fit to live."[17] Leading euthanasia administrator Viktor Brack told the court that one of his main tasks was to ensure that euthanasia was being carried out "in a humane" manner.[18]

Before and after *Roe v. Wade*, pro-abortion rhetoric—like the euthanasia semantics invoked by physicians preceding and during the Nazi era—has been heavily infused with humane rhetoric uttered by doctors professing the most honorable intentions. In 1972, psychiatrist Zigmond Lebenson described legally unencumbered abortion as "the practice of humanitarian medicine at its very best."[19] Several years later, Dr. Michael Burnhill called first-trimester abortion "a consistently high quality humane service" that constitutes "a revolution in human rights."[20]

Although much of the benevolent language is applied mainly to justify first-trimester abortion, it is also intended to rationalize those abortions performed in the later stages of pregnancy. At the 2004 New York partial-birth abortion ban trial, Yale University Medical School obstetrics/gynecology chairman Dr. Charles Lockwood testified that, after twenty weeks from the last menstrual period, the injection of potassium chloride into the hearts of the unborn followed by dilation and evacuation (D&E) dismemberment abortion "was a more humane approach to the fetus" than D&E alone.[21]

The legalization of abortion in 1973 not only endowed the philanthropic images of abortion with immense legitimacy, but also opened up a more favorable climate for promoting magnanimous portrayals of euthanasia and assisted suicide. Geriatrics physician Howard Caplan declared that "euthanasia is a blessing" and called lethal injections "a truly humane" way to end the lives of "elderly demented" patients in "a vegetative state" and "borderline functional people."[22]

Bolstered by the expressions "humane treatment," "compassionate care," and "the most humane kind of treatment," ten physicians from leading medical schools and centers under the auspices of the Society for the Right to Die wrote an article published in the *New England Journal of Medicine* titled "The Physician's Responsibility toward Hopelessly Ill Patients," in which they supported the withholding of artificially administered nutrition and hydration and other forms of life-sustaining treatment from "patients with brain death," "patients in a persistent vegetative state," "severely and irreversibly demented patients," and "elderly patients with permanent mild impairment of competence" (sometimes described as "pleasantly senile").[23]

A Painless Release

The humanitarian rhetoric dominating medicalized killing in Nazi Germany gained much of its credibility from an incessantly projected portrayal of extermination as a "minimally painful" or "pain-free process" designed to "release" people from unbearable suffering. Karl Binding and Alfred Hoche's 1920 influential pro-euthanasia treatise maintained that "death would be a release" for "*those irretrievably lost as a result of illness or injury.*" Furthermore, they recommended establishing a Permissions Board to sanction "the release" and entrust the petitioner with "*bringing about the patient's release from his evil situation in the most expedient way.*"[24]

Comforting accounts of the killing procedures employed at the Hadamar Hospital were presented during the Hadamar Trial in 1945. Hadamar director Alfons Klein asserted, "Those who had death stare into their face were given an injection of mercy to relieve them of their incurable and painful suffering." Chief Hadamar physician Adolf Wahlmann declared, "The method of injection is a completely painless method."[25]

Nurses relied on the same kind of soothing terminology to rationalize their participation in the extermination of more than ten thousand patients in the psychiatric institutions of the Third Reich. "Releasing these patients from their suffering" comprised a central defense in the 1965 trial held in Munich of fourteen nurses charged with crimes against humanity for putting to death patients at the Meseritz-Obrawalde Hospital during the 1940s. Main defendant and nurse Luise Erdmann, accused of participating in the killing of 210 patients, testified, "I realized that incurable patients were to be released by giving them Veronal or another medication.... I was aware of the fact that a person was killed, but I didn't see it as a murder, but as a release."[26]

Similar consoling rhetoric is intended to convey the image of contemporary abortion as a basically painless procedure, not only for the aborting woman but also for the unborn victim. According to Nurse Charlotte K. Schuster's idea of magnanimity, "both the patient with the unwanted pregnancy and the unwanted product of her conception deserve the release of abortion and the dignity of decent care."[27] A similar perception bolstered Dr. Peter Adam's defense of research involving cutting off the heads of living aborted humans ranging in age from twelve to twenty-two weeks' gestation. "The fetus," he asserted, "doesn't have the neurological development for consciousness or pain."[28]

Such responses fly in the face of recent decades of clinical and research experience with prematurely born infants, many of them twenty-two to twenty-three gestational weeks of age, who have exhibited hormonal reactions to painful stimuli and receive anesthesia for required surgery. Dr. Kanwaljest Anand, a world expert on the subject of pain in the fetus and newborn infant, concluded, "It is my opinion that the human fetus possesses the ability to experience pain from 20 weeks of gestation, if not earlier, and the pain perceived by a fetus is possibly more intense than that perceived by term newborns or older children."[29] The last thing abortion doctors wish to convey is anything that undermines their carefully constructed image as compassionate healers carrying out painless, humane services.

The American euthanasia movement is also replete with reassuring statements justifying the destruction of vulnerable human lives after birth. It features identical rhetoric dressed up in idyllic images of killing as a peaceful, painless "release" from unbearable suffering. It is incorporated in both past and present linguistic versions of euthanasia advocacy. Medical doctors can be found in the forefront of its most ardent promoters.

In 1939, the *New York Times* reported on the draft of a legislative
bill proposed by the Euthanasia Society of America (ESA) to legalize
"the painless killing of incurables."[30] ESA treasurer Charles Nixdorff
wrote to the editor pointing out the "misleading and sinister" conno-
tations associated with the *Times*' use of such words as "death" and
"killing." He suggested instead the phrases "merciful release" and "his
release" as more appropriate ways of portraying euthanasia in order to
allay any fears about what the society proposed.[31]

By the end of the twentieth and into the twenty-first century, the
American euthanasia movement had fully embraced the polemics of
killing patients as a painless way of releasing them from suffering.
Geriatric surgeon Dr. John Wrable called active euthanasia "an easy,
painless way of dying."[32] Dr. Jack Kevorkian's career of serial killings
began with implementation of a homemade assisted suicide device
touted as ensuring "a painless way of ending the suffering" of his first
victim, Janet Adkins, a fifty-four-year-old woman in the early stages
of Alzheimer's disease.[33]

During a 2005 *New York Times* interview, Dutch pediatrician Eduard Verhagen furnished an exceedingly tranquil portrayal of what
happens to infants with spina bifida who are injected with a deadly intravenous drip of morphine and midazolan. "The child goes to sleep"
and "it stops breathing," he revealed. "But it's beautiful in a way.... It
is after they die that you see them relaxed for the first time."[34]

Despite the actual prolonged and agonizing ordeal associated with
death by starvation and dehydration, the rhetoric of a gentle, peaceful, painless release from this life was in full swing in the portrayals
of Terri Schiavo's imposed starvation-dehydration death at a Florida
hospice on April 1, 2005, thirteen and a half days after the removal of
her feeding tube. No one resorted to this imagery more persistently
than Michael Schiavo's attorney George Felos. "She died about 9 a.m.,
cradled in her husband's arms," he announced. "Mrs. Schiavo died a
calm, peaceful, gentle death."[35] On NBC's *Today* television program,
Felos even invoked that old standby—"release"—to describe what
happened: "It was a very, very calm release. Mrs. Schiavo died with
dignity."[36]

Deliverance from Suffering

The linguistic charade of "deliverance" concealed the killing of Nazi psychiatric patients under the cover of condolence letters sent to relatives of the deceased containing phony death notices, expressions of sympathy, and reassurances about the merciful nature of the patient's demise. A letter to the wife of a patient killed at the Hadamar Hospital read, "Since your husband suffered from a grave and incurable mental illness, you must regard his death as a form of deliverance."[37] A sampling of letters from other killing centers contained similar wording. One typical letter stated, "One can understand his death as deliverance, as it delivered him from his suffering and spared him from institutionalization for life. May this thought be solace to you."[38]

A Nazi propaganda film, *Mentally Ill*, used the deliverance euphemism to present a highly sanitized version of the destruction process in an actual euthanasia institution. During one scene showing a doctor observing the operation of a gasometer, the film's narrator reveals how "the tortured and distorted inhuman form of the unfortunate suffering from incurable mental illness is smoothed into repose through the peace of a gentle death which finally brings the salvation of deliverance."[39]

In addition, the word "deliverance" constituted part of the defense invoked at the Nuremberg Doctors' Trial. Dr. Karl Brandt testified that "euthanasia ... was right. Death can mean deliverance. Death is life—just as much as birth."[40]

Contemporary pro-abortion semantics likewise incorporates the deliverance designation. In 1995, geneticist Dr. Dru Carlson sent a letter to US Representative Patricia Schroeder containing a highly cosmetized depiction of Dr. James McMahon's partial-birth abortion procedure as a gentle, painless, humane, and dignified form of deliverance:

> Dr. McMahon is caring, and gentle, and ultimately life-affirming in his approach to the abortion procedure.... He uses ultrasound guidance to gently deliver the fetal body.... There is no struggling of the

fetus; quite the contrary, from my personal observation I can tell you that the end is extremely humane and rapid. He provides dignity for all his patients: the mother's, the father's, the extended family's and finally to the fetuses themselves. He does not "mangle" fetuses, rather they are delivered intact.[41]

"Deliverance" has further emerged as a favorite code word in the vocabulary of contemporary euthanasia advocates for eliminating vulnerable postnatal individuals throughout the human life span. In the fall of 1973, *Newsweek* reported that the deliberate withholding of life-sustaining treatment from "defective" infants was a commonplace practice in hospital delivery rooms among doctors who "simply decide on their own that death is the kindest deliverance."[42]

In pro-euthanasia circles, smothering with a plastic bag—commonly known as "the bag technique" or "the exit bag"—is listed among the methods incorporated under the reassuring classification of "self-deliverance." Before the Denver Hemlock Society in 1996, a panel of speakers, including founder Derek Humphry, addressed the topic of "Avoiding Failed Attempts at Self-Deliverance." Humphry provided detailed instructions on the use of the bag technique as a backup method of self-deliverance when other methods fail.[43]

Although organized medicine has yet to place its official stamp of approval on physician-induced mercy killing, the pressure to do so continues to mount. Perhaps it is only a matter of time before the American Medical Association will define lethal substances given by doctors as a humane and painless method of "releasing" or "delivering" from suffering terminal and other vulnerable patients. The 1986 AMA policy statement sanctioning the withholding or withdrawing of nutrition and hydration from patients may well represent a quantum leap in this direction.[44]

The transformation of past and current medicalized killing before and after birth into humane, painless medical procedures carried out by decent, compassionate health care providers has gone a long way toward facilitating and sustaining the perpetrators in their own eyes and in the eyes of the public alike. While much of the charitable rhetoric has been and still is expressed on behalf of the victims in particular or humanity in general, it is the perpetrators, and not the victims, who are often meant to be the major beneficiaries. In his research on the Holocaust, Raul Hilberg concluded, "The 'humaneness' of the destruction process was evolved not for the benefit of the victims but for the welfare of the perpetrators."[45] This insight may well be just as valid today as it was during the darkest days of the Third Reich.

Such an acknowledgment is evident in the testimony of Yale University Law School professor and ardent abortion advocate Priscilla Smith before a congressional hearing of September 9, 2015, on an investigation of Planned Parenthood's profiteering from the sale of aborted body parts. It began when committee chairman Representative Bob Goodlatte read to her the portion of a US Supreme Court decision describing the D&E abortion procedure in which "the fetus dies just as a human adult or child would, bleeds to death as it's torn from limb to limb." He then asked Smith, "Is this a humane way to die?" She replied, "it is a very humane procedure and it protects the woman, her health and safety more than any other procedure."[46]

Some common portrayals of past and current perpetrators as decent health professionals carrying out benevolent medical procedures are recounted in table 14.

TABLE 14. PROFILES IN THE DECENCY OF MEDICAL EXECUTIONERS AND THEIR BENIGN DESTRUCTIVE PRACTICES

Before and during the Third Reich	Contemporary Society
DECENT PERPETRATORS	
"Decent fellows." *(Heinrich Himmler's glorification of Holocaust perpetrators, 1943)*	"A decent man." *(An environmentalist's praise of abortionist Dr. Henry Morgentaler, 2009)*
"He was the most decent colleague I met there [at Auschwitz]." *(Former Nazi doctor's remembrance of Dr. Josef Mengele, 1980)*	"A human being who is upright and honorable and decent." *(National Abortion Federation portrayal of abortionist Dr. Phillip Stubblefield, 1985)*
"We know them to be decent men." *(Federation of German Chemists' praise of I. G. Farben Corporation directors on trial at Nuremberg for complicity in concentration camp atrocities, 1948)*	"Decent, competent practitioners." *(Feminist writer Rickie Solinger's glorification of physicians who performed most of the illegal abortions in pre-Roe America, 2002)*
The Attributes of Benevolent Destructive Procedures	
HUMANENESS	
"This was a humane act." *(Dr. Albert Trzebinski's justification for administering lethal injections to children, 1945)*	"A . . . high quality humane service." *(Dr. Michael Burnhill's portrayal of abortions performed in the first trimester, 1975)*
"A more humane way." *(A public health physician's justification for using poison instead of shooting as the preferred method of killing patients with disabilities in 1945)*	"A more humane approach." *(Dr. Charles Lockwood's justification supporting the injection/dismemberment combination as the preferred method of performing late-term abortions, 2004)*
"The most humane form of death." *(Dr. Karl Brandt's report to Hitler in support of gassing as a method of extermination, early 1940s)*	"The most humane kind of treatment." *(Right-to-Die-Society doctors' portrayal of withholding treatment from cognitively impaired patients, 1984)*
A PAINLESS RELEASE	
"The patient's release." *(Professors Binding and Hoche's treatise on justifying euthanasia for unworthy lives, 1920)*	"The release of abortion." *(Nurse Charlotte Schuster's view on the deserved outcome of unwanted pregnancy, 1972)*
"A completely painless method." *(Dr. Adolf Wahlman's characterization of deadly injections administered at the Hadamar Hospital, 1945)*	"A painless way of ending the suffering." *(Dr. Jack Kevorkian's rationale for the implementation of his homemade assisted-suicide device, 1990)*
"A release." *(Nurse Luise Erdmann's justification for killing patients in the Third Reich, 1965 trial)*	"It was a very, very calm release." *(Attorney George Felos's description of Terri Schiavo's imposed starvation death, 2005)*
DELIVERANCE	
"Death can mean deliverance." *(Dr. Karl Brandt's defense of euthanasia presented at the Nuremberg Doctors' Trial, 1947)*	"Death is the kindest deliverance." *(Doctors' justification for denying medical treatment to infants born with disabilities, 1973)*
"A form of deliverance." *(The condolence letter covering up the killing of a patient at the Hadamar Hospital, 1944)*	"Fetuses . . . are delivered intact." *(Dr. Dru Carlson's description of Dr. James McMahon's partial-birth abortion procedure, 1995)*
"The salvation of deliverance." *(Nazi propaganda film depiction of gassing in euthanasia institutions, 1942)*	"Self-deliverance." *(Hemlock Society's classification for smothering patients with a plastic bag, 1996)*

PART III

CHALLENGING DESTRUCTIVE
MEDICAL RHETORIC

CHAPTER 15

Graphic Exposures of Mass Destruction

The destruction of millions—whether the expendables of the Third Reich or the unwanted unborn today—could not have been implemented successfully unless the benevolent language and images fabricated to conceal their fate had extended beyond the domain of the perpetrators to penetrate the public conscience. The establishment media has often served as an indispensable ally in the creation and maintenance of such large-scale killing enterprises by disseminating the euphemistic rhetoric to a vast audience. The strictly controlled media under the Nazi regime played a major role in stifling any information about what was actually happening to the victims of the Holocaust, and the media of the free world at that time failed to challenge this semantic masquerade. Not until the liberation of the concentration camps did the media of the Allied forces finally provide the long overdue coverage, especially through the widespread circulation of photographs and films documenting the massacre.

Largely because of the abysmal failure of today's media elite to provide unvarnished accounts of what abortion does to the unwanted unborn, an alternative media has arisen to tell the inconvenient truth about the contemporary medical assaults directed against human lives before birth. Its proponents cut through the dominant media blackout on the killing with such compelling graphic evidence as photographs, films, public exhibitions of enlarged photomurals, sketches, and other visual aids. Abortionists and their vociferous defenders try to discredit the veracity of these powerful images, just as Holocaust deniers persist in their attempts to undermine the authenticity of the Nazi concentration camp photographs. A comparison of the pictures of Holocaust victims and those of contemporary aborted victims provides indispensable visual insights into how some of history's most horrendous atrocities are being repeated against today's least visible and most vulnerable individuals.

Camouflaging the Nazi Holocaust

Throughout World War II, the massive annihilation of Jews, Gypsies, Poles, people with physical and mental disabilities, and other vulnerable populations in Nazi concentration camps and euthanasia hospitals continued unabated. Deceptive rhetoric—much of it consisting of sanitized and compassionate medical terminology—prevented the world from comprehending the enormity of the atrocities being perpetrated. An extensive corruption of language and reality helped facilitate a monumental cover-up of unprecedented proportions.

When the Nazis took over control of the government in 1932, Germany, a country of some sixty-six million people, was the world's leading producer of the printed word. The range and diversity of publications surpassed any other county. This prodigious output included seven thousand periodicals in all fields of knowledge and interest, thirty thousand books published annually, and more than forty-seven hundred daily and weekly newspapers. In addition, the local small-town and political party presses flourished. Eighty-one percent of the newspapers were family owned.[1]

The Nazi government succeeded in reducing this diverse and highly autonomous system of mass communications to the level of parrots and puppets of the Ministry of Propaganda. Images of Jews and others as insignificant or subhuman elements dominated the content of news accounts. Nowhere could be found words about or pictures of those destroyed in the concentration camps. Instead, the German people were fed a steady diet of congenial characterizations of individuals being "removed" from ghettoes and "evacuated" to "the East" for "resettlement" in "labor," "concentration," "recreation," or "resettlement" camps.

A German newspaper editor, Fritz Fiala, wrote a highly positive article on life at Auschwitz that appeared in newspapers throughout Europe. In it, the Jews were said to have their own rabbis, doctors, and officials. There was mention made of warm water, a children's kitchen, and an abundant supply of food. Also featured were pictures showing a Jewish coffee house, a group of smiling nurses, and well-nourished young men. The overall image of loving concern conveyed was expressed in a quotation allegedly coming from one of the inmates interviewed: "I wish the whole world knew with how much humanity Germany has treated us here."[2]

As the killing escalated in the eastern territories, so did the positive spin concocted by the German media. A host of articles published in German-language periodicals "painted life on the 'Jewish reservations' to the east in the rosiest colors."[3] Completely absent were any pictorial remnants of gas chambers, crematoria, or mass graves.

Despite the flood of disinformation, the underground press of Poland sent out reports and dispatches with details about death camp operations to neutral and democratic countries.[4] Many members of the Allied press, including Britain and the United States, refused to believe the horrendous revelations. The systematic destruction of millions was considered unthinkable, something preposterous on both the psychological and technical levels. Furthermore, during World War I, some of the Allied nations were guilty of spreading false stories concerning German atrocities involving the torture of children, the dismembering of bodies, and the use of asphyxiating gas against hundreds of thousands of victims. When reports of mass murder and the use of poisonous gas began circulating in the early 1940s, the Western press was therefore inclined to view them as simply "atrocity propaganda," closely akin to the fake atrocity stories of World War I.[5]

Masking the Medical Extermination of the Unborn

Leading up to and ever since the 1973 US Supreme Court *Roe v. Wade* decision, the American mainstream media establishment—similar to the media in the Third Reich—has become a pervasive agent for circulating the euphemistic semantics blanketing the mass killing of another group of vulnerable victims—unwanted human lives before birth. The contemporary media elite encompasses those who control and operate the institutions of popular culture—major publishing houses; reporters, broadcasters, columnists, editors, bureau chiefs, and executives involved in the collection and construction of the news; and writers, artists, producers, and celebrities in the television and moviemaking industries. A group of studies found that 90 percent of these gatekeepers of information who determine what ideas, perceptions, interpretations, attitudes, and values are allowed into the public domain are avid proponents of the most extreme abortion position: abortion on demand under the veneer of pro-choice rhetoric. An even greater proportion of individuals in the world of filmmaking—97 percent—are wedded to this viewpoint.[6]

Like their media counterparts in the Nazi regime who covered up genocide with benign characterizations of people being cared for in hospitals and resettlement camps, today's gatekeepers of public information specialize in transmitting the most benevolent portrayals of abortion. A typical example of the crucial role played by the press in concealing the destructive nature of abortion is a *St. Louis Post-Dispatch* story on the opening of an abortion facility that highlights pictures of roomy and attractive interiors. One scene shows women decorating a room, while another focuses on smiling staff members seated in a beautifully furnished reception area. Also emphasized is a picture of a procedure room supplied with medical equipment.[7] Nowhere could be found even a semblance of graphics depicting the mangled remains of aborted preborn infants. The dominant impression projected is a wholly idyllic one of empathetic health care professionals offering tender loving care in a pleasant and comforting environment.

The main difference between the media coverage in the Third Reich and in contemporary American society is that under the Nazis the media was *forced* to cover up the destruction of unwanted human lives, while today's media elite *voluntarily* camouflages the killing of the unwanted inside the womb.

The Allied Media Exposé of Concentration Camp Barbarities

It wasn't until Allied forces liberated Buchenwald, Dachau, Nordhausen, and other camps in April 1945 that the terrible truth about the massive annihilation of lives deemed "unworthy of life" became starkly evident. The widespread skepticism about the authenticity of the horrors disappeared abruptly as the liberators witnessed scenes which seemed unimaginable. Jack Hallett, one of the Dachau liberators, saw "a stack of bodies that ... looked like cordwood stacked up, and ... closer inspection found people whose eyes were still blinking maybe three or four deep inside the stack."[8]

Special tours of the camps showing the evidence of Nazi barbarism were conducted for arriving troops, dignitaries, members of the press, and German citizens who lived in nearby towns. Correspondent Gene Currivan furnished details about what people from the neighboring city of Weimer encountered on a tour of Buchenwald. One of the most shocking sights was a scientific laboratory containing "shelves of bottles filled with various organs of the human body. In one was half a human head ... [that] once belonged to a prisoner, as did all the other human parts displayed. In another room were a dozen death masks, skulls and shrunken human heads." During another tour, the visitors passed by "a trailer stacked high with withered, starved, naked bodies" before entering "a crematory with the most modern ovens." Each oven had "the remains of at least two bodies that had not yet been sifted into the chamber below."[9]

In addition to the numerous eyewitness accounts of Nazi tyranny uncovered upon liberation of the camps, Allied military photographers took still and motion pictures to document what words alone could not begin to convey. The visual evidence collected at the killing sites focused on the most graphic images of "fields and mounds of corpses, corpses in open graves and on trucks. Often it is impossible to make out which parts of the body belonged to which contorted corpse. The takes regularly change between panning shots to stress the huge number of corpses and medium close-ups that show most of them as mutilated."[10]

When the Soviet Army liberated Auschwitz, the largest of the Nazi death camps, numerous pictures were taken of the victims, including dead inmates lying throughout the camp compound, bodies and body parts crammed together in piles, and mass graves filled with hundreds of prisoners who died or had been killed by the SS. Memorable scenes were filmed of a funeral held on February 28, 1945, "of people found dead in Auschwitz when it was liberated and those who died there after the liberation." One photograph focused on a long, solemn procession of people carrying white wooden coffins on their shoulders. Another segment showed the coffins surrounding the graveside ready to be lowered into an enormous grave.[11]

Newspapers throughout the world published the horrific pictures. The *Newspaper World* acknowledged that the British press set out "deliberately to shock the public by publication, above all, of pictures of atrocities."[12] The *News Chronicle* revealed that it decided to print the pictures "because it is right that the world should see at close quarters indisputable truth of Germany's crimes against the human race."[13] The journal *Editor and Publisher* reported that an essential way of exposing such unbelievable atrocities was to "Print the pictures and lots of them."[14]

The Alternative Media Exposé of Abortion Atrocities

Today, a growing number of individuals, groups, and organizations serve as an alternative media, utilizing a wide range of strategies and sources for challenging the beneficent images of abortion imposed by the media elite and replacing them with graphic portrayals of the aborted victims. Some of these disseminators of truth-telling about the horrors of abortion are former abortionists or people who had previously worked in the abortion industry. Others are members of pro-life organizations engaged in research exposing the abortion industry. They transmit their findings to the public via verbal testimony, photographs, films, television, videos, DVDs, and the Internet.

In 1982, a pro-life organization headquartered in California produced a brochure highlighting the photos taken in the Los Angeles County Coroner's Office of some of the more than sixteen thousand aborted bodies found in a huge metal storage container. Most of them showed the effects of dismemberment and salt-poisoning abortion.[15]

A year later, it was brought to public attention that aborted humans were being burned along with stray cats and dogs in the Wichita, Kansas, city incinerator. This ghastly practice ended after a photographer was called in by the alarmed incinerator attendant to take pictures of the blood-soaked aborted bodies ready for disposal in the incinerator flames.[16]

From the late 1980s until the present, university professor and Citizens for a Pro-Life Society (CPLS) director Dr. Monica Migliorino Miller has worked tirelessly in bringing to public awareness the horrendous plight of the unwanted unborn. Her efforts began in early spring 1987, when she and a group of pro-life activists encountered forty-three broken fetal bodies stuffed inside cardboard boxes and thrown into garbage dumpsters on top of a loading dock behind an abortion clinic in downtown Chicago. "Despite the small size of the remains," Miller recalled, "the tiny hands, feet, ribs, eyes floating free of their sockets, and sometimes even an intact face were plainly visible through the plastic windows of the specimen bags." After several additional experiences involving the removal of aborted human beings from these dumpsters, she recounted how profoundly her mind had become "forever etched with the memory of hundreds of dismembered, broken bodies—with blood, intestines, and torn skin."[17]

Miller and the members of her organization have taken numerous photographs that not only graphically document the violence of abortion but also highlight the humanity of the victims:

> The powerful closeup lenses we learned to use revealed the beauty and poignancy of these fetal humans that no amount of crushing or dismemberment could entirely erase.... The photographs also were important because they proved that these children actually did live, however briefly, and were killed by a horrendous violence that literally trampled their humanity.... Our photos are meant to shake people into the reality of abortion.[18]

For the past several decades, Dr. Miller's efforts at organizing public funerals for thousands of aborted babies is intended to place an additional spotlight on the inherent dignity and worth of the tiny victims. The pictures accompanying these solemn ceremonies further heighten the intrinsic value of those being buried. In July 2009, Citizens for a Pro-Life Society produced a five-minute video, *Requiem for the Disappeared*, highlighting the burials of twenty-three aborted humans retrieved in March and April 2008 from the trash dumpsters located in back of three Michigan abortion facilities.[19]

While highly unusual, some segments of the mega media have even provided revealing pictorial coverage of the abortion burial ceremonies. When the more than sixteen thousand aborted bodies discovered outside Los Angeles in 1982 were finally buried in 1985, some enlarged autopsy photos of them were displayed on placards and banners throughout the graveside service. The October 7, 1985, edition of the *Los Angeles Times* published the picture of a solemn procession of pallbearers carrying the coffins past a poster-size autopsy photo of an aborted male, twenty-seven to twenty-nine weeks' gestation. His most prominent features—an agonized facial expression, a clenched fist, and legs partially torn away from the torso—are all clearly visible in the *Times'* graphic rendition.[20]

A burial service in Tallahassee, Florida, on August 5, 1988, containing 721 aborted bodies inside seven white coffins attracted several local television and newspaper reporters. Dominating the front page of the *Tallahassee-Democrat* was a picture showing several men carefully lowering one of the coffins into a grave, where a man with outstretched arms and hands is reaching up to receive it.[21]

The vivid coverage of the solemn burials of preborn humans killed by abortion is reminiscent of the photos of villagers who participated in providing decent burials for those exterminated in the Nazi concentration camps.

One of the undercover videos released by the Center for Medical Progress documenting the methods used by Planned Parenthood doctors in profiting off the selling of aborted bodies for research features pictures of the body parts ready for harvesting. On April 7, 2015, investigators posing as buyers from a fetal tissue procurement company met with Dr. Savita Ginde, vice president and medical director of Planned Parenthood of the Rocky Mountains in Denver, to discuss a potential partnership involving the sale of harvested fetal organs. Afterward, the investigators were taken into the abortion clinic laboratory, where Dr. Ginde and her medical assistants displayed the "quality" of the fetal body parts available. The extremely casual, clinical way the Planned Parenthood employees talked about sorting through the delicate, clearly recognizable legs, hearts, heads, and other organs is intended to give the impression they were involved in the strictly technical task of identifying and assessing leftover commodities instead of remaining completely oblivious to the stark evidence of destroyed human lives staring them in the face:

> MEDICAL ASSISTANT: I just want to see one leg, there's a foot....
> BUYER: Is that the heart?
> MEDICAL ASSISTANT: I think so, here's the heart....
> DR. GINDE: Do people do stuff with eyeballs?
> BUYER: Oh yeah. Although eyeballs, they generally want more developed than this.... The cal[varium, head], there was, first there was a brain in here.
> DR. GINDE: [It got] blasted out. Here's some organs for you ... a stomach, kidney, heart, adrenal. I don't know what else is in there.
> MEDICAL ASSISTANT: I don't see the legs.[22]

Throughout the duration of these observations, the video focuses on forceps poking around the aborted body parts located in glass plates plus enlarged graphic portrayals of a partially dismembered "11.6 fetus" and a "12 week fetus," both "prepared for procurement."

Public Exhibitions of Enlarged Nazi Atrocity Photographs

Besides the extensive publication of Nazi concentration camp pictures in newspapers, newsreels, and films, another prominent method of circulation was through the placement of enlarged photos on billboards. The *New York Times* reported on a plan developed by the information services of Britain and the United States in cooperation with the Allied Supreme Headquarters that consisted of a photographic layout of scenes at both Buchenwald and Belsen "reproduced on large boards for display in every community in conquered Germany at points where inhabitants will be compelled to view them as they go to and from their homes."[23]

London news organizations designed special exhibitions of the enlarged pictures. On April 26, 1945, the *World's Press News* revealed that crowds three and four persons deep thronged the windows of the London News Agency in Fleet Street throughout the day to observe a public display of "enlarged pictures dealing with Buchenwald and other horror camps."[24] Under the title "Seeing Is Believing," the *Daily Express* on May 1, 1945, arranged at its reading rooms in London an exhibit of photographs from Belsen, Buchenwald, and Norhausen. The reaction of visitors who viewed the display on the first day was described as that of "shocked silence." Many of them no longer had any reservations about the authenticity of the horrifying pictorial evidence: "I believe it's true. I can see with my own eyes. Pictures don't lie."[25]

American newspapers were also instrumental in constructing for public display billboard-size photos of the Nazi concentration camp atrocities. On May 29, 1945, the *St. Louis Post-Dispatch* mounted, for public exhibition in an adjoining annex, twenty-five enlargements of Army Signal Corps, Associated Press, and official British photographs of these barbarities. The pictorial display—titled "Lest We Forget"— attracted "a continuous stream of spectators," with almost five thousand persons having viewed the exhibition on the first day alone. An elderly man in attendance who had three sons in the armed services declared, "Atrocities are horrible, but it's all true. We must let the people know the truth about what happened."[26]

The exhibit of enlarged concentration camp pictures moved to Washington, DC, where it opened on June 30, 1945, at the Library of Congress under the co-sponsorship of the *St. Louis Post-Dispatch* and the *Washington Evening Star*. The *Post-Dispatch* reported that the first weekend of showing marked a total attendance of 10,814, with 5,229 persons appearing on Washington's hottest day of the year notwithstanding.[27] According to the *Washington Sunday Star*, a picture of visitors viewing a photomural depicting the bodies of concentration camp victims on the back of a large truck had a profound effect:

Solemn hundreds filed through the halls of the library, their attention arrested by grisly photographic proof of German savagery. Life-size pictures of starved and butchered men spoke more eloquently than words what went on inside of Nazi concentration camps. Sentiment from all lips was the same: These pictures, and the Army Signal Corps movies of the slaughter, should be shown to all Americans as a deterrent to future wars.[28]

Another especially arresting photo showed people looking at Library of Congress photomurals that contained a huge number of Nazi atrocity corpses stretched out and stacked up for disposal.

Public Exhibitions of Enlarged Abortion Atrocity Photographs

Besides documenting the reality of abortion through such graphic means as films, videos, DVDs, and the Internet, a number of pro-life activist organizations have constructed huge pictures of aborted fetal bodies for display in the public square. The Chicago-based Pro-Life Action League raises awareness about the injustice of abortion through public protests such as the annual Face the Truth Tours, during which large graphic abortion signs are displayed on busy streets "showing what abortion does to the unborn child."[29] Among the giant photos exhibited are the remains of a victim aborted at ten to twelve weeks, with a tiny but perfectly formed hand and foot still intact; the dismembered body of a little boy named Malachi, aborted at twenty-one weeks; and the severed head of a little girl with her jaw torn away during a third trimester abortion. On June 19, 2009, seventy Action League members held abortion signs depicting the broken body of "Baby Malachi" with the caption "Abortion is not health care."[30] This message was delivered in downtown Chicago across from the Hyatt Regency Hotel, where the yearly convention of the American Medical Association was being held.

Attorney and former Pennsylvania state legislator Gregg Cunningham has led the way in employing poster-size atrocity pictures as a means of linking abortion with various types of historical brutalities. As executive director of the Center for Bio-Ethical Reform (CBR), he created the Genocide Awareness Project (GAP), a huge mobile twenty-four-panel outdoor display featuring six-foot-by-thirteen-foot photomurals showing abortion adjacent to Holocaust photos and photos of such widely recognized forms of genocide as the slavery of black people in the antebellum American South and the annihilation of Native Americans on the frontier.[31] Ever since its inception in 1998, the traveling GAP has been seen by millions of students on hundreds of college campuses.

Many students reported being surprised, shocked, and stunned by the horrendous scenes depicted, responses closely resembling those who viewed the public displays of Nazi concentration camp photos in 1945. An article in the *Carolina Review* provided a graphic account of the GAP display at the University of North Carolina, Chapel Hill: "Tiny human arms, complete with miniature human fingers but severed at the shoulder, appeared like they had been chopped in blenders. Other pictures revealed tiny bodies covered in blood in the palm of a gloved hand."[32] A common reaction came from a student who stated, "I never knew that they chopped up babies like that."[33]

Refuting the Attempts to Discredit the Visual Evidence of Nazi Atrocities

Despite the unique power of the Nazi atrocity pictures to definitively document the sheer depravity and horrifying aftermath of exterminating human lives on an assembly-line basis, some individuals continue to deny that these atrocities ever happened. This extreme dismissal of the most irrefutable visual evidence has evolved into an organized movement of Holocaust deniers who perpetuate the outlandish canard that the murder of six million European Jews never occurred and the Holocaust was a hoax fabricated by Jews to gain preferential treatment and financial reparations. Aside from Holocaust deniers, others have vilified the atrocity photos by declaring them unfit for public viewing owing to their repulsive features. These denials and denunciations have been repudiated vigorously by those who have utilized the alarming but nonetheless indispensable factual images as a means of conveying what actually happened to the victims of Nazi tyranny.

The Institute of Historical Review was established to place a respectable academic and intellectual face on the Holocaust denial propaganda. One of its first projects was a 1979 Revisionist Convention that took place on the Northrup College campus in Los Angeles. Some of the world's most prominent Holocaust deniers presented papers "arguing that there had been no Holocaust and no gas chambers; that all the camp photographs had been faked; that the Jews (alas) were still alive."[34]

Conferences on Holocaust denial continue to persist into the twenty-first century. A prime example is a two-day gathering of Holocaust deniers in Tehran during the second week of December 2006. While the purpose of the conference was billed as an opportunity to "debate" the Holocaust, the speakers labeled the Holocaust a concoction fabricated to justify the occupation of Palestine and creation of the state of Israel. Conference exhibiters characterized "as a myth" one poster "with three photographs [that] showed dead bodies and described accounts of their gassing." Replacement captions described the pictures of these corpses as depicting "victims of a typhus epidemic in Europe, not of the Nazi death machine."[35]

Inveterate Holocaust denier Udo Walendy has written extensively on how "the German nation is maligned through the use of forged atrocity photographs." He attributed the horrific camp conditions depicted in these pictures to external circumstances instead of any Nazi-imposed practices and accused the Allies of deliberately mislabeling the photos of heaps of dead bodies in the Nordhausen camp as if they were "slave laborers" whose deaths were caused by "starvation, overwork and beatings," when in reality "these dead concentration camp inmates were victims of an Allied air raid." Walendy even tried to discredit two of the most authenticated icons of atrocity uncovered by the Allied liberation forces at Buchenwald—a preserved shrunken human head and flayed human skin covered with tattoos. He dismissed them as frauds, claiming that the head was of South American origin and came from a German anthropological museum, while the tattooed skin was "either of imitation leather or animal hide fabric or pasteboard."[36]

The accusations of photo fraud made by Holocaust deniers against the pictures of the concentration camp abominations have been definitively refuted. Those who took the pictures were not only eyewitnesses to the atrocities, but many of them were also highly trained professional photographers. The Allied forces went to great lengths to prove that the pictures and films were not fabricated but told the undeniable truth about an unprecedented atrocity of gigantic proportions. At General Dwight Eisenhower's invitation, delegations from the US Congress and the American press visited the camps "to see for themselves the evidence of Nazi atrocities" and "to prevent ... a recurrence of the notion popular after the last war that atrocities were items of propagandistic manufacture." Each delegation "scrupulously excluded rumor and hearsay" from its inspection and "confined its evidence to what it saw and personal testimony obtained from prisoners."[37]

Refuting the Attempts to Discredit the Visual Evidence of Abortion Atrocities

Just as Holocaust deniers attack the authenticity of photos depicting the Nazi death camp victims, contemporary physician abortionists and their defenders assault the veracity of pictures showing the bodies of aborted humans. Those in the forefront of the movement to discredit the visual evidence of abortion atrocities have even adopted some of the Holocaust deniers' debunking techniques, such as accusing those who display the aborted baby pictures of mislabeling the victims, doctoring the photos, and staging the gruesomeness of the scenes highlighted.

The widespread distribution of medical illustrations depicting each phase of the brain-sucking destruction procedure based on partial-birth specialist Dr. Martin Haskell's instructional paper presented before the National Abortion Federation in 1992 set off an alarm, resulting in a campaign of vilification aimed at undermining their authenticity. During one of the debates over the Partial-Birth

Abortion Ban Act in the US House of Representatives, the National Abortion Federation sent a letter to the House members that castigated the drawings as "graphic, misleading ... intentionally inflammatory and provocative."[38] Representative Zoe Lofgren reduced the illustrations to the trivial level of "cartoon charts," while Representative Nita Lowey called them "graphic pictures and sensationalized language and distortions."[39]

Despite these and other assaults on the drawings, their veracity was fully validated by impeccable sources. Dr. Watson Bowes, professor of maternal and fetal medicine at the University of North Carolina and coeditor of *Obstetrical and Gynecological Survey*, wrote in a letter to Congressman Charles Canady, "Having read Dr. Haskell's paper, I can assure you that these drawings accurately represent the procedure therein."[40] Even partial-birth abortionist Dr. Martin Haskell admitted to *American Medical News* staff writer Diane Gianelli that the drawings were accurate "from a technical standpoint."[41]

Numerous charges of photo fakery have also been directed against the Center for Bio-Ethical Reform's Genocide Awareness Project traveling photomural exhibit comparing abortion to historical forms of genocide. In response to the GAP display of abortion images on the Bowling Green State University campus, a *Bowling Green News* op-ed titled "Pro-Life Group Using Scare Tactics, Lies" accused CBR of mislabeling "older fetuses" by "mark[ing] them as younger." This allegation relied entirely on the statement of an abortion clinic worker who maintained, "The signs that say nine to 10 weeks are false" since "at that age, a fetus is still microscopic."[42] Another frequently promulgated accusation put forth is that the CBR photos depict stillborn or miscarried fetuses and not aborted babies.

CBR director Gregg Cunningham revealed how readily these allegations of photo fraud can be rebutted. Regarding the oft-repeated contention that the pictures of aborted fetuses displayed are "younger than they are advertised as being," he indicated, "Every one of our photos includes some common object which acts as a size reference. When CBR conducts GAP, we carry medical textbooks which can be used by skeptics to confirm the accuracy of the age captions on our aborted baby pictures." In addition, Cunningham relies on affidavits from photographers, technical experts, and former abortionists such as Dr. Anthony P. Levatino to validate the authenticity of the photographs. With respect to the claim that the photos of the aborted bodies—many of them partially mutilated and burned—are simply the result of miscarriages, he pointed out that "neither stillbirth nor miscarriage will tear off a baby's arms and legs, or rip off its head and face or scald its skin with chemical burns. The bodies of the babies in our pictures all display the unmistakable injuries of abortion."[43]

Responding to the Offensive Nature of Nazi and Abortion Atrocity Photos

When the pictures and films of Nazi barbarities were released to the public, some people objected, not necessarily because they disputed the veracity of the images projected. Their displeasure was based mainly on the contention that the scenes depicted were considered too offensive and nauseating for public exposure. During the Holocaust, Nazi officials had already established a similar justification for issuing communiqués against taking and showing pictures of those exterminated. According to these directives, "Photographs ... of such abominable excesses" were considered "offensive to the innermost German sense of honor" and "were looked upon as undermining the decency and discipline in the armed forces."[44]

British newspapers nevertheless overrode these objections, stressing the necessity of showing even the most despicable visual evidence of unimaginable atrocities. The *Daily Mirror* dubbed the assertion that "pictures [of camp atrocities] ought not to be published because they are nauseating to children" a false argument: "One reason for publishing [them] is to protect the children. It is better that they should be 'nauseated' now than mutilated later on."[45]

The American media, for the most part, followed the British media dictum that "this is no time to be squeamish," since an essential way to prevent humanity from suffering such tortures again is "to tell the story now so graphically that the world can never forget it."[46]

Today's practitioners and proponents of abortion extensively resort to the castigation of aborted baby pictures as offensive, disgusting, and an unwarranted violation of etiquette. Senator Barbara Boxer complained that such pictures "should never be shown in front of the pages who sit here."[47] Congresswoman Patricia Schroeder led an unsuccessful attempt to ban the illustrations from being shown in the US House of Representatives because, she claimed, they constituted "a breach of decorum."[48]

Some students and others likewise resort to the epithets "offensive" and "disgusting" as a means of repudiating the giant Genocide Awareness Project murals shown on college campuses depicting "actual photos of decapitated, dismembered, disemboweled bodies of aborted babies to publicly unmask the deception of 'choice.'" In 2005, a Western Carolina University student said of the display, "It's disgusting, disturbing, I can't even look at it."[49] When the GAP exhibit appeared on the University of Cincinnati campus during the fall of 2007, the student paper referred to its use of "primal and unnecessarily emotionally charged images" as "blatantly offensive to much of the populace."[50]

Center for Bio-Ethical Reform staff members have repeatedly exposed the hypocrisy of individuals who complain about the repulsive and disgusting abortion pictures but fail to be repulsed or disgusted by the act of abortion itself. When a University of Memphis professor characterized the placement of pictures of aborted humans next to a picture of Holocaust victims as "incredibly offensive" and a form of "hate speech," CBR director Cunningham responded, "If showing these babies is 'hate,' what is killing them?"[51]

CBR underscores, in particular, how the use of these admittedly revolting and shocking pictures continues a legacy of graphic truth-telling pioneered by human rights movements of the past. Cunningham asserted, "Ugly photos are the agency through which social reformers have outlawed every great evil from child labor to racial injustice." Stephanie Gray, director of Canadian CBR, emphasized that one of the things successful social reform movements throughout history "all had in common was that they dramatized an injustice with shocking imagery."[52]

Those who try to censor the graphic images of abortion because they are deemed offensive, disgusting, and an unwarranted violation of etiquette are resorting to a language of denigration that bears a close resemblance to the designations "offensive to the innermost German sense of honor" and "abominable excesses" employed in the Third Reich as a basis for banning the production and distribution of photos taken of the executed victims. The real reason for suppressing the pictures of aborted fetal humans has nothing to do with impropriety or poor taste. In today's visually oriented world, the public is bombarded with no-holds-barred, gruesome images of accidents, murders, massacres, and disasters of every stripe. Newspapers, magazines, television, films, and the Internet exhibit no qualms whatsoever about depicting the most graphic forms of violence imaginable.

Why, then, hold back on showing the violence of abortion? The answer is related to the awesome power of pictures to expose the deceptive rhetoric constructed to cover up what actually happens to unwanted unborn children. What is really offensive and disgusting is not what the pictures and films depicting abortion so explicitly disclose, but what has been allowed to happen to the victims portrayed in them. Equally offensive are the heavy-handed tactics used to repress the unadorned visual documentation clearly at odds with the relentless flow of benign descriptions of abortion transmitted to the public by the media elite.

Today's gatekeepers of what the public is allowed to view are not so much concerned about protecting their consumers' sensitivities as they are with propagating their own set of myths and distortions. Just as the Nazi press corps knew fully well how detrimental the pictures of death camp atrocities were to the cause of National Socialism, so too are members of the contemporary mainstream media elite acutely aware of how damaging the pictures of abortion barbarities are to the pro-abortion cause. They realize that such irrefutable evidence of mass killing not only threatens the respectability and legitimacy of the abortion industry, but also calls into question the very credibility of a media establishment so fully implicated in helping to perpetuate the destruction of millions of unwanted human lives before birth.

History Repeats: A Pictorial Comparison
of Abortion and Holocaust Victims

Aside from the smaller size of the aborted bodies, the pictures of contemporary abortion victims and Holocaust victims reveal a number of commonalities. The most significant similarity involves the alarming reality that all of the individuals depicted have been deliberately and systematically destroyed—today, overwhelmingly by physicians in the practice of medicine, and in the Third Reich, many were killed by medical professionals who administered the Nazi euthanasia program and death selections at Auschwitz. The utter brutality of assembly-line extermination is strikingly apparent in the photos of entangled and stacked corpses, mangled and dismembered bodies, clenched fists, and agonized facial expressions. As one views the comparative gallery of horrific images, the charade of abstract and euphemistic terminology devised to mask the execution of millions—present and past—becomes starkly evident to all but the most desensitized viewer.

Many of the photographs of aborted fetal bodies have come from pro-life sources or are the result of rare newspaper coverage. Most of the photographs of Nazi atrocities were compiled by Allied photographers upon liberation of the concentration camps.

CHAPTER 16

The Urgency of a Full-Scale Physicians' Crusade against Killing before and after Birth

Nothing less than a Herculean effort on the part of physicians is long overdue in order to offset two powerful destructive forces. The first— and most deeply embedded—is the widespread acceptance of abortion as a legitimate medical procedure. The other involves the ever growing attempts to transform physician-assisted suicide and euthanasia into justifiable types of medical treatment. In short, what is required is a full-fledged physicians' crusade against all forms of killing. Fortunately, a model for such a course of action is already part of the historical record. During the latter half of the nineteenth century, the American Medical Association mounted a triumphant campaign against the destruction of unborn human lives. This crusade against killing inside the womb contains indispensable insights and strategies for waging a successful campaign in opposition to the prevailing contemporary AMA policy highly supportive of abortion as a positive, valid medical procedure.

The Original Physicians' Crusade against Killing the Unborn

The uncompromising commitment of American medicine on behalf of the most defenseless human lives was first formally expressed in the American Medical Association's policy statement on abortion of 1859. After two years of studying the problem of criminal abortions, an AMA committee unequivocally condemned the practice of induced abortion at all stages of pregnancy, with the sole exception being when the mother's or unborn child's life was at stake. At several points in the report, the committee used the most blunt language in castigating abortion, referring to it as the "death of thousands," "the slaughter of countless children now steadily perpetrated in our midst," "such unnecessary and unjustifiable destruction of human life," and "such unwarrantable destruction of human life."[1]

The AMA made it abundantly clear that it opposed abortion, not because it was a hazardous surgical procedure for the pregnant woman, but because it was a fatal one for the unborn child. The committee's statement on the reason for its strong opposition to abortion declared, "No simple offence against public morality and decency, no mere misdemeanor, no attempt upon the life of the mother, but the wanton and murderous destruction of her child."[2]

Furthermore, the American Medical Association chose to speak out against abortion in every phase of development because of the commonly held misconceptions about the nature of prenatal life and what abortion does to that life: "a wide-spread popular ignorance of the true character of the crime—a belief, even among mothers themselves, that the foetus is not alive till after the period of quickening." The AMA report labeled this contention an error "based, and only based, upon mistaken and exploded medical dogmas."[3]

The whole issue of when human life begins and whether life in the womb is really human even early in gestation had been scientifically answered by the mid-1850s.[4] American medicine therefore felt obligated to set the record straight, especially since many of the unfounded assumptions and misconceptions about human life before birth had been perpetuated by physicians: "If, as is also true, these great, fundamental, and fatal flaws of the law are owing to doctrinal errors of the profession in a former age, it devolves upon us, by every bond we hold sacred, by our reverence for the fathers in medicine, by our love for our race, and by our responsibility as accountable beings, to see these errors removed and their grievous results abated."[5]

The AMA committee on abortion was not merely content to challenge a well-entrenched and unscientific theory about the onset of viable human life not occurring until after quickening, but also intended to expose abortion for what it really is—"the slaughter of countless children." Its resolutions, passed unanimously, called upon physicians as an important part of their professional responsibility to condemn abortion and persuade state legislatures to pass laws strongly protective of human life even at its most vulnerable stages:

> *Resolved*, That while physicians have long been united in condemning the act of producing abortion at every period of gestation, except as necessary for preserving the life of either mother or child, it has become the duty of this Association, in view of the prevalence and increasing frequency of the crime, publicly to enter an earnest and solemn protest against such unwarrantable destruction of human life.
>
> *Resolved*, That in pursuance of the grand and noble calling we profess, the saving of human lives, and of the sacred responsibilities thereby devolving upon us, the Association present this subject to the attention of the several legislative assemblies of the Union....
>
> *Resolved*, That the Association request the zealous cooperation of the various State Medical Societies in pressing this subject upon the legislatures of their respective States.[6]

In 1871, the AMA again felt compelled to issue another public pronouncement against abortion. The association continued to refute the false contention "that life does not exist in the foetus because no motion is felt" with a citation from *Archbold's Criminal Practice and Pleadings*:

> It was generally supposed that the foetus becomes animated at the period of quickening; but this idea is exploded. Physiology considers the foetus as much a living being immediately after conception as at any other time before delivery, and its future progress but as the development and increase of those constituent principles which it then received. It considers quickening as a mere adventitious event, and looks upon life as entirely consistent with the most profound foetal repose and consequent inaction. Long before quickening takes place, motion, the pulsation of the heart, and other signs of vitality, have been distinctly perceived, and, according to approved authority, the foetus enjoys life long before the sensation of quickening is felt by the mother. Indeed, no other doctrine appears to be consonant with

reason or physiology but that which admits the embryo to possess vitality from the very moment of conception.[7]

The AMA report contains numerous non-euphemistic accounts of abortion, and it is again apparent that the victims highlighted are not pregnant women but their preborn offspring. The targets of abortion are described as "those innocent and helpless victims" whose "resting-place is rudely invaded and that which would grow and ripen into mankind is cut off from existence by the hand of an educated assassin," standing at the bedside "ready to proceed to the work of destruction." Abortionists are portrayed as "presenting their poisoned cups and using their stilettoes to spill the blood of human victims, to take the lives of innocent, of unborn infants."[8] The association was manifestly emphatic in its steadfast stance against the killing of the unborn at all stages of development:

> "Thou shalt not kill." This commandment is given to all, and applied to all without exception.... and it matters not at what stage of development his victim may have arrived—it matters not how small or how apparently insignificant it may be—it is a murder, a foul unprovoked murder; and its blood, like the blood of Abel, will cry from earth to Heaven for vengeance.[9]

The rest of the report is replete with the most graphic language denouncing the horrendous nature of abortion: "This evil," "the horrid crime of foeticide," "this wholesale destruction of unborn infants," "the greatest curse which could befall the human family," "this crime in all its hideous deformity."[10]

A considerable portion of the AMA's severest criticism was directed not against abortionists in general, but *physician abortionists* in particular:

> There we shall discover an enemy in the camp; there we shall witness as hideous a view of moral deformity as the evil spirit could present. There we shall find ... men who cling to a noble profession only to dishonor it; men who seek not to save, but to destroy; men known not only to the profession, but to the public, as abortionists.... Yes, it is false brethren we have most to fear; men who are false to their profession, false to principle, false to honor....
>
> These modern Herods, like their prototype, have a summary

mode of dealing with their victims. They perform the triple office of Legislative, Judiciary, and Executive, and, to crown the tragedy, they become the executioners....

Yet these monsters of iniquity are permitted to stalk abroad in open day, carrying worse than contagion with them, poisoning wherever they are permitted to touch, invading the very sources of life, and fattening on the blood of their victims. And yet the profession of medicine remains inactive—that profession which is styled an honorable one; that profession so far-famed for its charity and benevolence, whose mission on earth is to do as much good and as little evil as possible to the human family—that profession, in the face of these evils, tolerates in its midst these men, who, with corrupt hearts and blood-stained hands, destroy what they cannot reinstate, corrupt souls ... and yet all is done under the aegis, under the cloak, of that profession.[11]

Also exceedingly noteworthy is the harsh manner in which the association recommended dealing with physician abortionists:

Every practicing physician in the land (as well as every good man) has a certain amount of interest at stake in this matter.... The members of the profession should form themselves into a special police to watch, and to detect, and bring to justice these characters. They should shrink with horror from all intercourse with them, professionally or otherwise. These men should be marked as Cain was marked; they should be made the outcasts of society.

It is time that the seal of reprobation were placed on these characters by all honest men; it is time that respectable men should cease to consult with them, should cease to speak to them, should cease to notice them except with contempt.[12]

At the end of this remarkably vivid and strongly worded document, the AMA enacted six forceful resolutions directed toward the attention of the medical, legal, educational, and religious professions:

Resolved, That we repudiate and denounce the conduct of abortionists, and that we will hold no intercourse with them either professionally or otherwise, and that we will, whenever an opportunity presents, guard and protect the public against the machinations of these characters by pointing out the physical and moral ruin which follows in their wake.

Resolved, That in the opinion of this Convention, it will be unlawful and unprofessional for any physician to induce abortion or premature labor, without the concurrent opinion of at least one respectable consulting physician, and then always with a view to the safety of the child—if that be possible.

Resolved, That we respectfully and earnestly suggest to private teachers and professors in public institutions the propriety of adopting, according to their judgment, the means best suited for preserving their pupils, and those who may hereafter come under their care, from the degrading crime of abortion.

Resolved, That we respectfully call the attention of the clergy of all denominations to the perverted views of morality entertained by a large class of females—aye, and men also—on this important question, and the ruin which has resulted and continues to result daily to the human family from such views.

Resolved, That we respectfully solicit the different medical societies, both State and local, to send delegates to the clergymen in their respective districts to request their aid in so important an undertaking.

Resolved, That it becomes the duty of every physician in the United States, of fair standing in his profession, to resort to every honorable and legal means in his power to crush out from among us this pest of society.[13]

The resolution pertaining to the enlistment of clergy in the AMA's movement against abortion is particularly significant insofar as it reveals how physicians, not the clergy, led the moral crusade against prenatal killing. Doctors were the ones responsible for getting the clergy involved, not the other way around. The nature and thrust of medical leadership are understandable when one considers the fact that by the 1850s doctors had acquired indisputable scientific evidence that the inhabitant in the womb was human from conception onward and abortion constituted nothing less than the destruction of a bona fide human being. The AMA thus felt compelled to communicate this finding to the clergy so that the Judeo-Christian prohibition against killing could be extended to a class of individuals that up to that time had not been fully recognized as genuine members of the human race. Members of the clergy were enlisted to join physicians in a highly influential campaign directed toward updating the law to reflect the most recent scientific knowledge about human life before birth and the concomitant need for the legal protection of individuals at all phases of prenatal development.

Of all the words ever written on the subject of abortion, none have denounced the destruction of unborn humans more passionately and absolutely than the AMA anti-abortion policy statements of 1859 and 1871. Not even the most avid contemporary right-to-life proponents have surpassed the severity with which these denunciations were expressed. The rationale for the use of such forthright language is set forth in the statement of 1871:

> If in the foregoing report our language has appeared to some strong and severe, or even intemperate, let the gentlemen pause for a moment and reflect on the importance and gravity of our subject, and believe that to do justice to the undertaking, free from all improper feeling or selfish considerations, was the end and aim of our efforts. We had to deal with human life. In a matter of less importance we could entertain no compromise. An honest judge on the bench would call things by their proper names. We could do no less.[14]

By taking an uncompromising stand in defense of the most defenseless human lives in the strongest possible terms, the AMA enhanced the physician's role as a healer par excellence. This served notice that educated assassins of the unborn would no longer be tolerated as part of legitimate American medical practice. Practically speaking, the resolutions of 1859 and 1871 had a profound impact. Historian James Mohr dubbed the period 1859-80 a veritable "physicians' crusade against abortion" and concluded that this crusade was so successful that it produced "the most important burst of anti-abortion legislation in the nation's history. At least forty anti-abortion statutes of various kinds were placed upon state and territorial lawbooks during that period." Moreover, he found, "The anti-abortion policies sustained in the United States through the first two-thirds of the twentieth century had their formal legislative origins, for the most part, in the wave of tough laws passed in the wake of the doctors' crusade and the public response their campaign evoked."[15]

AMA Repudiation of the Physicians' Crusade
against Prenatal Killing

The highly influential AMA-led crusade in opposition to killing the unborn was seriously undermined, largely owing to the extensive medical agitation in support of the legalization of abortion for an expanding list of indications from the 1940s through the late 1960s. On June 21, 1967, at the annual meeting of the American Medical Association, the House of Delegates, the association's 242-member policy-making body, adopted a statement in support of abortion according to the following stipulations:

1. There is documented medical evidence that continuance of the pregnancy may threaten the health or life of the mother, or
2. There is documented medical evidence that the infant may be born with incapacitating physical deformity or mental deficiency, or
3. There is documented medical evidence that continuance of a pregnancy, resulting from legally established statutory or forcible rape or incest may constitute a threat to the mental or physical health of the patient;
4. Two other physicians chosen because of their recognized professional competency have examined the patient and have concurred in writing; and
5. The procedure is performed in a hospital accredited by the Joint Commission on Accreditation of Hospitals.[16]

Thus the American Medical Association, far and away the nation's largest medical body (216,000 members in 1967), went on record in favor of medicalized killing, so long as the method of destruction was safely carried out in a scientific manner by credentialed executioners in the antiseptic setting of an accredited hospital.

Furthermore, the 1967 AMA statement erroneously concluded that doctors had supported the passage of strong laws against abortion during the second half of the nineteenth century because "[the] majority of these laws were enacted about 100 years ago when the technique of evacuating the uterus entailed an appreciable [maternal] morbidity and mortality."[17] The AMA in 1967 therefore came out in favor of extensive abortion law liberalization because it maintained that, owing to advances in medicine, abortion had been transformed into a safe procedure when performed by a licensed physician.

This position, however, stands in stark contradiction to the explicit rationale the AMA gave in 1859 for its support of stringent abortion laws—the laws were enacted not because abortions were hazardous procedures that threatened the life of the mother, but because they constituted "the wanton and murderous destruction of her child."[18] The 1871 AMA espousal of anti-abortion legislation employed an identical justification—physician abortionists were castigated as "monsters of iniquity" and "modern Herods" not for endangering pregnant women, but for perpetrating the "wholesale destruction of unborn infants."[19]

In sharp contrast to their statements of 1859 and 1871, the 1967 AMA statement characterized as "conscientious physicians" those "who believe that ... the interruption of an unwanted pregnancy, no matter what the circumstances, should be solely an individual matter between the patient and her doctor." Moreover, the AMA stressed that its abortion policy was "designed to afford ethical physicians the right to exercise their sound medical judgment concerning therapeutic abortion just as they do in reaching any other medical decision."[20]

Other prominent organizations of health professionals helped pave the way for a climate increasingly receptive to unrestricted abortion. In 1968, the American College of Obstetricians and Gynecologists came out in favor of "social and economic factors in determining whether an abortion should be performed."[21] Also in 1968, the American Public Health Association passed a resolution urging "that access to abortion be accepted as an important means of securing the right to spacing and choosing the number of children wanted."[22]

On June 25, 1970, for the first time in the 123-year history of the American Medical Association, the House of Delegates, by a vote of 103 to 73, enacted resolutions that de facto transformed the decision to kill unborn humans into a private matter between the physician and the pregnant woman. The key resolution stated:

> *Resolved,* That abortion is a medical procedure and should be performed only by a duly licensed physician and surgeon in an ac-

credited hospital acting only after consultation with two other physicians chosen because of their professional competency and in con-
formance with standards of good medical practice and the Medical
Practice Act of his state.[23]

The Restoration of a Physicians' Crusade against
All Forms of Killing

The passion, outrage, and vigorous action exhibited by AMA physicians during the second half of the nineteenth century in their crusade against the killing of unborn humans is in dire need of a vast
reinvigoration today. Chapter 17 reveals how current AMA policies
against medical involvement in killing prisoners on death row and
in opposition to physician-assisted suicide and euthanasia also orig-
inated from campaigns mounted by physicians at the highest rungs
of mainstream medicine. The long-standing anti-capital punishment
policy is likely to remain intact. The AMA stance against assisted suicide and euthanasia, however, is already under siege by some physicians and state medical associations. Although California, Colorado,
Montana, Oregon, Washington, and Vermont are the only states in
which physician-assisted suicide is legal, other states are being subjected to an emboldened movement aimed at overturning laws against
physician-assisted suicide and eventually euthanasia, under the guises
of patient autonomy and compassion.

Whether a contemporary full-scale physicians' crusade against
killing the vulnerable—before as well as after birth—ever gets off
the ground will greatly depend on doctors first becoming conversant
with the history of the AMA's anti-abortion policies of 1859 and 1871,
which denounced the killing of the unborn as immoral, unethical,
and despicable. Next, doctors will need to confront how profoundly
the AMA pro-abortion policies of 1967 and 1970 reversed the previous
statements. There is a giant gap indeed between the definition of abortion as an "unwarrantable destruction of human life" stance of 1859
and the abortion as a "medical procedure" position of 1970. The early
statements placed organized medicine steadfastly behind the doctor
as a healer and preserver of human life, while the recent positions set

the doctor up as a paid executioner of unwanted human lives. Chapter 17 focuses on the significance of the do-no-harm and healing imperatives embodied in the Hippocratic Oath as a central philosophical basis for waging another doctors' long-overdue campaign in opposition to killing.

The extreme contradictions between past and contemporary AMA policy statements on abortion highlighted in table 15 demonstrate how drastically the state of medical ethics regarding the value of human life before birth has deteriorated.

TABLE 15. THE AMERICAN MEDICAL ASSOCIATION ON ABORTION: AN ANATOMY OF CONTRADICTORY POLICIES

Past AMA Positions	Revised AMA Positions
WHEN DOES HUMAN LIFE BEGIN?	
1871: "No other doctrine appears to be consonant with reason or physiology but that which admits the embryo to possess vitality from the very moment of conception."	1967 and 1970: Neither AMA abortion policy statement includes any references to the scientific fact that human life begins at conception.
WHAT IS ABORTION?	
1859: "The slaughter of countless children . . . unwarrantable destruction of human life." 1871: "This wholesale destruction of unborn infants . . . it is a murder, a foul unprovoked murder."	1967: "The induced termination of pregnancy . . . the interruption of pregnancy." 1970: "A medical procedure . . . the decision to interrupt pregnancy . . . pregnancy termination."
WHAT SHOULD THE ETHICS OF ABORTION BE?	
1871: " 'Thou shalt not kill.' This commandment is given to all without exception . . . and it matters not at what stage of development his victim may have arrived."	1967: "This is a personal and moral consideration which in all cases must be faced according to the dictates of the conscience of the patient and her physician."
WHO SHOULD PERFORM ABORTIONS?	
1871: "It will be unlawful and unprofessional for any physician to induce abortion."	1970: "Abortion . . . should be performed only by a duly licensed physician."
WHY DID DOCTORS OPPOSE ABORTION IN NINETEENTH-CENTURY AMERICA?	
1859: "No attempt upon the life of the mother, but the wanton and murderous destruction of her child."	1967: "The technique of evacuating the uterus entailed an appreciable [maternal] morbidity and mortality."
WHO ARE PHYSICIAN ABORTIONISTS?	
1871: "Men who cling to a noble profession only to dishonor it . . . the executioners . . . modern Herods."	1967: "Conscientious physicians . . . conscientious practitioners . . . ethical physicians . . . prominent physicians."
WHAT SHOULD BE DONE TO PHYSICIAN ABORTIONISTS?	
1871: "These men should be marked as Cain was marked; they should be made the outcasts of society."	1967: They should be permitted to perform abortions as long as they take place "in an accredited hospital."

Toward a Revitalization of the Hippocratic Ethic in the Face of Widespread Assaults on the Hippocratic Oath

Although medical participation in mass destruction is often justified on the basis of conformity to authority—either as an instrument of the law or others—there is one preeminent authority doctors must reject in order to rationalize sustained involvement in killing: Hippocrates, "the Father of Medicine." First promulgated almost twenty-five hundred years ago, the Hippocratic Oath explicitly condemns killing before and after birth. Hippocrates presents a formidable challenge to doctors who are intent on perverting medical skills for destructive ends. He cannot be so easily dismissed as just another religious fanatic trying to impose his sectarian views on everyone else. Hippocrates was a pagan who truly believed in the sanctity of all human lives and made this the centerpiece of his oath. The medical killers of the Third Reich persistently assailed the integrity of the Hippocratic Oath, while an alarming segment of doctors today continue to do likewise for the purpose of endowing their assaults on unwanted and vulnerable victims with enhanced legitimacy.

The Hippocratic Oath: Its Origin and Significance

For millennia, the role of medicine has been clear and uncontested. The physician as a healer fully dedicated to the promotion of life and health has a long-standing tradition of overwhelming support.

This was not always so. In primitive times, the sorcerer, owing to a specialized knowledge of harmful and beneficial substances, was an unusual type of physician: he prescribed and administered drugs designed to heal some and kill others. In a culture dominated by ignorance and superstition, the sorcerer physician combined the dual task of curing those afflicted by mysterious forces and eliminating those defined as causing their afflictions. According to an analysis by anthropologist Margaret Mead in 1972, "Throughout the primitive world the doctor and the sorcerer tended to be the same person. He with the power to kill had the power to cure, including specially the undoing of his own killing activities. He who had power to cure would necessarily also be able to kill."[1]

It wasn't until a greater understanding of the natural causes of diseases began to replace superstition that the doctor as both healer and killer was called into question. A significant challenge came in the form of a treatise titled "The Sacred Disease," in which Hippocrates maintained that epilepsy and other illnesses were not due to such malignant forces as evil spirits, angry gods, or unscrupulous enemies, but arose from material causes.[2] For this and other reasons, Hippocrates became know as the "wisest and the greatest practitioner of his art" and the "most important and most complete medical personality of antiquity."[3]

One of Hippocrates's most profound and enduring legacies to the medical profession in particular and civilization in general is the Hippocratic Oath, formulated in the fourth century BC. It states in part:

> I swear by Apollo Physician and Asclepius.... I will apply dietetic measures for the benefit of the sick according to my ability and judgment; I will keep them from harm and injustice. I will neither give a deadly drug to anybody if asked for it, nor will I make a suggestion to this effect. Similarly I will not give to a woman an abortive remedy.

In purity and holiness I guard my life and my art.... Whatever houses I may visit, I will come for the benefit of the sick, remaining free of
all intentional injustice.[4]

Anthropologist Mead concluded that the Hippocratic Oath
marked a turning point in the history of medicine: "For the first time
in our tradition," it effectuated "a complete separation between curing
and killing."[5] This meant that never again would physicians be expected or allowed to kill anyone in any manner as part of their range of
professional tasks. From this point on, doctors were to be entirely and
preeminently healers of the sick. The oath's central principle—*primum non nocere*, first of all do no harm—is the very cornerstone of humane medical practice, an unwavering beacon that has guided doctors
for millennia. Because physicians had been so heavily invested in killing as well as healing before the time of Hippocrates, it is not surprising that the oath contains explicit prohibitions of both abortion and
euthanasia. Hippocrates was insistent on removing physicians from
association with all forms of destruction whether they involved killing
the child before birth or the adult during the terminal stages of existence. There are no exceptions or qualifications to the sanctity-of-life
ethic so deeply etched in the oath. It is a total, categorical commitment intended to protect, care for, and cure individuals at all phases
of the human life cycle. Mead underscores this point:

With the Greeks the distinction was made clear. One profession, the
followers of Asclepius, were to be dedicated completely to life under
all circumstances, regardless of rank, age, or intellect—the life of a
slave, the life of the Emperor, the life of a foreign man, the life of a
defective child.[6]

The oath provided the doctor with a code for professional conduct
of the highest ethical standards. It was meant to confer on the physician the kind of professional independence needed to withstand attempts by others to reinstate the dark age of exterminative medicine.
With Hippocrates and his oath, the course of civilized medicine was
set with conspicuous clarity—the doctor as a servant, protector, and
healer of the sick and never again as an instrument to be exploited by
the state, any pressure group, or individual bent on distorting medical

skills for destructive purposes. This, in Mead's assessment, is "a priceless possession which we cannot afford to tarnish," especially in light of the fact that "society always is attempting to make the physician into a killer—to kill the defective child at birth, to leave sleeping pills beside the bed of a cancer patient."[7]

An authoritative commentary by Hippocratic scholar Dr. Herbert Ratner in the early 1970s highlighted the importance of Hippocrates and his oath for the establishment of medicine as a learned profession dedicated to the service of humanity and its significance for keeping medicine true to its healing tradition:

> In the golden age of ancient Greece, medicine emerged as the prototype of the learned professions. The contribution of Hippocrates, the father of medicine, was to incorporate the rights of the patient, as well as the obligations of the physician, into the Oath.
>
> Hippocrates' profound grasp of the nature of a learned profession serving one of man's basic needs makes the Hippocratic Oath one of the great documents and classics of man, a fact not only signified by its universal inclusion in collections of the great books of western civilization, but by the universal veneration accorded it by physicians, singly and collectively, through the ages.[8]
>
> It is the Oath—a code of ethics which holds steadfast to a moral obligation in conformity with the definitive nature of a learned profession (here medicine)—which is the prime protector of the purity of the medical art. By imposing on its members an obligation to remain resolute against the assault of a sick society, the Oath, properly constituted, becomes the one hope of preserving the unconfused role of the physician as healer.[9]

Although the Hippocratic Oath possesses a definite transcendent quality—being sworn before the gods and goddesses of ancient Greek culture—Hippocrates's antipathy toward killing did not arise mainly out of an overtly religious foundation; it came from a primarily medical orientation. He viewed any kind of killing as completely foreign to the role of the physician. With Hippocrates, the commandment "Thou Shall Not Kill"—an injunction meant to transcend all races, religions, and creeds—was finally extended to the highly appropriate province of medical practice.

Medical Assaults on the Hippocratic Oath
in the Third Reich

The involvement of doctors in the destruction and experimental exploitation of unwanted human beings in the Third Reich and in the countries under Nazi occupation was the culmination of a pernicious erosion of respect for human life. An integral part of this process was an unrelenting onslaught on the sanctity-of-life core intrinsic to the Hippocratic Oath.

As early as 1920, Nazi euthanasia forerunners Professor Karl Binding and Dr. Alfred Hoche constructed an elitist edifice for advocating the destruction of "life unworthy of life" and declaring the Hippocratic Oath to be outdated. According to Dr. Hoche, "Not even the Hippocratic Oath, with its generalities, is operative today."[10]

Medical participation in many aspects of the Holocaust constituted the most radical departure from the do-no-harm principle embodied in the Hippocratic Oath. The attack against Hippocratic ethics was in evidence at the Nuremberg Doctors' Trial. The prosecution declared that all twenty-three health care professionals—twenty of them physicians— "violated the Hippocratic commandments which they had solemnly sworn to uphold and abide by, including the fundamental principles never to do harm—'primum non nocere.'"[11]

Nuremberg defendant Dr. Georg Weltz—charged with participating in the destruction-inducing high-altitude and freezing experiments—rejected the Hippocratic Oath as a pertinent moral guide for the medical profession:

> Q: The prosecutor has reproached all the defendants with violating the Hippocratic oath. I should like to have your personal attitude as a physician toward this subject.
>
> A: The Hippocratic oath ... is the professional oath of a certain profession which pledges allegiance to certain principles. It is an honorable historical document which, however, does not altogether fit present times. If it is to be applied today its wording has to be changed very extensively....
>
> At the university at which I studied it was not customary that persons take such an oath when they were being graduated.... It is a

matter of course that we must recommend to our patients a number of measures of which we know in advance under certain conditions they can be harmful.[12]

Dr. Karl Brandt—a leader in administering the Nazi euthanasia program and experimental atrocities on non-consenting victims—testified, "The oath of Hippocrates ... which calls upon the doctor to not to give to a patient poison even on the patient's request ... can no longer be maintained in this form. I am convinced that if this Hippocrates were alive today he would formulate his oath differently." Dr. Brandt proceeded to malign the oath for stating that "patients and sufferers are not to be given any poison," calling a doctor who "asserts such a thing" as perpetrating "either a lie, or a hypocrisy." He contended, "There is no doctor today who does not give a suffering patient narcotics, and tries to make the final hour of a dying patient easier." Such a practice, Brandt claimed, "is against the oath of Hippocrates," and he therefore concluded that "One may hang a copy of the Oath of Hippocrates in one's office but nobody pays any attention to it."[13]

Another basic moral principle explicitly embodied in the Hippocratic Oath—the condemnation of abortion—was extensively violated by Reich physicians, particularly when treating women residing in countries under German occupation and eastern female workers exploited as slave laborers for the Nazi war effort. Soon after the invasion of Poland in the fall of 1939, a Nazi decree was issued focusing on abortion as one of the key devices for reducing the Polish population:

> All measures serving birth control are to be admitted or to be encouraged. Abortion must not be punishable in the remaining territory. Abortives and contraceptives may be publicly offered for sale in every form without any police measures being taken.... Institutes and persons who make a business of performing abortions should not be prosecuted by the police.[14]

By August 1942, Secretary Martin Bormann set forth the Nazi population-control policies, which included the expansion of abortion and contraception to all populations under the control of the Ministry of the Occupied Territories of the East:

The Slavs are to work for us. Insofar as we do not need them, they may die. Therefore, compulsory vaccination and German health services are superfluous. The fertility of the Slavs is undesirable. *They may use contraceptives or practice abortion*; the more the better. Education is dangerous. It is enough if they can count up to a hundred. At best an education which produces useful stooges for us is admissible.[15]

War Crimes and Crimes against Humanity

One of the major contributions made at the Nuremberg War Crimes Trials was underscoring how the involvement of Nazi doctors and like-minded perpetrators in the experimental exploitation and destruction of unwanted human lives before and after birth constituted unconscionable assaults on the physician's most fundamental healing imperative embodied in the Hippocratic Oath. The tribunals went a step further by castigating the medical-induced experimental atrocities, acts of euthanasia, and abortions as "war crimes" and "crimes against humanity."

During the first Nuremberg Trial—known as "The Medical Case" —the defendants were charged with committing both "war crimes and crimes against humanity." Those involved in perpetrating experimental atrocities were indicted under the count "war crimes":

Between September 1939 and April 1945 all of the defendants herein unlawfully, willfully, and knowingly committed war crimes ... involving medical experiments without the subjects' consent, upon civilians and members of the armed forces of nations then at war with the German Reich and who were in the custody of the German Reich, in exercise of belligerent control, in the course of which experiments the defendants committed murder, brutalities, cruelties, tortures, atrocities and other inhuman acts.[16]

Under the "crimes against humanity" count, some of the defendants were also charged with carrying out the systematic killing of aged, insane, incurably ill, and disabled patients in nursing homes, hospitals, and asylums:

Between September 1939 and April 1945 the defendants ... unlawfully, willfully, and knowingly committed crimes against humanity ...
involving the execution of the so-called "euthanasia" program of the
German Reich, in the course of which the defendants herein murdered hundreds of thousand of human beings, including German
civilians, as well as civilians of other nations.[17]

At the Eighth Nuremberg War Crimes Trial—*The United States
v. Ulrich Greifelt et al.* (the RuSHA-Race and Resettlement Office
Case)—one of the charges leveled against the defendants consisted of
"encouraging and compelling abortions on Eastern workers for the
purposes of preserving their working capacity as slave labor and of
weakening Eastern nations."[18] In his summation, prosecutor James
McHaney defined abortion as falling under both the "war crimes" and
"crimes against humanity" classifications:

> The performance of abortions on Eastern [Slavic] workers is a war
> crime, as defined in Article II (b) of Control Council Law No. 10. It
> is a violation of Article 48 of the Hague Regulations, which provides
> that family honor and rights must be respected. It is also an act of "ill
> treatment" of a civilian population.
> The performance of abortions on Eastern workers is also a crime
> against humanity.... It constitutes an "act of extermination," "perse-
> cution on racial grounds," and an "inhumane act".... Even under the
> assumption that her request was genuinely voluntary ... it constitutes
> a war crime and a crime against humanity."[19]

Therefore abortion as well as experimental atrocities and the extermination of those viewed as postnatal discards were defined as "war
crimes and crimes against humanity" that required nothing less than
the full-scale application of justice at the international level.

The Declaration of Geneva

Out of the ashes of medical involvement in the Nazi Holocaust,
the World Medical Association (WMA)—consisting of thirty-nine
national medical societies, including the American Medical Association—met in Geneva, Switzerland, in 1948. The extensive attacks
mounted against the Hippocratic Oath by the doctors at the Nurem-

berg Doctors' Trial prompted the WMA to adopt a modern reaffirmation of Hippocratic ethics dubbed "The Declaration of Geneva" or
"The Geneva Code." It asserted in part:

> At this time of being admitted as a member of the medical profes-
> sion: I solemnly pledge myself to consecrate my life to the service
> of humanity.... I will practice my profession with conscience and
> dignity; the health of my patient will be my first consideration....
> I will maintain the utmost respect for human life from the time of
> conception. Even under threat, I will not use my medical knowledge
> contrary to the laws of humanity.[20]

The declaration thus retained the do-no-harm and sanctity-of-life
principles embodied in the classic Hippocratic Oath. The phrase "I
will maintain the utmost respect for human life from the time of conception" placed the physician in the role of a healer unequivocally
dedicated to the service of *all* human beings, both born and unborn,
from the *earliest* phase of their existence. This point was again underscored when the World Medical Association enacted the International
Code of Medical Ethics at a meeting in London in 1949. It stated, "A
doctor must observe the principles of *The Declaration of Geneva* ap-
proved by the World Medical Association" and reiterated that "A doctor must always bear in mind the importance of preserving life from
conception until death."[21]

The WMA was perfectly clear regarding its rationale for adopting
the Geneva Code—it was a reminder of the barbarities perpetrated
by physicians in the Third Reich and "a check upon any repetition,
anywhere in the world, of the German doctors' descent into savagery."
The association recommended further that this "modern version" of
the Hippocratic Oath "be read by every doctor on receipt of his diplo-
ma." Philosopher Albert Deutsch emphasized, "May those who recite
it as they enter the noble Hippocratic fellowship ever recall the deeds
that necessitated its drafting—determined never to let such things
happen again."[22]

The Hippocratic Oath under Siege in the United States

One would think that, after what happened in Nazi Germany, doctors would never again participate in any activities even remotely associated with killing or conducting lethal experiments on vulnerable subjects. One would think that reassertion of the do-no-harm and sanctity-of-life provisions in the Hippocratic Oath and the Declaration of Geneva would suffice to deter present-day physicians from repeating the crimes against humanity committed by the German doctors. One would think that the oath and its modern counterpart would help doctors resist any efforts to turn them into instruments of destruction.

How quickly memory fades with the passage of time! What has happened, deplorably, is just the opposite. Instead of abandoning their destructive practices, many contemporary physicians have decided to attack the oath and along with it the reputation of Hippocrates. Their efforts are motivated primarily by a need to rationalize participation in the modern destruction of the unwanted unborn and the growing assaults against those after birth deemed lives not worth living. It would be untenable to continue doing away with the unwanted at the current assembly line rate and still retain an oath so clearly opposed to such destructive operations.

American proponents of abortion have attempted to discredit Hippocrates and his oath with rhetoric and arguments strikingly reminiscent of the semantics and justifications invoked by Nazi doctors to rationalize their participation in the Holocaust. A widespread way of dismissing the significance of the oath has been through repeated assertions about its being out of touch with modern mainstream medicine and a changing society. The 1973 US Supreme Court decision in *Roe v. Wade* that legalized abortion set the stage by reducing the Hippocratic Oath to the status of a rigid, outmoded piece of secular dogma.[23] By the end of the 1970s and into the 1980s, the assaults upon the Hippocratic Oath had become standard fare. According to St. Louis abortionist Dr. Bolivar Escobedo, "The Hippocratic Oath is nothing but a ritual or symbolic act that bears no legal force."[24] Middle-trimester abortionist Dr. William Petersen relegated the oath to the status of an antiquated tradition. It was "carried down from olden times," he stressed, adding that "many of our old traditions have been changed by present-day demands."[25]

The outdated nature ascribed to the Hippocratic Oath is a theme not confined to only those doctors who perform abortions; it has become one of contemporary medicine's most intransigent narratives supported by a broad spectrum of professionals, including medical policymakers, professors at leading medical schools and institutions, and medical ethicists. Today's advocates of physician-assisted suicide and euthanasia attack the Hippocratic Oath largely because of its opposition to physicians who prescribe or even suggest the administration of deadly drugs to patients. "The reality is that most doctors never even read the Hippocratic oath," maintained Hemlock Society founder Derek Humphry. "It's totally out of synchronization with modern life."[26] Physician, business executive, and ethics instructor Ralph Thompson declared, "The Hippocratic oath is obsolete.... The oath's didactic references to abortion and euthanasia are too simplistic to be useful."[27] Dr. Richard Momeyer of Miami University in Oxford, Ohio, goes so far as to view the wording in the Hippocratic Oath as flexible enough to permit physician-assisted suicide: "Within the Hippocratic tradition that emphasizes the exercising of medical skills for patient benefit, physicians may even cooperate with requests for physician-assisted suicide."[28]

One of the Hippocratic Oath's most prominent debunkers is physician-assisted suicide proponent Dr. Sherwin Nuland, a Yale University medical professor and best-selling author. The *New England Journal of Medicine* supplied editorial space for him to dismiss the oath as simply a collection of long-standing, synoptic sayings out of touch with the real needs of patients and of little more than symbolic value: "To seek refuge in ancient aphorisms is to turn away from the unique needs of each of our patients who have entrusted themselves to our care."[29]

The relentless assaults on the Hippocratic Oath—particularly its do-no-harm and absolute respect-for-human-life provisions—have had a profound impact upon the oaths taken at medical school graduations. A content analysis of oaths administered in American and

Canadian medical schools during the closing decade of the twentieth century revealed that only 8 percent prohibited abortion and only
14 percent prohibited euthanasia. The authors of this study noted a
great paradox in their findings insofar as "the administration of oaths
to medical graduates has steadily increased throughout this century,
while the content of those oaths has steadily shifted away from the
basic tenets of the original Hippocratic Oath."[30] The 2007 analysis
of medical oaths by Erich Loewy, emeritus medical professor at the
University of California, Davis, thus concluded, "The old Hippocratic
Oath is no longer suitable for modern times."[31]

In his observation heralding the death of the Hippocratic ideals,
Dr. Imre Loefler summed up the oath's extensive deconstruction by
acknowledging, "The Hippocratic oath, particularly in respect to its
three most essential principles—the sanctity of life, the privacy of patients, and the 'do-no-harm' command—is increasingly subverted,
ignored, altered, reinterpreted."[32]

The Declaration of Geneva—the other ethical statement sometimes invoked at medical school graduations—has suffered a similar
process of radical deconstruction. Originally touted "the new Hippocratic Oath" by the World Medical Association in 1948, it employed
modern phraseology to reaffirm—not depart from—the do-no-harm,
sanctity-of-life components of Hippocratic ethics, especially its two
sentences proclaiming, "I will maintain the utmost respect for human
life from the time of conception. Even under threat, I will not use my
medical knowledge contrary to the laws of humanity."[33]

Despite the honorable intentions motivating these compelling
vows, Trinity Evangelical Divinity School professor and ethics scholar
Nigel M. De S. Cameron, in *The New Medicine: Life and Death after
Hippocrates*, concluded that this revised, modernistic wording already
contained the seeds of demise through supplanting the transcendent
thrust of the Hippocratic Oath with "a pallid affirmation made by the
physician in the presence of man alone" and replacing the categorical
prohibitions of abortion and euthanasia with vague affirmations of
"respect" and "honor," which "invite revision and amendment."[34]

Several stratagems have evolved with the express purpose of undermining the declaration's expression of utmost respect for human

life from conception. Dr. Mary Arneson recalled, "I did take the Declaration of Geneva except for omitting the words 'from the time of
conception,' which struck me as hypocritical when my medical education had included a rotation at an abortion clinic."[35] In an address
to a University of Arizona medical school honor society, Dr. Louis
Weinstein asserted that "to become the Healer I wish to be I must
expand my thinking." His idea of expanded thinking included an
all-encompassing redefinition of "respect" that embraces the entire
curing-killing spectrum: "I shall have the highest respect for human
life and remember that it is wrong to terminate life in certain circumstances, permissible in some, and an act of supreme love in others."[36]

At its Forty-Sixth General Assembly in 1994, one of the WMA's basic ethical principles—"I will maintain the utmost respect for human
life from the time of conception"—had been truncated to "I will maintain the utmost respect for human life from its beginning."[37] Given
the large number of physicians who continue to deny or ignore the
scientific fact that human life begins at conception, this inordinate deconstruction leaves wide latitude for not only the acceptance of abortion, but also the increasing range of destructive experiments on human embryos and fetuses whose lives have been rendered superfluous.

The Hippocratic Foundation of Organized Medicine's Opposition to Capital Punishment

Ironically, while the do-no-harm moral core of the Hippocratic Oath has been repeatedly watered down and shredded by medical
practitioners and proponents of abortion, euthanasia, and assisted
suicide, this same moral center has been steadfastly proclaimed by
the American Medical Association and leading medical groups as
the central rationale for the condemnation of medical involvement in
state-ordered executions. This began in the late 1970s when Oklahoma
and Texas became the first states to mandate lethal injection as the
preferred method for carrying out death sentences.

An influential article in the January 24, 1980, issue of the *New England Journal of Medicine* established the historical and ethical ground-
work for opposition to medical participation in capital punishment by

drug injection. "This new method of capital punishment ... presents the most serious and intimate challenge in modern American history to active medical participation in state-ordered killing of human beings," declared the authors, Harvard Medical School professors William Curran and Ward Casscells. "Unlike any other methods, this procedure requires the direct application of biomedical knowledge and skills in a corruption and exploitation of the healing profession's role in society."[38]

The authors are crystal clear about the ethical underpinnings for their critique: "The Hippocratic Oath itself is the foundation of this position. Its essential purpose was to identify the Greek group of physicians as healers who would never kill or harm their patients." Moreover, Curran and Casscells invoked pertinent passages from the oath: "I will use treatment to help the sick according to my ability and judgment, but never with a view to injury and wrong-doing. Neither will I administer a poison to anyone when asked to do so nor will I suggest such a course." They also highlighted a quotation from the modern reaffirmation of the Hippocratic Oath, the Declaration of Geneva: "Even under threat, I will not use my medical knowledge contrary to the laws of humanity."[39]

Also in 1980, the American Psychiatric Association (APA)—building on the Hippocratic heritage—asserted in its statement against medical involvement in capital punishment, "The physician's serving the state as an executioner, either directly or indirectly, is a perversion of medical ethics and of his or her role as a healer and comforter."[40]

As an increasing number of states switched to the lethal injection protocol for state-ordered executions, the AMA, other medical groups, and influential physicians responded by reaffirming the Hippocratic-based prohibition against medical participation in this form of medicalized killing. In 1993, the AMA's Council on Ethical and Judicial Affairs underscored the "Oath of Hippocrates" as the key ethical source for issuing a report stating that "physicians as professionals committed to 'first of all do no harm,' *primum non nocere*, could not ethically participate in executions." This pronouncement served as a basis for enactment of the resolution, "A physician, as a member of a profession dedicated to preserving life when there is hope of doing so, should not be a participant in a legally authorized execution." It also quoted key passages from the Hippocratic Oath to reinforce this commitment:

> I will use treatment to help the sick according to my ability and judgment, but never with a view to injury and wrong-doing. Neither will I administer a poison to anyone when asked to do so nor will I suggest such a course.[41]

Well into the first decade of the twenty-first century, all thirty-eight states with the death penalty have come to rely on lethal injections, with thirty-five of them allowing physician participation in executions, while seventeen actually require it.[42] The American Medical Association, its affiliates, and like-minded medical groups are thus ever poised to cite the doctor-as-healer imperative embodied in the Hippocratic Oath as a basis for combating attempts by various states to employ medical personnel in carrying out legally authorized executions.

The AMA's Hippocratic-Based Campaign against Euthanasia and Physician-Assisted Suicide

The American Medical Association also has a long-standing policy prohibiting medical involvement in mercy killing and euthanasia. In June 1977, the AMA's Council on Ethical and Judicial Affairs (CEJA) stated that "mercy killing or euthanasia ... is contrary to public policy, medical tradition, and the most fundamental measures of human value and worth."[43]

A CEJA report, *Decisions near the End of Life*, adopted by the House of Delegates of the AMA at its 1991 annual meeting, declared, "Physicians must not perform euthanasia or participate in assisted suicide." The rationale for the council's "prohibition against physicians killing their patients" is "based on a commitment that medicine is a profession dedicated to healing, and that its tools should not be used to cause patients' deaths."[44]

Throughout the remainder of the 1990s, the Hippocratic Oath was repeatedly cited as the premier authority underlying organized medicine's opposition to physician-assisted suicide. "For nearly 2,500 years, physicians have vowed to 'give no deadly drug if asked for it, [nor] make a suggestion to this effect,'" former AMA president Dr. Lonnie Bristow testified in 1996 before a US congressional committee. "The AMA believes that 'physician-assisted suicide' is unethical and fundamentally inconsistent with the pledge physicians make to devote themselves to healing and to life."[45]

During its October 1996 term, the US Supreme Court heard oral arguments pertaining to lower court rulings in New York and Washington States that sanctioned a constitutional right to die with the aid of a physician. The American Medical Association—in conjunction with the American Nurses Association, the American Psychiatric Association, a host of state medical societies, and other prominent medical organizations and related groups—submitted an *amicus curiae* (friend of the court) legal brief to the US Supreme Court supporting the constitutionality of state laws prohibiting physician-assisted suicide. The ethical rationale underlying the brief's opposition to physician-assisted suicide was explicitly based on the doctor-as-healer tenet embodied in the Hippocratic Oath:

> The power to assist in intentionally taking the life of a patient is antithetical to the central mission of healing that guides both medicine and nursing....
>
> The ethical prohibition against physician-assisted suicide is a cornerstone of medical ethics. Its roots are as ancient as the Hippocratic Oath that a physician "will neither give a deadly drug to anybody if asked for it, nor ... make a suggestion to this effect," and the merits of the ban have been debated repeatedly in this nation since the late nineteenth century.... Physician-assisted suicide remains "fundamentally incompatible with the physician's role as healer, would be difficult or impossible to control, and would pose serious societal risks."[46]

Reasserting the Hippocratic Oath's Moral Center Prohibiting Abortion

The Hippocratic Oath's moral core—the physician as a healer and never a killer—is adamantly expressed especially in the American Medical Association's long-standing condemnation of medical participation in capital punishment. It is therefore urgent that the AMA and other medical groups extend their unwavering Hippocratic-founded prohibition of medical involvement in state-ordered executions to also encompass prohibition of medical participation in state-sanctioned feticide. Such extension can be readily accomplished in at least two ways. First, after invoking the Hippocratic Oath's statement "Neither will I administer a poison to anyone when asked to do so nor will I suggest such a course," the AMA could reinsert the oath's original anti-abortion stricture: "Similarly, I will not give to a woman an abortive remedy." Second, if the AMA prefers the Declaration of Geneva as its moral compass, it could reinsert the declaration's original equality-of-life passage: "I will maintain the utmost respect for human life from the time of conception."

Under current conditions passing for medical ethics, either proposed change is highly unlikely. A glaring paradox thus remains: Why does the American Medical Association consider the Hippocratic Oath and the Declaration of Geneva as appropriate ethical standards for support of its prohibition against medical participation in a relatively small number of legally authorized executions, yet is blind to their relevance as a basis for opposition to the medical execution of millions before birth? The extreme contradiction between the AMA policies on capital punishment (repudiation of physicians as legal executioners of condemned criminals) and abortion (approval of physicians as legal executioners of the innocent unborn) cries out for confrontation and remediation.

Selective application of the Hippocratic Oath and its modern counterpart, the Declaration of Geneva, to castigate only certain types of medical killing belies a serious violation of the healing thrust intrinsic to these fundamental codes of medical ethics. Both were intended to remove the doctor from involvement in all forms of killing, inside and outside the womb.

Despite the highly selective versions of the Hippocratic Oath that continue to be disseminated by leading medical organizations and other elitist sources, some eminent physicians subscribe to a view of the unadulterated Hippocratic Oath as reflecting the embodiment of medical wisdom, particularly its unswerving commitment to the "essential activity of healing the sick." One of the most influential doctors in the vanguard of attempting to restore its healing, life-affirming essence is Dr. Leon Kass, a renowned medical professor and biomedical ethicist, as well as a former chairman of the US President's Council on Bioethics.

Dr. Kass's categorical opposition to killing is expressed in an article published in *The Public Interest* titled, "Neither for Love Nor Money: Why Doctors Must Not Kill." He views this opposition as directly related to the Hippocratic Oath's deeply embedded healing imperative that "The central core of medicine: to heal, to make whole, is the doctor's primary business" and "despite enormous changes in medical technique and institutional practice ... the center of medicine has not changed: it is as true today as it was in the days of Hippocrates that the ill desire to be whole."[47] In another publication, Kass emphasized that the Hippocratic Oath leaves no room for any act of medicalized killing: "The doctor refuses to participate directly in ending a life, whether one in the fullness of days or on the way to birth. To protect life, to maintain and support it, to restore it to wholeness is the common principle.... It can be derived from the inner meaning of medicine itself, especially if one remembers that the doctor is nature's cooperative ally and not its master." Dr. Kass called into question "whether physicians who perform abortions are truly physicians" and added that "one must wince at the monstrous because self-contradictory union that is the obstetrician-abortionist."[48]

A growing number of doctors have become greatly alarmed about how organized medicine's unqualified appropriation of the watered-down versions of the Hippocratic Oath's categorical prohibitions against the taking of human life has contributed to the spread of a veritable abortion culture—a mockery of medicine in which millions of unborn lives have been snuffed out under the pretext of a valid medical procedure. They also remain troubled about the increasing pressure being exerted by medical proponents and practitioners of physician-assisted suicide and euthanasia to change the AMA's Hippocratic-founded opposition to these methods of terminating the lives of vulnerable patients.

To counter the pervasive hypocrisy within elitist medical circles over the genuine meaning of the Hippocratic Oath's do-no-harm provisions, concerned physicians have established organizations of doctors and medical ethicists committed to the absolute respect, care, and protection of all human lives intended in the original Hippocratic code of ethical medical practice. One of the leading activists was the late Dr. Joseph Stanton, a Tufts University medical professor and founder of the Value of Life Committee, a group created to counter the 1973 US Supreme Court's decision in *Roe v. Wade*, which was an assault on the Hippocratic Oath. After extensive feedback from prominent scholars, physicians, and authors of textbooks on medical ethics, Stanton and Value of Life Committee colleagues published in April 1995 an updated reaffirmation of the Hippocratic Oath. Its unequivocal commitment to human life incorporates the following statement:

> I WILL FOLLOW that method of treatment which according to my ability and judgment I consider for the benefit of my patient and abstain from whatever is harmful or mischievous. I will neither prescribe nor administer a lethal dose of medicine to any patient even if asked nor counsel any such thing nor perform act or omission with direct intent deliberately to end a human life. I will maintain the utmost respect for every human life from fertilization to natural death and reject abortion that deliberately takes a unique human life.[49]

Other pro-life organizations such as the American Right to Life likewise rely upon the Hippocratic Oath for providing the prime ethical principle against abortion. During the fifth century BC, "Hippocrates, considered the father of medicine, also acknowledged the immorality of killing an unborn child" according to the pronouncements "never do harm" and "I will not ... cause an abortion." Although medical schools "still commonly administer a Hippocratic pledge but sadly, in pro-abortion cultures, they have removed the promise to not kill an unborn child" and have replaced it "by vague generalities." For most doctors, then, "the taking of the oath is not meaningful ... but just something that happens." Therefore "when the oath you take doesn't really say much of anything, it can't be of much use as an ethical guide." Nevertheless, "moms intuitively knew to talk about the 'baby' in their womb" while "today, 4D ultrasound shows for all to see what has always been known, the precious humanity of the preborn child. So good doctors all remember the Hippocratic pledge to first do no harm."[50]

Return of the Hippocratic Oath to its genuine, unequivocal pro-life position remains a daunting challenge given the widespread assaults on or the distorted versions of the oath that dominate medical organizational policy statements and medical school graduation oath-taking ceremonies. According to the Christian Medical and Dental Associations (CMDA), many doctors still remain ambivalent about or even opposed to the wholesale killing of the unborn. The CMDA's vice president for governmental relations, Jonathan Imbody—backed up by the technology of sonograms personalizing the humanity of life before birth—put forth the Hippocratic Oath as an indispensable source for welcoming and protecting today's youngest and most vulnerable individuals:

> Abortion violates every human instinct. For doctors, abortion also contradicts the professional oath that has marked medicine since the 4th century BC, when Hippocratic physicians began reassuring their patients, "I will not give to a woman an abortive remedy."
>
> Most physicians who view a sonogram displaying the movements of the unborn child will experience an instinctive urge to protect that young person. To suppress that vital instinct is to sacrifice an essential part of our own humanity. The first step in restoring that loss is to follow the ancient physicians in resolving to "first, do no harm." The next step is to welcome every new life into the world as if it were our own. Our lives and the lives of our unborn children are inseparable.[51]

Another group strongly committed to the Hippocratic Oath's sanctity-of-life ethic is the twenty-five-hundred-member American Association of Pro-Life Obstetricians and Gynecologists (AAPLOG). Its mission statement affirms "that we, as physicians, are responsible for the care and well being of both our pregnant woman patient and her unborn child"; "that elective disruption/abortion of human life at any time from fertilization onward constitutes the willful destruction of an innocent human being"; and "that this procedure will have no place in our practice of the healing arts."[52] The main theme of the AAPLOG's 2016 educational conference is aptly "Hippocratic Medicine: The Means to Health and Human Flourishing."[53]

The Prospects for a Hippocratic Restoration

Becoming conversant with how the subversion of the Hippocratic Oath has been instrumental in fueling the Nazi Holocaust and is facilitating today's medical assaults on vulnerable victims affords a prime teaching moment for doctors to get in touch with the genuine ethical roots of their professional raison d'être. The inevitable effect has the potential for leading physicians to an unqualified commitment to the do-no-harm, sanctity-of-life principles embodied in the oath and its modern counterpart, the Declaration of Geneva. This means that physicians must assume their indispensable role as guardians and healers of human life at all stages of development.

Amid the mountains of evidence of atrocities against the most basic moral precepts in the Hippocratic Oath committed by doctors on trial at Nuremberg, American medical science consultant Dr. Andrew Ivy testified before the court in 1947 as to the indispensability of Hippocratic ethics:

> Q: Several of the defendants have pointed out in this case that the oath of Hippocrates is obsolete today. Do you follow that opinion?
>
> A: I do not. The moral imperative of the oath of Hippocrates I believe is necessary for the survival of the scientific and technical philosophy of medicine.[54]

Almost two years after testifying at the Nuremberg Doctors' Trial, Dr. Ivy elaborated upon the enormous impact that the moral imperative of the Hippocratic Oath has had on the scientific and technical philosophy of medicine:

> Though I had been in medicine for thirty years, I realized, for the first time at the Nürnberg Trials, the full meaning and importance of the contributions of Hippocrates and his school to medicine and human welfare.
>
> Hippocrates contributed the scientific philosophy of medicine as we know it today when he taught that disease is due to material causes and not to evil spirits, witches or the wrath of gods. He contributed a technical philosophy when he taught that diligence, accuracy, thoroughness in observation and skill were essential for success in the practice of a science and art of medicine. He apparently realized

that a scientific and technical philosophy of medicine could not survive through the ages unless it was associated with a sound moral philosophy. One cannot conceive of a sound society with medicine that does not have a sound moral philosophy.[55]

Time will tell whether the efforts of some doctors and medical groups to invoke the uncensored Hippocratic Oath as a foundation for opposition to abortion constitute a revolution in the making or not. Such efforts face a formidable obstacle that consists of a firmly entrenched acceptance of abortion in which an increasing number of physicians and biomedical scientists not only participate in the wholesale destruction of unwanted unborn humans, but also are complicit in exploiting their remains for an ever expanding array of experimental and commercial enterprises. The assaults on the Hippocratic Oath have helped facilitate an era of unrestrained killing by the very profession that had once been so uncompromisingly dedicated to human life at all stages of development.

A monumental endeavor will be required to galvanize medical opinion in the direction of a full-fledged recommitment to the Hippocratic provisions protective of all human lives, before as well as after birth. Long overdue is a call for members of the medical profession to muster the ethical fortitude necessary to challenge the malaise and mentality responsible for transforming many mainstream medical practitioners into agents of death and destruction. The Hippocratic Oath provides a compelling philosophic and moral basis for restoring doctors to their time-honored position as healers above all.

Table 16 furnishes an historical and contemporary sketch of the Hippocratic Oath, some of the most egregious assaults on its most basic principles, and the application of its do-no-harm moral imperative as a bulwark against medical participation in killing vulnerable human lives inside and outside the womb.

TABLE 16. MILESTONES IN MEDICAL ETHICS, THEIR VIOLATIONS, AND A RESTORATION OF THE HIPPOCRATIC ETHIC

BEFORE HIPPOCRATES
The physician in the role of a sorcerer functioned as both a killer and a healer.

THE HIPPOCRATIC OATH (460–377 BC)
Establishment of the doctor as an exclusive healer and never again as a killer.

THE THIRD REICH (1933–45)
The key role of doctors in the massive extermination of lives considered devoid of value.

THE NUREMBERG WAR CRIMES TRIALS (1946–49)
The denunciation of experimental atrocities, euthanasia, and abortion as constituting "war crimes" and "crimes against humanity."

THE DECLARATION OF GENEVA (1948)
Reaffirmation of the physician as a healer from the time of conception.

CONTEMPORARY SOCIETY (1973–present)
The extensive participation of doctors in destroying millions of unwanted unborn humans and an increasing number of vulnerable individuals after birth.

The Hippocratic Oath under Assault

THE THIRD REICH	THE UNITED STATES
"Not even the Hippocratic Oath . . . is operative." (*Dr. Alfred Hoche, 1920*)	"The Hippocratic ethic is obsolete." (*Dr. Ralph Thompson, 2004*)
"One may hang a copy of the Oath of Hippocrates in one's office but nobody pays any attention to it." (*Dr. Karl Brandt, 1947*)	"The reality is that most doctors never even read the Hippocratic oath. It's totally out of synchronization with modern life." (*Derek Humphry, 1986*)
"The Oath of Hippocrates . . . which calls upon the doctor to not to give to a patient poison even on the patient's request . . . can no longer be maintained in this form." (*Dr. Karl Brandt, 1947*)	"Within the Hippocratic tradition that emphasizes . . . medical skills for patient benefit, physicians may even cooperate with requests for physician-assisted suicide." (*Dr. Richard Momeyer, 1995*)
"An honorable historical document which does not altogether fit present times." (*Dr. Georg Weltz, 1947*)	"The old Hippocratic Oath is no longer suitable for modern times." (*Dr. Erich Loewy, 2007*)

A Revival of the Inclusive Hippocratic Oath

"The ethical principles of the medical profession worldwide should be interpreted to unconditionally condemn this new form of capital punishment [lethal injection]. The Hippocratic Oath itself is the foundation of this position. Its essential purpose was to identify the Greek group of physicians as healers who would never kill their patients."
(*Drs. William Curran and Ward Cassells, 1980*)

"The ethical prohibition against physician-assisted suicide is a cornerstone of medical ethics. Its roots are as ancient as the Hippocratic Oath that a physician 'will neither give a deadly drug to anybody if asked for it, nor . . . make a suggestion to this effect.'"
(*Legal brief submitted to US Supreme Court by the AMA and other health care groups, 1996*)

"Abortion violates every human instinct. For doctors, abortion also contradicts the professional oath that has marked medicine since the 4th century BC, when Hippocratic physicians began reassuring their patients, 'I will not give to a woman an abortive remedy.'"
(*Jonathan Imbody, Christian Medical and Dental Associations, 2007*)

Conclusion

A major responsibility for today's massive destruction of prenatal human beings must be placed on the shoulders of influential physicians who promote, mandate, and implement the killing of the unborn as well as scavenge their remains for experimental exploitation in full accord with the policies established by influential medical organizations. Upstanding doctors—and not the so-called back-alley butchers—committed much of the mayhem against the unborn even when abortion was illegal and played a leading role in many of the propaganda campaigns aimed at abolishing laws opposed to abortion.

The decline of medical ethics today is starkly epitomized in the fact that the destruction of human life before birth is now ranked among the most frequently performed medical and surgical procedures. Under the cover of technology, ideology, and terminology, medical doctors continue to violate the ethics of humanity and their professional raison d'être by killing unborn human lives at a staggering rate. The mentality powering the transformation of killing into a form of valid medical practice was evident as far back as a 1972 statement released by one hundred obstetrics professors from leading American medical schools in support of legalizing abortion on demand: "For the first time, except perhaps for cosmetic surgery, doctors will be expected to do an operation simply because the patient asks that it be done. Granted, this changes the physician's traditional role, but it will be necessary to make this change if we are to serve the new society in which we live."[1]

The doctor's traditional role was radically altered to encompass the destruction of the most vulnerable human beings. Dr. Herbert Ratner's incisive exposé of this mentality contains considerable relevance today as well: "The notion of . . . exterminative medicine, in which the physician serves as killer is as monstrous as expecting the learned profession of law to serve injustice, or of the ministry to serve vice and sin, and to promote hell as well as heaven."[2]

The World Health Organization (WHO) has incorporated some of the major deceptive linguistic expressions uncovered in this book as vehicles for transforming the destruction of the unborn into an international human right. Its publication *Safe Abortion: Technical and Policy Guidance for Health Care Systems* (2012) abounds with medicalized characterizations of feticide as "procedures," "regimens," forms of "treatment," and "good-quality care" performed by "health-care providers" and "health-service providers" who are simply "emptying" the "products of conception" and the "contents of the uterus" within a "health-care facility" or a "service-delivery site." The WHO's portrayal of "the safest and most effective surgical technique for later abortion" is likewise devoid of any references to what is in fact a grotesque destruction process involving the literal dismemberment of unborn victims and extracting their mutilated bodies with forceps. The exceedingly benign version promulgated by the WHO refers to this type of abortion as merely a "dilatation and evacuation" procedure that results in "evacuating the uterus."[3]

A growing number of physicians and medical groups are also in the vanguard of a movement to legalize physician-assisted suicide and euthanasia. Assisted-suicide practices in Europe have become so permissive that doctors routinely euthanize not only terminally ill patients but also the chronically ill, the elderly who are "tired of life," young children, and those with mental illnesses. Thousands of patients under Belgium's euthanasia law have been killed by their doctors without consent.[4] In the United States, only six states have legalized assisted suicide. As of the end of March 2015, however, legislators in twenty-five states have introduced new bills to legalize doctor-prescribed suicide. Bioethics scholar Wesley J. Smith described the assisted suicide movement as "indefatigable" and "now more energized than any other time in recent years."[5]

Although things appear bleak and time is running out for the survival of a truly humane social order where all human lives are considered of inestimable value, an opportunity still exists to alter the devastating course of events. Grassroots resistance to the medical destruction of millions persists. According to data compiled by the activist pro-life organization Operation Rescue, there were 2,176 surgical abortion clinics operating nationwide in 1991. By the end of November 2013, the number of abortion facilities had dropped to 616, a 72 percent decline.[6] Despite the avalanche of doctor-prescribed suicide bills introduced in state legislatures, none have been enacted so far, in large part owing to the steadfast opposition from some leading medical groups.

Nevertheless, the task of educating the medical profession and public alike regarding the dignity and intrinsic worth of human life at all stages of development and the harsh realities of what abortion, experimental exploitation, assisted suicide, and euthanasia do to this life still remains a formidable undertaking. Nothing less than a revolution in attitudes, language, perceptions, and values is long overdue. At the most fundamental level, such a revolution requires *calling things by their proper names*, a principle steadfastly articulated by the American Medical Association in its 1871 justification for condemning abortion in the strongest possible language: "We had to deal with human life. In a matter of less importance we could entertain no compromise. An honest judge on the bench would call things by their proper names. We could do no less."[7]

The violation of this basic principle has long served to entrench the concealment of medicalized killing beneath a relentless barrage of degrading designations and soothing abstractions. In his classic essay "Politics and the English Language," George Orwell warned that "as soon as certain topics are raised the concrete melts into the abstract," which perpetuates "the defense of the indefensible" through "the invasion of one's mind by ready-made phrases" that are "designed to make lies sound truthful and murder respectable." Furthermore, because the purpose underpinning this language of obfuscation consisting "largely of euphemism, question-begging and sheer cloudy vagueness" is "to name things without calling up mental images of them," Orwell favored "put[ting] off using words as long as possible" and "get[ting] one's meaning as clear as one can through pictures and sensations."[8] Consequently, accentuating the striking similarities between the photographs of contemporary unborn abortion victims and Holocaust victims contributes an indispensable graphic dimension for bolstering the imperative to call things by their proper names.

The exercise of raw medical power against human lives before and after birth must come to an end. Persistent appeals and challenges are in dire need of being addressed to members of the medical profession:

- to cease their war on the unwanted unborn and their mounting assaults on the vulnerable born;
- to lay down their curettes, forceps, and other instruments distorted for lethal purposes;
- to pull the plugs on their suction machines;
- to remove the deadly solutions from their syringes;
- to destroy their poisonous pills;
- to protect, care for, and heal human lives whatever their status, condition, or stage of development.

Doctors need to become reacquainted with the ancient roots of their profession and dedicate themselves to the sanctity-of-life ethic embodied in the Hippocratic Oath, a document that explicitly condemns killing inside and outside the womb and is the very cornerstone of civilized, ethical medicine.

The evidence compiled in this study contains an abundance of disquieting revelations for documenting how fully implicated physicians were in the Holocaust and other atrocities, as well as how today's medical participation in abortion, euthanasia, and assisted suicide replicates some of history's darkest chapters. Also relevant here is the closeness of the contemporary methods employed to destroy vulnerable individuals before as well as after birth. A prime example is Dr. Katharine Sheehan's injection of digoxin into the fetal heart to cause fetal demise and Dr. Jack Kevorkian's injection of potassium chloride to stop the heart of a patient with a disability.

The numerous destructive parallels covered in this book stand little chance of exposure, let alone examination, unless the whole domain of past and present medical-imposed killing—so thoroughly obscured under a thick blanket of deceptive rhetoric, prestigious practitioners, and sanitized settings—is opened up for extensive scrutiny, challenge, and action. Becoming conversant with these findings constitutes an indispensable step toward halting the current appalling state of affairs so aptly captured in the compelling admonition attributed to philosopher George Santayana: "Those who do not remember the past are doomed to repeat it."

NOTES

Introduction

1. Doe v. Bolton, 410 U.S. 222 (1973).

2. Ivan Illich, *Medical Nemesis: The Expropriation of Health* (New York: Pantheon Books, 1976), 3, 271.

3. Jacob Neusner, "Matters of Opinion: Israeli's Holocaust," *Christianity Today,* October 26, 1998, 1.

4. Trevor Stokes and Art Caplan, "German Doctors Apologize for Holocaust Horrors," NBC News, May 24, 2012, https://www.nbcnews.com/health/health-news/german-doctors-apologize-holocaust-horrors-flna793850.

5. Willard Gaylin and Marc Lappe, "Fetal Politics: The Debate on Experimenting with the Unborn," *Atlantic* (May 1975): 66.

6. "Abortions Reported Denied to Hundreds of Thousands," *St. Louis Post-Dispatch*, October 8, 1975, 13D.

7. Edwin Black, *War against the Weak: Eugenics and America's Campaign to Create a Master Race* (New York: Four Walls Eight Windows, 2003).

8. "A New Ethic for Medicine and Society," editorial, *California Medicine* 113 (September 1970): 67–68.

Chapter 1. The Methods of Medicalized Killing

1. "The Maidanek Horror," *New York Times*, August 31, 1944, 16.

2. Drew Middleton, "Films Back Charge of German Crimes," *New York Times*, February 20, 1946, 6.

3. Robert H. Abzug, *Inside the Vicious Heart: Americans and the Liberation of Nazi Concentration Camps* (New York: Oxford University Press, 1985), 128.

4. Affidavit of Zdenka Nedvedove-Nejedla, MD, in *Trials of War Criminals before the Nuernberg Military Tribunals*, 15 vols. (Washington, DC: US Government Printing Office, 1949), 1:400–402 (hereafter cited as *War Crimes Trials*).

5. Affidavit of Sofia Maczka, doctor of medicine, *War Crimes Trials*, 1:402–5.

6. "Transcript of the Proceedings in Case 1," in *The Medical Case*, vol. 1 of *War Crimes Trials*, 1:931 (deposition of Gustawa Winkowska, January 2, 1947).

7. Richard Ough, "Abortion, Ethics and the Church: A Doctor's Testimony," *Church Times*, September 5, 1975, 4.

8. National Abortion Federation v. Ashcroft, 287 F. Supp. 2d 525 (S.D.N.Y. 2003).

9. National Abortion Federation v. Ashcroft, 287 F. Supp. 2d 525 (S.D.N.Y. 2003).

10. Micaiah Bilger, "Authorities Find More Bodies of Aborted Babies on Property of Abortionist Who Kept 2,246 as Trophies," LifeNews.com, October 9, 2019, https://www.lifenews.com/2019/10/09/authorities-find-more-bodies-of-aborted-babies-on-property-of-abortionist-who-kept2246-as-trophies/.

11. Eugen Kogon, Hermann Langbein, and Adalbert Rückerl, eds., *Nazi Mass Murder: A Documentary History of the Use of Poison Gas*, trans. Mary Scott and Caroline Lloyd-Morris (New Haven, CT: Yale University Press, 1993), 28.

12. Kogon et al., *Nazi Mass Murder*, 59.

13. Kogon et al., *Nazi Mass Murder*, 175.

14. Kogon et al., *Nazi Mass Murder*, 200.

15. Robert S. Galen et al., "Fetal Pathology and Mechanism of Fetal Death in Saline-Induced Abortion: A Study of 143 Gestations and Critical Review of the Literature," *American Journal of Obstetrics and Gynecology* 120 (October 1, 1974): 352–54.

16. The People of the State of California v. William Baxter Waddill Jr., West Orange County Judicial District, State of California, Case No. 77W2085, April 18, 1977, 39–40.

17. "Do It Yourself: Carbon Monoxide," Mercitron, accessed July 4, 2020, http://mercitron.exblog.jp/.

18. Michael Burleigh, *Death and Deliverance: "Euthanasia" in Germany, 1900–1945* (Cambridge: Cambridge University Press, 1994), 241.

19. Burleigh, *Death and Deliverance*, 240–41.

20. Leon Poliakov, *Harvest of Hate: The Nazi Program for the Destruction of the Jews of Europe*, rev. ed. (New York: Schocken Books, Holocaust Library, 1979), 274.

21. Dr. Miklos Nyiszli, *Auschwitz: A Doctor's Eyewitness Account*, trans. Tibere Kremer and Richard Seaver (Greenwich, CT: Fawcett Crest, 1960), 30, 73.

22. James Bopp, "The Death of Infant Doe," *National Right to Life News*, May 20, 1982, 1, 8.

23. Richard H. Gross et al., "Early Management and Decision-Making for the Treatment of Myelomeningocele," *Pediatrics* 72 (October 1983): 450–53.

24. "Feeding Withdrawal Gets Conditional Nod," *American Medical News*, March 28, 1986, 1.

25. "Feeding Withdrawal Gets Conditional Nod."

26. Terri's Family: Mary and Robert Schindler with Suzanne Schindler Vitadamo and Bobby Schindler, *A Life That Matters: The Legacy of Terri Schiavo—A Lesson for Us All* (New York: Warner Books, 2006), 4.

27. "Transcript of the Proceedings in Case 1," in *The Medical Case*, vol. 1 of *War Crimes Trials*, 1:1214 (testimony of Eugen Kogon).

28. Robert Jay Lifton, *The Nazi Doctors: Medical Killing and the Psychology of Genocide* (New York: Basic Books, 1986), 350–51.

29. Bernd Naumann, *Auschwitz: A Report on the Proceedings against Robert Karl Ludwig Mulka and Others before the Court at Frankfurt*, trans. Jean Steinberg (New York: Frederick A. Praeger, 1966), 137.

30. Naumann, *Auschwitz*, 138.

31. Harold M. Schmeck, "Twin Found Defective in Womb Reported Destroyed in Operation," *New York Times*, June 18, 1981, A1, A19; Matt Clark with Linda R. Prout, "A Choice in the Womb," *Newsweek*, June 29, 1981, 86.

32. Thomas D. Kerenyi and Usha Chitkara, "Selective Birth in Twin Pregnancy with Discordancy for Down's Syndrome," *New England Journal of Medicine* 304 (June 18, 1981): 1527.

33. Planned Parenthood Federation v. Ashcroft, 320 F. Supp. 2d 957 (N.D. Cal. 2004).

34. Mitchell S. Goldbus et al., "Selective Termination of Multiple Gestations," *American Journal of Medical Genetics* 31 (1988): 341.

35. "Death by Doctor," *60 Minutes*, November 22, 1998.

36. Roger S. Magnusson, *Angels of Death: Exploring the Euthanasia Underground* (New Haven, CT: Yale University Press, 2002), 195, 205, 240.

37. Earl W. Kintner, ed., *The Hadamar Trial: Trial of Alfons Klein and Others* (London: William Hodge, 1949), 166.

38. Kintner, *Hadamar Trial*, 174–76, 181.

39. Andrea Sachs, "Abortion Pills on Trial," *Time*, December 5, 1994, 46.

40. Richard U. Hausknecht, "Methotrexate and Misoprostol to Terminate Early Pregnancy," *New England Journal of Medicine* 333 (August 31, 1995): 537.

Chapter 2. Advances in Medicalized Killing Proficiency

1. Earl W. Kintner, ed., *The Hadamar Trial: Trial of Alfons Klein and Others* (London: William Hodge, 1949), 177.

2. Kintner, *Hadamar Trial*, 167.

3. "Transcript of the Proceedings in Case 1," in *The Medical Case*, vol. 1 of *Trials of War Criminals before the Nuernberg Military Tribunals*, 15 vols. (Washington, DC: US Government Printing Office, 1949) (hereafter cited as *War Crimes Trials*), 7391–92 (testimony Dr. Hermann Pfannmueller).

4. Irene Strzelecha, "Hospitals," in *Anatomy of the Auschwitz Death Camp*, ed. Yisrael Gutman and Michael Berenbaum (Bloomington: Indiana University Press, 1994), 389.

5. Extract from a sworn statement by Dr. Erwin Schuler (Ding), July 20, 1945, concerning euthanasia with phenol injection, in *War Crimes Trials*, 1:687.

6. Robert S. Galen et al., "Fetal Pathology and Mechanism of Fetal Death in Saline-Induced Abortion: A Study of 143 Gestations and Critical Review of the Literature," *American Journal of Obstetrics and Gynecology* 120 (October 1, 1974): 352.

7. Yuvol Yaron et al., "Selective Termination and Elective Reduction in Twin Pregnancy: 10 Years Experience at a Single Centre," *Human Reproduction* 13, no. 8 (1998): 2302.

8. Derek Humphry, *Final Exit: The Practicalities of Self-Deliverance and Assisted Suicide for the Dying*, 3rd ed. (New York: Delta, 2002), 163–65.

9. Michael Burleigh, *Death and Deliverance: "Euthanasia" in Germany, 1900–1945* (Cambridge: Cambridge University Press, 1994), 133–34.

10. Joseph Wechsberg, ed. *The Murderers among Us: The Wiesenthal Memoirs* (New York: McGraw-Hill, 1967), 315.

11. Dr. Miklos Nyiszli, *Auschwitz: A Doctor's Eyewitness Account*, trans. Tibere Kremer and Richard Seaver (Greenwich, CT: Fawcett Crest, 1960), 45.

12. Extract from Schuler (Ding) statement, in *War Crimes Trials*, 1:687.

13. Testimony regarding Josef Klehr's techniques of proficient killing can be found in Bernd Naumann, *Auschwitz: A Report on the Proceedings against Robert Karl Ludwig Mulka and Others before the Court at Frankfurt*, trans. Jean Steinberg (New York: Frederick A. Praeger, 1966), 295.

14. Raul Hilberg, *The Destruction of the European Jews*, 3rd ed., 3 vols. (New Haven, CT: Yale University Press, 2003), 3:922.

15. Pamela Zekman and Pamela Warrick, "Dr. Ming Kow Hah: Physician of Pain," *Chicago Sun-Times*, November 15, 1978, 1, 4–5.

16. Usha Citkara et al., "Selective Second-Trimester Termination of the Anomalous Fetus in Twin Pregnancies," *Obstetrics and Gynecology* 73 (May 1989): 693.

17. Planned Parenthood Federation v. Ashcroft, 320 F. Supp. 2d 957 (N.D. Cal. 2004).

18. Roger S. Magnusson, *Angels of Death: Exploring the Euthanasia Underground* (New Haven, CT: Yale University Press, 1993), 23, 148.

19. Nicole Veash, "Abortion: The Right to Choose an Abortion—In Your Lunch Break," *The Independent*, October 15, 1997; "Out to Lunch," *Wall Street Journal*, July 22, 1997, A14.

20. Gitta Sereny, *Into That Darkness: From Mercy Killing to Mass Murder* (London: Andre Deutsch, 1974), 201.

21. Claude Lanzmann, *Shoah: An Oral History of the Holocaust. The Complete Text of the Film* (New York: Pantheon, 1985), 103–4.

22. John F. McDermott and Walter F. Char, "Abortion Repeal in Hawaii: An Unexpected Crisis in Patient Care," *American Journal of Orthopsychiatry* 41 (July 1971): 623; Walter F. Char and John F. McDermott, "Abortion and Acute Identity Crisis in Nurses," *American Journal of Psychiatry* 128 (February 1972): 956.

23. William J. Sweeney with Barbara Lang Stern, *Woman's Doctor: A Year in the Life of an Obstetrician-Gynecologist* (New York: William Morrow, 1973), 207.

24. Suzanne T. Poppema with Mike Henderson, *Why I Am an Abortion Doctor* (Amherst, NY: Prometheus Books, 1996), 22.

25. Peter Korn, *Lovejoy: A Year in the Life of an Abortion Clinic* (New York: Atlantic Monthly Press, 1996), 254.

26. Alexander Mitscherlich and Fred Mielke, *Doctors of Infamy: The Story of the Nazi Medical Crimes*, trans. Heinz Norden (New York: Henry Schuman, 1949), 101.

27. "Affidavit, Nuremberg Doc. No. 3816-PS, Prosecution Exhibit 370," in *The Medical Case*, 1600.

28. "Ending Early Pregnancy the Natural Way," Early Abortion Options, accessed September 28, 2020, https://earlyabortionoptions.com/early-abortion-options/.

29. "Your Early Abortion Options: Aspiration Abortion," Early Options, accessed July 4, 2020, http://www.earlyabortionoptions.com/abortion-method/aspiration-abortion/.

30. Matthew J. Franck, "The Court of the Problem: Terri Schiavo and Supreme Court Precedent," *National Review*, March 30, 2005.

31. "Interview with Michael Schiavo and George Felos," *Larry King Live*, October 27, 2003.

Chapter 3. When Killing Goes Awry

1. Earl W. Kintner, ed., *The Hadamar Trial: Trial of Alfons Klein and Others* (London: William Hodge, 1949), 147–48.

2. Henry Friedlander, *The Origins of Nazi Genocide: From Euthanasia to the Final Solution* (Chapel Hill: University of North Carolina Press, 1995), 170.

3. Olga Lengyel, *Five Chimneys: A Woman Survivor's Story of Auschwitz* (Chicago: Ziff-Davis, 1947), 73.

4. Bernd Naumann, *Auschwitz: A Report on the Proceedings against Robert Karl Ludwig Mulka and Others before the Court at Frankfurt*, trans. Jean Steinberg (New York: Frederick A. Praeger, 1966), 267.

5. Usha Chitkara, "Selective Second-Trimester Termination of the Anomalous Fetus in Twin Pregnancies," *Obstetrics and Gynecology* 73 (May 1989): 692.

6. Richard L. Berkowitz et al., "Selective Reduction of Multifetal Pregnancies in the First Trimester," *New England Journal of Medicine* 318 (April 21, 1988): 1045.

7. Mary K. McKinney, Steven B. Tuber, and Jennifer I. Downey, "Multifetal Pregnancy Reduction: Psychodynamic Implications," *Psychiatry* 59 (Winter 1996): 401.

8. Roger S. Magnusson, *Angels of Death: Exploring the Euthanasia Underground* (New Haven, CT: Yale University Press, 2002), 241, 203.

9. Naumann, *Auschwitz*, 137.

10. Alexander Mitscherlich and Fred Mielke, *Doctors of Infamy: The Story of the Nazi Medical Crimes*, trans. Heinz Norden (New York: Henry Schuman, 1949), 86.

11. Thomas D. Kerenyi, Nathan Mandelman, and David H. Sherman, "Five Thousand Consecutive Saline Inductions," *American Journal of Obstetrics and Gynecology* 116 (July 1, 1973): 598.

12. Berkowitz et al., "Selective Reduction," 1044, 1046.

13. Magnusson, *Angels of Death*, 88.

14. Magnusson, *Angels of Death*, 149–50.

15. Jankiel Wiernik, "One Year in Treblinka," in *The Death Camp Treblinka: A Documentary*, ed. Alexander Donat (New York: Holocaust Library, 1979), 164.

16. Gunther Schwarberg, *The Murders at Bullenhuser Damm: The SS Doctor and the Children*, trans. Erna Baber Rosenfeld and Alvin H. Rosenfeld (Bloomington: Indiana University Press, 1984), 97.

17. The People of the State of California vs. William Baxter Waddill Jr., West Orange County Judicial District, State of California, Case No. 77W2085, April 11, 1977, 141–55.

18. Court of Common Pleas, First Judicial District of Pennsylvania, Criminal Trial Division, *Report of the Grand Jury*, No. 0009901–2008 (Philadelphia: First Judicial District of Pennsylvania, January 14, 2011), 4–5.

19. Court of Common Pleas, *Report of the Grand Jury*, 4–5.

20. Claudia Morain, "Out of the Closet on the Right to Die," *American Medical News*, December 12, 1994, 14–15; Clyde H. Farnsworth, "Vancouver AIDS Suicides Botched," *New York Times*, June 14, 1994, C12.

21. Stephen Jamison, "When Drugs Fail: Assisted Deaths and Not-So-Lethal Drugs," in *Drug Use in Assisted Suicide and Euthanasia*, ed. Margaret P. Batten and Arthur G. Lipman (New York: Pharmaceutical Press/Hayworth Press, 1996), 231–32.

22. Raul Hilberg, *The Destruction of the European Jews*, 3rd ed., 3 vols. (New Haven, CT: Yale University Press, 2003), 3:957.

23. G. M. Gilbert, *The Psychology of Dictatorship* (New York: Ronald Press, 1950), 246.

24. Eugen Kogon, Hermann Langbein, and Adalbert Ruckerl, eds. *Nazi Mass Murder: A Documentary History of the Use of Poison Gas*, trans. Mary Scott and Caroline Lloyd-Morris (New Haven, CT: Yale University Press, 1993), 164–65.

25. Liz Jeffries and Rick Edmonds, "Abortion: The Dreaded Complication," *Philadelphia Inquirer*, August 2, 1981, 4, 5.

26. Planned Parenthood Federation v. Ashcroft, 320 F. Supp. 2d 957 (N.D. Cal. 2004).

27. Carhart v. Ashcroft, 331 F. Supp. 2d 805 (D. Neb. 2004).

28. National Abortion Federation v. Ashcroft, 330 F. Supp. 2d 436 (S.D.N.Y. 2004).

29. Derek Humphry, "Oregon's New Assisted Suicide Law Gives No Sure Comfort to Dying," letter to the editor, *New York Times*, December 3, 1994, 22.

30. B. D. Onwuteaka-Philipsen et al., "Attitudes of Dutch General Practitioners and Nursing Home Physicians to Active Voluntary Euthanasia and Physician-Assisted Suicide," *Archives of Family Medicine* 4 (1995): 951–55.

Chapter 4. Body Disposal

1. G. M. Gilbert, *Nuremberg Diary* (New York: Farrar, Straus, 1947), 250.

2. Dr. Miklos Nyszli, *Auschwitz: A Doctor's Eyewitness Account*, trans. Tibere Kremer and Richard Seaver (Greenwich, CT: Fawcett Crest, 1960), 46–47.

3. Olga Lengyel, *Five Chimneys: A Woman Survivor's True Story of Auschwitz* (Chicago: Ziff-Davis, 1947), 75.

4. Extract from the field interrogation of Kurt Gerstein, April 26, 1945, describing the mass gassing of Jews and other "Undesirables," in *Trials of War Criminals before the Nuernberg Military Tribunals*, 15 vols. (Washington, DC: US Government Printing Office, 1949), 1:869 (hereafter cited as *War Crimes Trials*).

5. National Abortion Federation v. Ashcroft, 330 F. Supp. 2d 436 (S.D.N.Y. 2004).

6. National Abortion Federation v. Ashcroft, 330 F. Supp. 2d 436 (S.D.N.Y. 2004).

7. National Abortion Federation v. Ashcroft, 330 F. Supp. 2d 436 (S.D.N.Y. 2004).

8. Extract from the field interrogation of Kurt Gerstein, in *War Crimes Trials*, 1:866-67.

9. Shmuel Spector, "Aktion 1005—Effacing the Murder of Millions," *Holocaust and Genocide Studies* 5, no. 2 (1990): 157–73.

10. Claire Vitucci, "Fetus Burial," *Associated Press*, October 10, 1998.

11. George F. Will, "54 Babies," *Washington Post*, December 3, 1998, A23.

12. Alexander Mitscherlich and Fred Mielke, *Doctors of Infamy: The Story of the Nazi Medical Crimes*, trans. Heinz Norden (New York: Henry Schuman, 1949), 105.

13. The Jewish Black Book Committee, *The Black Book: Nazi Crimes against the Jewish People* (New York: Duell, Sloan and Pearce, 1946), 388.

14. Lengyel, *Five Chimneys*, 16.

15. Troy Newman with Cheryl Newman, *Their Blood Cries Out*, 2nd ed. (Wichita, KS: Restoration Press, 2003), 62–66.

16. *Abortion: The Inside Story* (Chicago: Pro-Life Action League, 1995), video.

17. "Clinic Boss Admits Dumping Aborted Babies in Trash," *Mainichi Daily News*, Domestic Section, July 24, 2004, 8; "Yokahama Clinic Admits Dumping Aborted Fetuses in Garbage," *Kyodo News Service, Japanese Economic Newswire*, International News Section, July 23, 2004.

18. Henry Friedlander, *The Origins of Nazi Genocide: From Euthanasia to the Final Solution* (Chapel Hill: University of North Carolina Press, 1995), 98.

19. Spector, "Aktion 1005," 159.

20. Jewish Black Book Committee, *Black Book*, 389.

21. "Use of Disposal Sparks Abortion Fireworks," *Omaha World-Herald*, June 11, 1978.

22. "Politics Suggested in Fetal-Disposal Issue," *Up the Creek*, September 11–17, 1992.

23. Suzanne T. Poppema with Mike Henderson, *Why I Am an Abortion Doctor* (Amherst, NY: Prometheus Books, 1996), 163–64.

Chapter 5. Psychological Responses of Health Care Professionals to Participation in Killing

1. Robert Jay Lifton, *The Nazi Doctors: Medical Killing and the Psychology of Genocide* (New York: Basic Books, 1986), 197.

2. Raul Hilberg, *The Destruction of the European Jews*, 3rd ed., 3 vols. (New Haven, CT: Yale University Press, 2003), 1:343–44.

3. Hilberg, *Destruction of the European Jews*, 1:337.

4. Warren M. Hern and Billie Corrigan, "What about Us? Staff Reactions to D&E," *Advances in Planned Parenthood* 15, no. 3 (1980): 5.

5. Hern and Corrigan, "What about Us?," 7.

6. Diane M. Gianelli, "Abortion Providers Share Inner Conflicts," *American Medical News*, July 12, 1993, 3, 37.

7. Lisa H. Harris, "Second Trimester Abortion Provision: Breaking the Silence and Changing the Discourse," supplement, *Reproductive Health Matters* 16, no. 31 (2008): 76.

8. Gina Kolata, "The Job Nobody at the Fertility Clinic Wants," *New York Times*, August 26, 2001, 24.

9. Kenneth R. Stevens, "Emotional and Psychological Effects of Physician-

Assisted Suicide and Euthanasia on Participating Physicians," *Issues in Law and Medicine* 12, no. 3 (2006): 187.

10. Arthur E. Chin et al., "Legalized Physician-Assisted Suicide in Oregon—The First Year's Experience," *New England Journal of Medicine* 340 (February 18, 1999): 583.

11. Erin Hoover, "Doctor Who Assisted Suicide Shocked by the Suddenness," *Oregonian*, June 14, 1998, C2.

12. Lifton, *Nazi Doctors*, 443–44.

13. Ella Lingens-Reiner, *Prisoners of Fear* (London: Victor Gollancz, 1948), 74.

14. Hugh Gregory Gallagher, *By Trust Betrayed: Patients, Physicians, and the License to Kill in the Third Reich* (New York: Henry Holt, 1990), 20–21.

15. Francis J. Kane et al., "Emotional Reactions in Abortion Services Personnel," *Archives of General Psychiatry* 28 (March 1973): 410.

16. Norma Rosen, "Between Guilt and Gratification: Abortion Doctors Reveal Their Feelings," *New York Times Magazine*, April 17, 1977, 71, 73.

17. Roger S. Magnusson, *Angels of Death: Exploring the Euthanasia Underground* (New Haven, CT: Yale University Press, 2002), 114.

18. Magnusson, *Angels of Death*, 144.

19. Lifton, *Nazi Doctors*, 196, 309.

20. Lifton, *Nazi Doctors*, 196.

21. Hern and Corrigan, "What about Us?," 7.

22. Harris, "Second Trimester Abortion Provision," 76, 79, 80.

23. Steven K. Dobscha et al., "Oregon Physicians' Responses to Requests for Assisted Suicide: A Qualitative Study," *Journal of Palliative Medicine* 7 (June 2004): 451, 460.

24. Erich Fromm, "Man Would as Soon Flee as Fight," *Psychology Today* (August 1973): 39, 41.

25. Robert Jay Lifton, "Medicalized Killing in Auschwitz," *Psychiatry* 48 (November 1982): 294.

26. Lifton, *Nazi Doctors*, 442.

27. Lifton, *Nazi Doctors*, 194.

28. Alexander Mitscherlich and Fred Mielke, *Doctors of Infamy: The Story of the Nazi Medical Crimes*, trans. Heinz Norden (New York: Henry Schuman, 1949), 86.

29. Michael Burleigh, *Death and Deliverance: "Euthanasia" in Germany, 1900–1945* (Cambridge: Cambridge University Press, 1994), 159–60, 254.

30. Magda Denes, *In Necessity and Sorrow: Life and Death in an Abortion Hospital* (New York: Basic Books, 1976), 141.

31. Wendy Simonds, *Abortion at Work: Ideology and Practice in a Feminist Clinic* (New Brunswick, NJ: Rutgers University Press, 1996), 97.

32. Susan Squire, "The Gynecologist," *New York Woman* (February 1990): 79.

33. Magnusson, *Angels of Death*, 156, 242.

34. Bernd Naumann, *Auschwitz: A Report on the Proceedings against Robert Karl Ludwig Mulka and Others before the Court at Frankfurt*, trans. Jean Steinberg (New York: Frederick A. Praeger, 1966), 151, 154.

35. Bruno Bettelheim, "Foreword," in Dr. Miklos Nyiszli, *Auschwitz: A Doctor's*

Eyewitness Account, trans. Tibere Kremer and Richard Seaver (Greenwich, CT: Fawcet Crest, 1960), xiii.

36. Carole Joffe, *Doctors of Conscience: The Struggle to Provide Abortion before and after Roe V. Wade* (Boston: Beacon Press, 1995), 195, 174–75.

37. Simonds, *Abortion at Work*, 46.

38. Simonds, *Abortion at Work*, 68.

39. Sarah Kliff, "The Abortion Evangelist," *Newsweek*, August 24, 2009, 44–49.

40. "Northern California Planned Parenthood Counters Anti-Abortion Group's Undercover Videos," KPIX 5 News, August 9, 2015, http://sanfrancisco.cbslocal.com/2015/08/09/northern-california-planned-parenthood-counters-anti-abortion-groups-undercover-videos/.

41. Magnusson, *Angels of Death*, 156, 170, 209.

42. Peter Reagan, "Helen," *The Lancet* 353, no. 9160 (April 10, 1999): 1265–67.

Chapter 6. Experimental Exploitation of Death and Destruction

1. "Transcript of the Proceedings in Case 1," in *The Medical Case*, vol. 1 of *Trials of War Criminals before the Nuernberg Military Tribunals*, 15 vols. (Washington, DC: US Government Printing Office, 1949) (hereafter cited as *War Crimes Trials*), 1:6406 (testimony of Gerhard Rose).

2. "Transcript of the Proceedings in Case 1," 1:4048 (testimony of Karl Gebhardt).

3. Richard Sasuly, *I. G. Farben* (New York: Boni and Gaer, 1947), 126.

4. James A. Thompson et al., "Embryonic Stem Cell Lines Derived from Human Blastocysts," *Science* 282, no. 5391 (November 6, 1998): 1145–47.

5. "Session 6: Human Cloning 3, Policy Issues and Research Cloning," President's Council on Bioethics, January 18, 2002, https://bioethicsarchive.georgetown.edu/pcbe/transcripts/jan02/jan18session6.html.

6. Robert S. Schwartz, "The Politics and Promise of Stem-Cell Research," *New England Journal of Medicine* 355 (September 21, 2006): 119.

7. "Sound Compromise Emerges on Use of Human Embryos: Our View," *USA Today*, July 23, 2001, 14A.

8. "The Embryo Taboos," *New York Times*, July 15, 2001, 14.

9. "Affidavit of Sofia Maczka, 16 April 1946, Concerning Experimental Operations on Inmates of the Ravensbrueck Concentration Camp," in *War Crimes Trials*, 1:404–5.

10. Christian Humpel et al., "Human Fetal Neocortical Tissue Grafted to Rat Brain Cavities Survives, Leads to Reciprocal Nerve Fiber Growth, and Accumulates Host IgG," *Journal of Comparative Neurology* 340 (February 1994): 337–38.

11. "Harvard's Stem Cell Care," *Boston Globe*, June 8, 2006, A14.

12. Nicholas Wade, "What's Next: Rare Hits and Heaps of Misses to Pay For," *New York Times*, November 9, 2010, D1.

13. David Prentice, "Written Testimony of David A. Prentice, PhD: Update on

Progress of Kansas' Midwest Stem Cell Therapy Center Research," Charlotte Lozier Institute, February 8, 2016, https://lozierinstitute.org/written-testimony-of-david-a-prentice-ph-d-update-on-progress-of-kansas-midwest-stem-cell-therapy-center-research/.

14. "Extract from the Closing Brief against Defendant Sievers: Freezing Experiments," in *War Crimes Trials*, 1:200.

15. "Report of 10 October 1942, On Cooling Experiments on Human Beings," in *War Crimes Trials*, 1:242.

16. Geoffrey Chamberlain, "An Artificial Placenta," *American Journal of Obstetrics and Gynecology* 100 (March 1, 1968): 624.

17. Chamberlain, "Artificial Placenta."

18. Robin McKie, "Men Redundant? Now We Don't Need Women Either. Scientists Are Developing an Artificial Womb That Allows Embryos to Grow Outside the Body," *The Observer*, February 10, 2002, 7.

19. "Death after Cooling in Water: Practical and Theoretical Considerations," in *War Crimes Trials*, 1:236.

20. Chamberlain, "Artificial Placenta," 624.

21. "Report from Mrugowsky to the Criminological Institute, 12 September 1944, Concerning Experiments with Aconitine Nitrate Projectiles," in *War Crimes Trials*, 1:635–36.

22. Tryphena Humphrey, "The Development of Human Fetal Activity and Its Relation to Postnatal Behavior," in *Advances in Child Development and Behavior*, ed. Hayne W. Reese and Lewis P. Lipsitt (New York: Academic Press, 1970), 1–57.

23. Humphrey, "Development of Human Fetal Activity," 23, 25.

24. Humphrey, "Development of Human Fetal Activity," 38, 39.

25. "Extracts from the Closing Brief against Defendants Ruff, Romberg, and Weltz," in *War Crimes Trials*, 1:101.

26. "First Interim Report on the Low-Pressure Chamber Experiments in the Concentration Camp of Dachau," in *War Crimes Trials*, 1:146–47.

27. Robert C. Goodlin, "Cutaneous Respiration in a Fetal Incubator," *American Journal of Obstetrics and Gynecology* 86 (July 1, 1963): 574.

28. Bela A. Resch et al., "Comparison of Spontaneous Contraction Rates of In Situ and Isolated Fetal Hearts in Early Pregnancy," *American Journal of Obstetrics and Gynecology* 118 (January 1, 1974): 73–74.

29. Bela A. Resch and Julius G. Papp, "Effects of Caffeine on the Fetal Heart," *American Journal of Obstetrics and Gynecology* 146 (May 15, 1983): 231–32.

30. Leo Alexander, *Neuropathology and Neurophysiology, Including Electro-Encephalography, in Wartime Germany*, Report No. 359 (Washington, DC: Office of the Publication Board, Department of Commerce, July 1945), 20.

31. Michael I. Shevell and Juergen Peiffer, "Julius Hallervorden's Wartime Activities: Implications for Science under Dictatorship," *Pediatric Neurology* 25, no. 2 (2001): 164.

32. "Letter from Sievers to Rudolf Brandt, 9 February 1942, and Report by Hirt Concerning the Acquisition of Skulls of Jewish-Bolshevik Commissars," in *War Crimes Trials*, 1:749.

33. J. Fishman et al., "Catechol Estrogen Formation by the Human Fetal Brain and Pituitary," *Journal of Clinical Endocrinology and Metabolism* 42 (1976): 177–80.

34. Peter A. J. Adam et al., "Oxidation of Glucose and D-B-OH-Butyrate by the Early Human Fetal Brain," *Acta Paediatrica Scandinavica* 64 (1975): 17, 18.

35. William L. Shirer, *The Rise and Fall of the Third Reich: A History of Nazi Germany* (New York: Simon & Schuster, 1960), 979.

36. "Affidavit of Defendant Fischer, 19 November 1946, Concerning Sulfanilamide Experiments Conducted in the Concentration Camp Ravensbrueck," in *War Crimes Trials*, 1:375.

37. "Transcript of the Proceedings in Case 1," 1:4222 (testimony of Fritz Fischer).

38. "Post-Abortion Fetal Study Stirs Storm," *Medical World News*, June 8, 1973, 21.

Chapter 7. Fronts for the Sanitization of Medicine's Dirty Work

1. Everett C. Hughes, "Good People and Dirty Work," *Social Problems* 10 (Summer 1962): 3; also idem, *The Sociological Eye: Selected Readings* (Chicago: Aldine and Atherton, 1971), 87.

2. Dr. Miklos Nyiszli, *Auschwitz: A Doctor's Eyewitness Account*, trans. Tibere Kremer and Richard Seaver (Greenwich, CT: Fawcett Crest, 1960), 46–47.

3. Carole Joffe, "What Abortion Counselors Want from Their Clients," *Social Problems* 26 (October 1978): 119.

4. Carole Joffe, "Abortion Work: Strains, Coping Strategies, Policy Implications," *Social Work* (November 1979): 488.

5. Sallie Tisdale, "We Do Abortions Here: A Nurse's Story," *Harper's Magazine* (October 1987): 68, 70.

6. These and other grisly details regarding Dr. Gosnell's grossly contaminated "House of Horrors" can be found in Court of Common Pleas, First Judicial District of Pennsylvania, Criminal Trial Division, *Report of the Grand Jury*, No. 0009901-2008 (Philadelphia: First Judicial District of Pennsylvania, January 14, 2011), 1–22.

7. Raul Hilberg, *The Destruction of the European Jews*, 3rd ed., 3 vols. (New Haven, CT: Yale University Press, 2003), 1:37.

8. Henry Friedlander, *The Origins of Nazi Genocide: From Euthanasia to the Final Solution* (Chapel Hill: University of North Carolina Press, 1995), 94–95.

9. Olga Lengyel, *Five Chimneys: A Woman Survivor's True Story of Auschwitz* (Chicago: Ziff-Davis, 1947), 14.

10. Dr. Gisella Pearl, *I Was a Doctor in Auschwitz* (New York: International University Press, 1948), 27.

11. Henri Rosencher, "Medicine in Dachau," *British Medical Journal* 2 (December 21, 1946): 953.

12. Dr. Elie A. Cohen, *Human Behavior in the Concentration Camp*, trans. M. H. Braaksma (New York: Grosset & Dunlap, the Universal Library, 1953), 261.

13. Robert Jay Lifton, *The Nazi Doctors: Medical Killing and the Psychology of Genocide* (New York: Basic Books, 1986), 169.

14. Lifton, *Nazi Doctors*, 170.

15. Abraham J. Rongy, *Abortion: Legal or Illegal?* (New York: Vanguard Press, 1933), 130.

16. Mary S. Calderone, "Illegal Abortion as a Public Health Problem," *American Journal of Public Health* 50 (July 1960): 949.

17. Pamela Dillett, "Inside an Abortion Clinic," *National Observer*, February 15, 1975, 18.

18. Helen Dudar, "Abortion for the Asking," *Saturday Review* (April 1973): 31.

19. Herbert McLaughlin, "Clinic Design Emphasizes Restraint to Minimize Patients' Tension," *Modern Hospital* (September 1973): 75.

20. Hilberg, *Destruction of the European Jews*, 3:1097.

21. Robert N. Proctor, *Racial Hygiene: Medicine under the Nazis* (Cambridge, MA: Harvard University Press, 1988), 133.

22. Proctor, *Racial Hygiene*, 189.

23. Hugh Gregory Gallagher, *By Trust Betrayed: Patients, Physicians and the License to Kill in the Third Reich* (New York: Henry Holt, 1990), 132.

24. "'A Total Cleanup': Himmler's Order, July 19, 1942," in *A Holocaust Reader*, ed. Lucy S. Dawidowicz (New York: Behrman House, 1976), 97.

25. Cathy Yarbrough, "Abortion Big Business in Atlanta," *Atlanta Constitution*, July 18, 1973, 3-B.

26. Planned Parenthood of New York City, *Abortion: A Woman's Guide* (New York: Abelard-Schuman, 1973), 22.

27. Wendy Simonds, *Abortion at Work: Ideology and Practice in a Feminist Clinic* (New Brunswick, NJ: Rutgers University Press, 1996), 70.

28. Joffe, "What Abortion Counselors Want," 119.

29. Helena Kubica, "The Crimes of Josef Mengele," in *The Anatomy of the Auschwitz Death Camp*, ed. Yisrael Gutman and Michael Berenbaum (Bloomington: Indiana University Press, 1994), 320–21.

30. Filip Müller, *Eyewitness Auschwitz: Three Years in the Gas Chambers*, ed. and trans. Susanne Flatauer (Chicago: Ivan R. Dee, 1999), 61.

31. Lengyel, *Five Chimneys*, 72, 73.

32. McLaughlin, "Clinic Design Emphasizes Restraint," 74–75.

33. Jeffrey Perlman, "Waddill Trial Has Heavy Impact," *Los Angeles Times*, May 15, 1978, Part I, p. 3.

34. Peter Korn, *Lovejoy: A Year in the Life of an Abortion Clinic* (New York: Atlantic Monthly Press, 1996), 7.

35. Barbara Reynolds, "They Loved Flowers, They Killed People," *USA Today*, April 21, 1983, 9A.

36. Fredric Wertham, MD, *A Sign for Cain: An Exploration of Human Violence* (New York: Macmillan, 1966), 187.

37. Jean-Francois Steiner, *Treblinka*, trans. Helen Weaver (New York: Simon and Schuster, 1967), 208–9.

38. Rosencher, "Medicine in Dachau," 953.

39. "Transcript of the Proceedings in Case 1," in *The Medical Case*, vol. 1 of *Trials of War Criminals before the Nuernberg Military Tribunals*, 15 vols. (Washington, DC: US Government Printing Office, 1949), 8600 (testimony of Paul Dorn).

40. Korn, *Lovejoy*, 7.

41. Kate Pickert, "What Choice?," *Time*, January 14, 2013, http://content.time.com/time/magazine/article/0,/7/,2132761,00.html.

42. Noah Bierman, Phil Long, and Amy Driscoll, "Final Moments: A Still Room, a Hug—Then the Last Breath," *Miami Herald*, April 1, 2005, 1A.

43. Rev. Frank Pavone, *Abolishing Abortion: How You Can Play a Part in Ending the Greatest Evil of Our Day* (Nashville, TN: Nelson Books, 2015), 29.

44. Lengyel, *Five Chimneys*, 71.

45. Alexander Donat, ed., *The Death Camp Treblinka: A Documentary* (New York: Holocaust Library, 1979), 307.

46. Daniel M. Ball, "An Abortion Clinic Ethnography," *Social Problems* 14 (Winter 1967): 299.

47. Mary K. Zimmerman, *Passage through Abortion: The Personal and Social Reality of Women's Experiences* (New York: Praeger, 1977), 180.

48. Verlyn Klinkenborg, "Violent Certainties," *Harper's Magazine* (January 1995): 45.

49. Lengyel, *Five Chimneys*, 14.

50. Eugen Kogon, Hermann Langbein, and Adalbert Rückerl, eds., *Nazi Mass Murder: A Documentary History of the Use of Poison Gas*, trans. Mary Scott and Caroline Lloyd-Morris (New Haven, CT: Yale University Press, 1993), 180.

51. Nyiszli, *Auschwitz*, 44.

52. Rudolf Hoess, *Commandant of Auschwitz: The Autobiography of Rudolf Hoess* (Cleveland: World Publishing Company, 1959), 173.

53. Korn, *Lovejoy*, 242.

54. Dudar, "Abortion for the Asking," 31.

55. Barbara Grizzuti Harrison, "Now That Abortion Is Legal," *McCall's* (November 1973): 70.

Chapter 8. Ideological Foundations
of Medicalized Killing

1. Aleksandr Solzhenitsyn, *The Gulag Archipelago, 1918–1956: An Experiment in Literary Investigation, I-II*, trans. Thomas P. Whitney (New York: Harper and Row, 1973–74), 173–74.

2. Henry Friedlander, *The Origins of Nazi Genocide: From Euthanasia to the Final Solution* (Chapel Hill: University of North Carolina Press, 1995), 197.

3. "A New Ethic for Medicine and Society," *California Medicine* 113 (September 1970): 67–68.

4. Leo Alexander, "Medical Science under Dictatorship," *New England Journal of Medicine* 241 (July 14, 1949): 44.

5. Richard Weikart, *From Darwin to Hitler: Evolutionary Ethics, Eugenics, and Racism in Germany* (New York: Palgrave Macmillan, 2004), 89.

6. Weikart, *From Darwin to Hitler*, 74.

7. Ernst Haeckel, *The Wonders of Life: A Popular Study of Biological Philosophy*, trans. Joseph McCabe (London: Watts, 1904), 22, 123, 124.

8. Daniel Gasman, *The Scientific Origins of National Socialism: Social Darwinism in Ernst Haeckel and the German Monist League* (New York: Elsevier, 1971), 93.

9. Karl Binding and Alfred Hoche, *Permitting the Destruction of Unworthy Life: Its Extent and Form*, trans. Walter E. Wright (Leipzig: Felix Meiner, 1920). [Reprinted in *Issues in Law and Medicine* 8 (February 1992): 246, 258, 260, 261.]

10. Michael S. Bryant, *Confronting the "Good Death": Nazi Euthanasia on Trial, 1945–1953* (Boulder: University Press of Colorado, 2005), 32–35.

11. Bryant, *Confronting the "Good Death,"* 38–39.

12. Bryant, *Confronting the "Good Death,"* 40–41.

13. "Extracts from the Closing Brief against the Defendant Karl Brandt," in *Trials of War Criminals before the Nuernberg Military Tribunals*, 15 vols. (Washington, DC: US Government Printing Office, 1949), 1:799–801 (hereafter cited as *War Crimes Trials*).

14. Robert N. Proctor, *Racial Hygiene: Medicine under the Nazis* (Cambridge, MA: Harvard University Press, 1988), 196, 197.

15. Proctor, *Racial Hygiene*, 6.

16. Guenter Lewy, *The Nazi Persecution of the Gypsies* (Oxford: Oxford University Press, 2000), 55.

17. Weikart, *From Darwin to Hitler*, 157.

18. "Abortion and Race Hygiene," *Journal of the American Medical Association* 105 (July 20, 1935): 213.

19. Leon Poliakov, *Harvest of Hate: The Nazi Program for the Destruction of the Jews of Europe*, rev. ed. (New York: Holocaust Library, 1979), 273.

20. "Circular, Signed by Kaltenbrunner, 9 June 1943, Concerning Interruption of Pregnancy of Female Eastern Workers," in *War Crimes Trials*, 4:1078.

21. "Letter from the Higher SS and Police Leader Southeast to the RKFDV, Katowice, 29 September 1944, Concerning a Pregnancy Interruption," in *War Crimes Trials*, 4:1085–86.

22. Edwin Black, *War against the Weak: Eugenics and America's Campaign to Create a Master Race* (New York: Four Walls Eight Windows, 2003), 25.

23. Christine Rosen, *Preaching Eugenics: Religious Leaders and the American Eugenics Movement* (New York: Oxford University Press, 2004), 77.

24. Black, *War against the Weak*, 52.

25. Martin S. Pernick, *The Black Stork: Eugenics and the Death of "Defective" Babies in American Medicine and Motion Pictures Since 1915* (New York: Oxford University Press, 1999), 95.

26. Margaret Sanger, *Woman and the New Race* (New York: Brentano's, 1920), 63.

27. Ian Dowbiggin, *A Merciful End: The Euthanasia Movement in Modern America* (New York: Oxford University Press, 2003), 198.

28. "Mercy Death Ready for Albany," *New York Times*, February 14, 1939, 2.

29. "'Mercy' Death Law Proposed in State," *New York Times*, January 27, 1939, 21.

30. Dowbiggin, *Merciful End*, 56.

31. Abraham J. Rongy, *Abortion: Legal or Illegal?* (New York: Vanguard Press, 1933), 51–54.

32. Fredrick J. Taussig, *Abortion Spontaneous and Induced: Medical and Social Aspects* (St. Louis: C. V. Mosby, 1936), 318, 320.

33. Mary S. Calderone, ed., *Abortion in the United States* (New York: Hoeber-Harper, 1958), 115.

34. "AMA Policy on Therapeutic Abortion," *Journal of the American Medical Association* 201 (August 14, 1967): 544.

35. Mark I. Evans, "Efficacy of Second-Trimester Selective Termination for Fetal Abnormalities: International Collaborative Experience among the World's Largest Centers," *American Journal of Obstetrics and Gynecology* 171 (July 1994): 90.

36. Amy Harmon, "Genetic Testing + Abortion = ???," *New York Times*, May 13, 2007, 4:4.

37. Amy Harmon, "In New Tests of Fetal Defects, Agonizing Choices for Parents," *New York Times*, June 20, 2004, A24.

38. Emily Brazelon, "The Place of Women on the Court," *New York Times Magazine*, July 12, 2009, 47.

39. Brazelon, "Place of Women on the Court."

40. Joseph Fletcher, "Indicators of Humanhood: A Tentative Profile of Man," *Hastings Center Report* 2 (November 1972): 1–3.

41. Raymond S. Duff and A. G. M. Campbell, "Moral and Ethical Dilemmas in the Special-Care Nursery," *New England Journal of Medicine* 289 (October 25, 1973): 890, 892.

42. Anthony Shaw, "Defining the Quality of Life," *Hastings Center Report* 7 (October 1977): 91–92.

43. Richard H. Gross et al., "Early Management and Decision Making for the Treatment of Myelomeningocele," *Pediatrics* 72 (October 1983): 450, 452–53, 456.

44. Helga Kushse and Peter Singer, *Should the Baby Live? The Problem of Handicapped Infants* (Oxford: Oxford University Press, 1985), 120.

45. Peter Singer, *Practical Ethics*, 2nd ed. (Cambridge: Cambridge University Press, 1993), 183.

46. Peter Singer, *Rethinking Life and Death: The Collapse of Our Traditional Ethics* (New York: St. Martin's Griffin, 1994), 190.

47. Eduard Verhagen and Pieter J. J. Sauer, "The Groningen Protocol—Euthanasia in Severely Ill Newborns," *New England Journal of Medicine* 352 (March 10, 2005): 959–62.

48. Robert Perlman et al., *Your Life, Your Choices: Planning for Future Medical Decisions: How to Prepare a Personalized Living Will* (Washington, DC: Department of Veterans Affairs, 1997).

49. Perlman et al., *Your Life, Your Choices*, 21.

50. Perlman et al., *Your Life, Your Choices*, 21.

51. Jim Towey, "The Death Book for Veterans: Ex-Soldiers Don't Need to Be Told They're a Burden to Society," *Wall Street Journal*, August 19, 2009, A13.

Chapter 9. The Quality-of-Life Ideology and Semantic Gymnastics

1. "A New Ethic for Medicine and Society," *California Medicine* 113 (September 1970): 67–68.

2. "New Ethic for Medicine and Society," 68.

3. "New Ethic for Medicine and Society," 68.

4. Fredric Wertham, MD, *A Sign for Cain: An Exploration of Human Violence* (New York: Macmillan, 1966), 153.

Chapter 10. The Imposition of Dehumanizing Labels

1. Raul Hilberg, *The Destruction of the European Jews*, 3rd ed., 3 vols. (New Haven, CT: Yale University Press, 2003), 1:13.

2. Helen Fein, *Accounting for Genocide: National Responses and Jewish Victimization During the Holocaust* (New York: Free Press, 1979), 8.

3. Clarissa Henry and Marc Hillel, *Of Pure Blood*, trans. Eric Mossbacher (New York: McGraw Hill, 1976), 32.

4. "Selected Letters of Doctor Friedrich Mennecke: Introduced and Annotated by Peter Chroust," in *Cleansing the Fatherland: Nazi Medicine and Racial Hygiene*, ed. Götz Aly, Peter Chroust, and Christian Pross, trans. Belinda Cooper (Baltimore: Johns Hopkins University Press, 1994), 250.

5. Götz Aly, "Medicine against the Useless," in *Cleansing the Fatherland*, 53.

6. "Letter from Sievers to Rudolf Brandt, 9 February 1942, and Report by Hirt Concerning the Acquisition of Skulls of Jewish-Bolshevik Commissars," in *Trials of War Criminals before the Nuernberg Military Tribunals*, 15 vols. (Washington, DC: US Government Printing Office, 1949), 1:749 (hereafter cited as *War Crimes Trials*).

7. Garrett Hardin, "Abortion—Or Compulsory Pregnancy?," *Journal of Marriage and the Family* 30 (May 1968): 250–51.

8. Amitai Etzioni, "A Review of the Ethics of Fetal Research," *Society* (March/April 1976): 72.

9. Wendy Simonds, *Abortion at Work: Ideology and Practice in a Feminist Clinic* (New Brunswick, NJ: Rutgers University Press, 1996), 84, 81.

10. Joseph Fletcher, "The Right to Die: A Theologian Comments," *Atlantic Monthly* (April 1968): 62.

11. Francis A. Schaeffer and C. Everett Koop, *Whatever Happened to the Human Race* (Old Tappan, NJ: Fleming H. Revell, 1979), 73.

12. Hilberg, *Destruction of the European Jews*, 3:1118.

13. Ernst Fraenkel, *The Dual State: A Contribution to the Theory of Dictatorship*, trans. E. A. Shils with Edith Lowenstein and Klaus Knorr (New York: Oxford University Press, 1941), 95.

14. George L. Mosse, *Toward the Final Solution: A History of European Racism* (New York: Howard Fertig, 1978), 210–11.

15. Michael Burleigh, *Death and Deliverance: "Euthanasia" in Germany, 1900–1945* (Cambridge: Cambridge University Press, 1994), 284, 285.

16. Hannah Arendt, *The Origins of Totalitarianism* (New York: Harcourt Brace Jovanovich, 1973), 290.

17. Richard L. Rubenstein, *The Cunning of History: Mass Death and the American Future* (New York: Harper and Row, 1975), 87.

18. Roe v. Wade, 410 U.S. 158, 162 (1973).

19. John Lachs, "Humane Treatment and the Treatment of Humans," *New England Journal of Medicine* 294 (April 8, 1976): 838–40.

20. Michael Tooley, *Abortion and Infanticide* (New York: Oxford University Press, 1983), 411.

21. A. Giubilini and F. Minerva, "After-Birth Abortion: Why Should the Baby Live?," *Journal of Medical Ethics* 39, no. 5 (2013): 261–63.

22. Richard Weikart, *From Darwin to Hitler: Evolutionary Ethics, Eugenics, and Racism in Germany* (New York: Palgrave Macmillan, 2004), 147.

23. Karl Binding and Alfred Hoche, *Permitting the Destruction of Unworthy Life: Its Extent and Form*, trans. Walter E. Wright (Leipzig: Felix Meiner, 1920). [Reprinted in *Issues in Law and Medicine* 8 (Fall 1992): 262.]

24. "Opening Statement of the Prosecution by Brigadier General Telford Taylor, 9 December 1946," in *War Crimes Trials*, 1:27.

25. Philippe Aziz, *Doctors of Death*, 4 vols., trans. Edouard Bizul and Philip Haentzler (Geneva: Ferni, 1976), 1:232.

26. Howard D. Kibel, "Staff Reactions to Abortion: A Psychiatric View," *Obstetrics and Gynecology* 39 (January 1972): 131.

27. Mary Anne Warren, "On the Moral and Legal Status of Abortion," *The Monist* 57 (January 1973): 58.

28. "Abortion Controversy—The Silent Scream," *Nightline*, February 12, 1985.

29. Carl Sagan and Ann Druyan, "Is It Possible to Be Pro-Life and Pro-Choice?," *Parade Magazine*, April 22, 1990, 6, 8.

30. George H. Ball, "What Happens at Conception?," *Christianity and Crisis*, October 19, 1981, 286.

31. Peter Singer, "Sanctity of Life or Quality of Life?," *Pediatrics* 72 (July 1983): 129.

32. W. T. Belfield, "Racial Suicide for Social Parasites," *Journal of the American Medical Association* 50 (January 4, 1908): 55–56.

33. Edwin Black, *War against the Weak: Eugenics and America's Campaign to Create a Master Race* (New York: Four Walls Eight Windows, 2003), 255.

34. George Williams Hunter, *A Civic Biology: Presented in Problems* (New York: American Book Company, 1914), 263.

35. Friedrich Wilhelm Nietzsche, *Twilight of the Idols and the Anti Christ*, trans. R. J. Hollingdale (Baltimore: Penguin, 1968), 88.

36. "The Jew as Global Parasite," in *The Holocaust: Selected Documents in Eighteen Volumes*, vol. 4, *Propaganda and Aryanization, 1938–1944*, ed. John Mendelsohn (New York: Garland, 1982), 86–90.

37. Michael H. Kater, *Doctors under Hitler* (Chapel Hill: University of North Carolina Press, 1989), 119.

38. Leon Poliakov, *Harvest of Hate: The Nazi Program for the Destruction of the Jews of Europe*, rev. ed. (New York: Schocken Books, Holocaust Library, 1979), 265.

39. Warren M. Hern, *Abortion Practice* (Philadelphia: J. B. Lippincott, 1984), 14–15.

40. Rosalind Pollack Petchesky, *Abortion and Women's Choice: The State, Sexuality, and Reproductive Freedom* (Boston: Northeastern University Press, 1984), 346.

41. Rachel Conrad Wahlberg, "The Woman and the Fetus: 'One Flesh'?," *New Women/New Church* (September-October 1987): 5.

42. Daniel Callahan, "On Feeding the Dying," *Hastings Center Report* 13 (October 1983): 22.

43. Robert Jay Lifton, *The Nazi Doctors: Medical Killing and the Psychology of Genocide* (New York: Basic Books, 1986), 16–17.

44. Irmgard Grube affidavit, "Transcript of the Proceedings in Case 1," in *The Medical Case*, vol. 1 of *War Crimes Trials*, 1:7569 (testimony Viktor Brack).

45. Aly, "Medicine against the Useless," in *Cleansing the Fatherland*, 49.

46. Robert N. Proctor, *Racial Hygiene: Medicine under the Nazis* (Cambridge, MA: Harvard University Press, 1988), 183.

47. "Shall This Child Die?," *Newsweek*, November 12, 1973, 70.

48. Lachs, "Humane Treatment," 838–40.

49. "To Feed or Not to Feed?," *Time*, March 31, 1986, 60; Mark Rust, "AMA Policy Cited in Coma Decisions," *American Medical News*, May 2, 1986, 1, 10.

50. Timothy E. Quill, "Terri Schiavo—A Tragedy Compounded," *New England Journal of Medicine* 352 (April 21, 2005): 1630.

51. Nicole Hahn Rafter, *White Trash: Eugenic Family Studies 1877–1919* (Boston: Northeastern University Press, 1988), 2; "White Trash: Eugenics as Social Ideology," *Society* 26 (December 1988): 44.

52. E. E. Southard, "The Feeble-Minded as Subjects of Research in Efficiency" (presented at the National Conference of Charities and Corrections, Baltimore, May 12–19, 1915).

53. Margaret Sanger, *The Pivot of Civilization* (Amherst, NY: Humanity Books, 1922, 2003), 130–33.

54. Binding and Hoche, *Permitting the Destruction of Unworthy Life*, 261.

55. Poliakov, *Harvest of Hate*, 112, 115.

56. Rolf Hochhuth, *A German Love Story*, trans. John Browjohn (Boston: Little, Brown, 1980), 18.

57. Lifton, *Nazi Doctors*, 179.

58. Nick Thimmesch, "Bizarre Cases of Abortions Gone Awry," *St. Louis Globe-Democrat*, June 19–20, 1982, 5B.

59. Seth Effron and Jane Floerchinger, "Wichita Bans Burning Fetuses in Incinerator," *Wichita Eagle-Beacon*, August 2, 1983, 2A.

60. "Forum: Ethics in Embryo," *Harper's Magazine*, September 1987, 38.

61. Adam Withnall, "Thousands of Unborn Foetuses Incinerated to Heat UK Hospitals," *Independent*, March 24, 2014, https://www.independent.co.uk/life-style/health-and-families/health-news/thousands-unborn-foetuses-incinerated-heat-uk-hospitals-9212863.html.

62. Dr. Eowyn, "Oregon's Covanta Plant Incinerates Aborted Babies to Generate Electricity," Fellowship of the Minds, April 24, 2014, https://fellowshipoftheminds.com/oregons-covanta-plant-incinerates-aborted-babies-to-generate-electricity.

63. Terry Mizrahi, *Getting Rid of Patients: Contradictions in the Socialization of Physicians* (New Brunswick, NJ: Rutgers University Press, 1986), 66.

64. Melvin Konner, *Becoming a Doctor: A Journey of Initiation in Medical School* (New York: Viking Press, 1987), 383.

65. Roger Jeffrey, "Normal Rubbish: Deviant Patients in Casualty Departments," *Sociology of Health and Illness* 1 (June 1979): 92, 94.

66. Leo Alexander, *Neuropathology and Neurophysiology, Including Electro-Encephalography, in Wartime Germany*, Report No. 359 (Washington, DC: Office of the Publication Board, Department of Commerce, July 1945), 20–21.

67. William E. Seidelman, "Mengele Medicus: Medicine's Nazi Heritage," *Millbank Quarterly* 66, no. 2 (1988): 226.

68. Lifton, *Nazi Doctors*, 341.

69. Lifton, *Nazi Doctors*, 361–62.

70. "Diary of Johann Paul Kremer," in *K L Auschwitz Seen by the SS: Hoss, Broad, Kremer*, trans. Constantine FitzGibbon and Krystyna Michalik (New York: Howard Fertig, 1984), 221, 222.

71. Lifton, *Nazi Doctors*, 293.

72. Eric S. Jacobson and Martha Goetsch, "Cytologic Identification of Trophoblastic Epithelium in Products of First-Trimester Abortion," *Obstetrics and Gynecology* 66 (July 1985): 124–26.

73. The verbatim transcript of this meeting—titled "Council of Europe, Parliamentary Assembly: Joint Hearing of the Legal Affairs Committee, the Sub-Committee on Bio-Ethics of the Committee on Social and Health Questions, and the Committee on Science and Technology"—is published in the journal *Human Reproduction* 1 (1986): 463–91. The references to Dr. Andersson's comments can be found on pages 485 and 489.

74. Peter Korn, *Lovejoy: A Year in the Life of an Abortion Clinic* (New York: Atlantic Monthly Press, 1996), 236–37.

75. "Investigative Footage," Center for Medical Progress, accessed August 31, 2020, http://www.centerformedicalprogress.org/cmp/investigative-footage/.

76. "Investigative Footage."

77. "Investigative Footage."

Chapter 11. Treatment for Disease

1. Steven Selden, *Inheriting Shame: The Story of Eugenics and Racism in America* (New York: Teachers College Press 1999), 4.

2. Edwin Black, *War against the Weak: Eugenics and America's Campaign to Create a Master Race* (New York: Four Walls Eight Windows, 2003), 57, 59, 75.

3. John F. Fitzgerald, "The Duty of the State toward Its Idiots and Feebleminded," *Albany Medical Annals* 22 (March 1901): 129.

4. Martin W. Barr, *Mental Defectives: Their History, Treatment and Training* (Philadelphia: P. Blakiston's Sons, 1913), 190.

5. Lothrop Stoddard, *The Rising Tide of Color against White World-Supremacy* (New York: Charles Scribner's Sons, 1922), 259–60.

6. Ernst Haeckel, *The Wonders of Life: A Popular Study of Biological Philosophy*, trans. Joseph McCabe (London: Watts, 1904), 122.

7. Daniel Gasman, *The Scientific Origins of National Socialism: Social Darwinism in Ernst Haeckel and the German Monist League* (New York: Elsevier, 1971), 93.

8. Adolf Hitler, *Mein Kampf,* trans. Ralph Manheim (Boston: Houghton Mifflin Company, 1971), 46, 58, 78, 233, 247, 248, 249, 253.

9. Robert N. Proctor, *Racial Hygiene: Medicine under the Nazis* (Cambridge, MA: Harvard University Press, 1988), 196.

10. Michael H. Kater, *Doctors under Hitler* (Chapel Hill: University of North Carolina Press, 1989), 178.

11. Robert Jay Lifton, *The Nazi Doctors: Medical Killing and the Psychology of Genocide* (New York: Basic Books, 1986), 15–16.

12. Proctor, *Racial Hygiene,* 214–15.

13. Donald Kenrick and Grattan Puxon, *The Destiny of Europe's Gypsies* (New York: Basic Books, 1972), 100.

14. "Disease of Unwanted Pregnancy," *Time,* September 15, 1967, 84.

15. Natalie Shainess, "Abortion Is No Man's Business," *Psychology Today* (May 1970): 20.

16. Joseph Fletcher, *Humanhood: Essays in Biomedical Ethics* (Buffalo, NY: Hoeber-Harper, 1958), 164.

17. Willard Cates, David A. Grimes, and Jack C. Smith, "Abortion as a Treatment for Unwanted Pregnancy: The Number Two Sexually-Transmitted Condition," *Advances in Planned Parenthood* 12, no. 3 (1978): 115–21.

18. Robert E. Hall, ed., *Abortion in a Changing World,* 2 vols. (New York: Columbia University Press, 1970), 1:46.

19. Sara Rimer, "An Abortion-Clinic Rounds: Forceps and Bulletproof Vest," *New York Times,* September 3, 1993, A12.

20. "Circular, 5 April 1943, Containing the Decree of Reich Health Leader Dr. Conti, Concerning the Interruption of Pregnancy of Female Eastern Workers," in *Trials of War Criminals before the Nuernberg Military Tribunals,* 15 vols. (Washington, DC: US Government Printing Office, 1949), 4:1094–95 (hereafter cited as *War Crimes Trials*).

21. "Transcript of the Proceedings in Case 1," in *The Medical Case,* vol. 1 of *War Crimes Trials,* 1:7392–94 (testimony Hermann Pfannmuller).

22. "Direct Examination of Heinrich Ruoff," in *The Hadamar Trial: Trial of Alfons Klein and Others,* ed. Earl W. Kintner (London: William Hodge, 1949), 176.

23. Lifton, *Nazi Doctors,* 307.

24. Kenrick and Puxon, *Destiny of Europe's Gypsies,* 148, 161.

25. Bernd Naumann, *Auschwitz: A Report on the Proceedings against Robert Karl Mulka and Others before the Court at Frankfurt,* trans. Jean Steinberg (New York: Frederick A. Praeger, 1966), 79, 140.

26. Cates et al., "Abortion as a Treatment," 119–20.

27. Franca Fruzzetti et al., "Use of Sulprostone for Induction of Preoperative Cervical Dilation or Uterine Evacuation: A Comparison of Different Treatment Schedules," *Obstetrics and Gynecology* 72 (November 1988): 704–8.

28. Suzanne T. Poppema with Mike Henderson, *Why I Am an Abortion Doctor* (Amherst, NY: Prometheus Books, 1996), 11, 138, 191–97, 201–5.

29. Rita L. Marker, "The Art of Verbal Engineering," *Duquesne Law Review* 35 (1996): 95.

30. George J. Annas, "'Culture of Life' Politics at the Bedside—The Case of Terri Schiavo," *New England Journal of Medicine* 352 (April 21, 2005): 1714.

31. Alan M. Altman et al., "Midtrimester Abortion with Laminaria and Vacuum Evacuation on a Teaching Service," *Journal of Reproductive Medicine* 30 (August 1985): 602.

32. Jeff Burbank, "Doctor Tells Nurse's View of Abortion," *Las Vegas Review-Journal*, November 1, 1990, 1A.

33. "Doctors of the Death Camps," *Time*, June 25, 1979, 68.

34. Lifton, *Nazi Doctors*, 18.

35. Rudolf Hoess, *Commandant of Auschwitz: The Autobiography of Rudolf Hoess*, trans. Constantine FitzGibbon (Cleveland, OH: World Publishing Co., 1959), 162–63.

36. Hannah Arendt, *Eichmann in Jerusalem: A Report on the Banality of Evil*, rev. ed. (New York: Viking Press, 1965), 69.

37. "Position Statement on Abortion," *American Journal of Psychiatry* 126 (April 1970): 1554.

38. Zigmund Lebensohn, "Legal Abortion as a Positive Mental Health Measure in Family Planning," *Comprehensive Psychiatry* 14 (March/April 1973): 95.

39. Thomas D. Kerenyi and Usha Chitkara, "Selective Birth in Twin Pregnancy with Discordancy for Down's Syndrome," *New England Journal of Medicine* 304 (June 18, 1981): 1525–27.

40. Kirk Johnson, "Webster v. Reproductive Health Services: the AMA Position," *Journal of the American Medical Association* 262 (September 15, 1989): 1522.

41. Edward Walsh, "No Legal Action Is Anticipated as Kevorkian Suicides Multiply," *Washington Post*, August 24, 1996, A2.

Chapter 12. Choice and Selection

1. Malkah T. Notman, "Pregnancy and Abortion: Implications for Career Development of Professional Women," *Annals of the National Academy of Sciences* 208 (March 15, 1973): 209.

2. Seth Mydans, "When Is an Abortion Not an Abortion?," *Atlantic Monthly* (May 1975): 72.

3. Elizabeth Kaye, "She Does Abortions: A Doctor's Story," *Mademoiselle* (February 1988): 151, 153.

4. "A Dear Colleague" membership campaign letter mailed to Wyoming physicians from Nancy Neufeld, coordinator for Physicians for Choice, December 2, 1983.

5. Carole Joffe, *Doctors of Conscience: The Struggle to Provide Abortion before and after Roe V. Wade* (Boston: Beacon Press, 1995), 207.

6. "APA Actions on Reproductive Rights," *American Journal of Psychiatry* 145 (May 1992): 723.

7. NARAL Pro-Choice America, "Directives on New Name," press release, January 6, 2003.

8. Douglas Johnson, "Unholy Messaging," National Review Online, October 7, 2008, https://www.nationalreview.com/2008/10/unholy-messaging-douglas-johnson/.

9. Derek Humphry, "Give the Dying Freedom of Choice," *USA Today*, November 16, 1988, 8A.

10. Steven Ertelt, "Hemlock Society Changes Name to Moderate Its Image," LifeNews.com, July 24, 2003, www.lifenews.com/2003/07/24/bio-16/.

11. The terminology employed by Compassion and Choices can be found on their website, accessed July 6, 2020, http://www.compassionandchoices.org.

12. "Organized Efforts Continue to Target States for Legalized Assisted Suicide," *Update: International Task Force on Euthanasia and Assisted Suicide* 23, no. 5 (2009): 1–2.

13. "Health Insurance Reform," Compassion and Choices, August 13, 2009, http://www.compassionandchoices.org/act/legislative_work/healthcare_reform.

14. Ernst Haeckel, *The History of Creation; Or the Development of the Earth and Its Inhabitants by the Action of Natural Causes*, trans. E. Ray Lankester, 4th ed., vol. 1 (New York: D. Appleton, 1892), 175–78.

15. "Selected Letters of Doctor Freidrich Mennecke: Introduction: Introduced and Annotated by Peter Chroust," in *Cleansing the Fatherland: Nazi Medicine and Racial Hygiene*, ed. Götz Aly, Peter Chroust, and Christian Pross, trans. Belinda Cooper (Baltimore: Johns Hopkins University Press 1994), 244.

16. Eugen Kogon, Hermann Langbein, and Adalbert Rückerl, eds., *Nazi Mass Murder: A Documentary History of the Use of Poison Gas*, trans. Mary Scott and Caroline Lloyd-Morris (New Haven, CT: Yale University Press, 1993), 174, 176.

17. Robert Jay Lifton, *The Nazi Doctors: Medical Killing and the Psychology of Genocide* (New York: Basic Books, 1986), 186.

18. Bernd Naumann, *Auschwitz: A Report on the Proceedings against Robert Karl Ludwig Mulka and Others before the Court at Frankfurt*, trans. Jean Steinberg (New York: Frederick A. Praeger, 1966), 155.

19. Thomas D. Kerenyi and Usha Chitkara, "Selective Birth in Twin Pregnancy with Discordancy for Down's Syndrome," *New England Journal of Medicine* 304 (June 18, 1981): 1525–27.

20. Mark I. Evans et al., "Selective First-Trimester Termination in Octuplet and Quadruplet Pregnancies: Clinical and Ethical Issues," *Obstetrics and Gynecology* 71 (March 1988): 293.

21. Mara Havistendahl, *Unnatural Selection: Choosing Boys over Girls, and the Consequences of a World Full of Men* (New York: Public Affairs, 2011), 24, 42, 46, 56, 150, 250.

22. Havistendahl, *Unnatural Selection*, xviii.

23. Ross Douthat, "160 Million and Counting," *New York Times*, June 25, 2011, A21.

24. J. Lorber, "Early Results of Selective Treatment of Spina Bifida Cystica," *British Medical Journal* 4 (October 27, 1973): 201–4.

25. Richard H. Gross et al., "Early Management and Decision Making for the Treatment of Myelemeningocele," *Pediatrics* 72 (October 1983): 450–53, 455, 456.

26. Gross et al., "Early Management and Decision Making," 450, 451, 456.

27. Naumann, *Auschwitz*, 150–51.

28. Leon Poliakov, *Harvest of Hate: The Nazi Program for the Destruction of the*

Jews of Europe, rev. ed. (New York: Schocken Books, Holocaust Library, 1979), 268.

29. Raul Hilberg, *The Destruction of the European Jews*, 3rd ed., 3 vols. (New Haven, CT: Yale University Press, 2003), 2:527.

30. Gerald Reitlinger, *The Final Solution: The Attempt to Exterminate the Jews of Europe, 1939–1945* (New York: A. S. Barnes, 1961), 243.

31. Judgment of the Tribunal, *Trials of War Criminals before the Nuernberg Military Tribunals*, 15 vols. (Washington, DC: US Government Printing Office, 1949), 2:250.

32. Götz Aly, "Medicine against the Useless," in Aly et al., *Cleansing the Fatherland*, 66–67.

33. Ana Montesguardo and Ivan E. Timor-Tritsch, "Transvaginal Multifetal Pregnancy Reduction: Which? When? How Many?," *Annals of Medicine* 25 (1993): 276.

34. Josef Shalev et al., "Selective Reduction in Multiple Gestations: Pregnancy Outcome after Transvaginal and Transabdominal Needle-Guided Procedures," *Fertility and Sterility* 52 (September 1989): 416–19.

35. S. Lipitz et al., "A Comparative Study of Multifetal Pregnancy Reduction from Triplets to Twins in the First versus Early Second Trimesters after Detailed Fetal Scans," *Ultrasound in Obstetrics and Gynecology* 18 (July 2001): 35–36.

36. Mark I. Evans, "The Truth about Multiple Births," *Newsweek*, March 2, 2009, www.ivfquestion.com/topic/essay-by-dr-mark-evans-in-this-weeks-newsweek.

37. Mark I. Evans et al., "What Are the Ethical and Technical Problems Associated with Multifetal Pregnancy Reduction?," *Clinical Obstetrics and Gynecology* 41 (March 1998): 47, 52.

38. Mark I. Evans, et al., "Fetal Reduction from Twins to a Singleton: A Reasonable Consideration?," *Obstetrics and Gynecology* 104 (July 2004): 102.

39. Ruth Padawar, "The Two-Minus-One Pregnancy," *New York Times Magazine*, August 14, 2011, 24–27.

40. Pearl S. Buck, "Foreword," in *The Terrible Choice: The Abortion Dilemma*, ed. Robert E. Cooke, MD, et al. (New York: Bantam Books, 1968), x.

Chapter 13. Distortions of the Evacuation Designation

1. Götz Aly, "Medicine against the Useless," in *Cleansing the Fatherland: Nazi Medicine and Racial Hygiene*, ed. Götz Aly, Peter Chroust, and Christian Pross, trans. Belinda Cooper (Baltimore: Johns Hopkins University Press, 1994), 48–50.

2. Hugh Gregory Gallagher, *By Trust Betrayed: Patients, Physicians, and the License to Kill in the Third Reich* (New York: Henry Holt, 1990), 111.

3. The Jewish Black Book Committee, *The Black Book: The Nazi Crime against the Jewish People* (New York: Duell, Sloan and Pearce, 1946), 329.

4. "Extracts from the Closing Brief of the Defendant Karl Brandt," in *Trials of War Criminals before the Nuernberg Military Tribunals*, 15 vols. (Washington, DC: US Government Printing Office, 1949), 1:826.

5. Raul Hilberg, *The Destruction of the European Jews*, 3rd ed., 3 vols. (New Haven, CT: Yale University Press, 2003), 2:421–22.

6. Eugen Kogon, Hermann Langbein, and Adalbert Ruckerl, eds. *Nazi Mass Murder: A Documentary History of the Use of Poison Gas*, trans. Mary Scott and Caroline Lloyd-Morris (New Haven, CT: Yale University Press, 1993), 154.

7. Hilberg, *Destruction of European Jews*, 2:544.

8. Gerald Reitlinger, *The Final Solution: The Attempt to Exterminate the Jews of Europe, 1939–1945* (New York: A. S. Barnes, A Perpetua Book, 1961), 491.

9. Philip S. Green, "Office Abortion: A Humane Approach to a Traumatic Experience," *Journal of the Medical Society of New Jersey* 77 (November 1980): 809, 810.

10. George J. L. Wulff and Michael Freiman, "Elective Abortion: Complications Seen in a Free-Standing Abortion Clinic," *Obstetrics and Gynecology* 49 (March 1977): 352–55.

11. P. G. Stubblefield, "Surgical Techniques of Uterine Evacuation in First- and Second-Trimester Abortion," *Clinics in Obstetrics and Gynecology* 13 (March 1986): 63–66.

12. Warren M. Hern, "Laminaria, Induced Fetal Demise and Misoprostol in Late Abortion," *International Journal of Obstetrics and Gynecology* 75 (2001): 281.

13. Planned Parenthood Federation v. Ashcroft, 320 F. Supp. 2d 957 (N.D. Cal. 2004).

14. Joe Ortwerth accessed information regarding Washington University's Family Planning Fellowship on June 28, 2008. For his exposure of the Washington University Family Planning Fellowship Program, see the *Missouri Family Policy Council Newsletter*, September 14, 2009.

15. Hilberg, *Destruction of European Jews*, 2:550.

16. Hilberg, *Destruction of European Jews*, 2:743.

17. Hilberg, *Destruction of European Jews*, 2:544.

18. Hilberg, *Destruction of European Jews*, 2:906.

19. Robert N. Proctor, *Racial Hygiene: Medicine under the Nazis* (Cambridge, MA: Harvard University Press, 1988), 211.

20. Hilberg, *Destruction of European Jews*, 3:1097.

21. Gallagher, *By Trust Betrayed*, 115.

22. Barbara Goldsmith, "The Woman Who Avenged the Children of Izieu," *Parade Magazine*, January 22, 1984, 4.

23. Warren M. Hern, *Abortion Practice* (Philadelphia: J. B. Lippincott, 1984), 107.

24. Warren M. Hern, "Serial Multiple Laminaria and Adjunctive Urea in Late Outpatient Dilatation and Evacuation Abortion," *Obstetrics and Gynecology* 63 (April 1984): 544.

25. T. P. Dutt et al., "Ultrasonic Assessment of Uterine Emptying in First-Trimester Abortions Induced by Intravaginal 15-methyl prostaglandin F2a methyl ester," *American Journal of Obstetrics and Gynecology* 133 (March 1, 1979): 484, 487.

26. Planned Parenthood Federation v. Ashcroft, 320 F. Supp. 2d 957 (N.D. Cal. 2004).

27. "Politics Suggested in Fetal-Disposal Issue," *Up the Creek*, September 11-17, 1992.

28. "What Are the Types of Abortion Procedures?," WebMD, accessed July 6, 2020, http://www.webmd.com/women/manual-and-vacuum-aspiration-for-abortion.

29. Hern, *Abortion Practice*, 107, 152, 153, 155.

30. National Abortion Federation v. Ashcroft, 330 F. Supp. 2d 436 (S.D.N.Y. 2004).

Chapter 14. Decent Perpetrators and
Their Humane Services

1. Helen Fein, *Accounting for Genocide: National Responses and Jewish Victimization During the Holocaust* (New York: Free Press, 1979), 25.

2. Fredric Wertham, MD, *A Sign for Cain: An Exploration of Human Violence* (New York: Macmillan, 1966), 171.

3. Benno Muller-Hill, "Genetics after Auschwitz," in *The Nazi Holocaust: Historical Articles on the Destruction of European Jews, 3. The "Final Solution," the Implementation of Mass Murder*, vol. 2, ed. Michael R. Marrus (Westport, CT: Meckler, 1989), 666.

4. Robert Jay Lifton, *The Nazi Doctors: Medical Killing and the Psychology of Genocide* (New York: Basic Books, 1986), 321, 322.

5. Nathan C. Nash, "Mengele an Abortionist, Argentine Files Suggest," *New York Times*, February 11, 1992, A8.

6. Lifton, *Nazi Doctors*, 114–15, 117.

7. Jerome E. Bates and Edward S. Zawadzki, *Criminal Abortion: A Study in Medical Sociology* (Springfield, IL: Charles C. Thomas, 1964), 95, 175–86.

8. Rickie Solinger, *Beggars and Choosers: How the Politics of Choice Shapes Adoption, Abortion, and Welfare in the United States* (New York: Hill and Wang, 2001), 52.

9. Andrew Scholberg, "How Abortionists See It—A View from the Inside," *The Interim*, January 6, 1986.

10. Tim Murray, "Mogenthaler Not So Much of a Hero?," *Canada: The Sinking Lifeboat* (blog), August 9, 2009, http://sinkinglifeboat.blogspot.com/2009/08/morgenthaler-not-so-much-of-hero.html.

11. Warren M. Hern, "Life on the Front Lines," *Women's Health Issues* 4 (Spring 1994): 48.

12. John H. Richardson, "The Last Abortion Doctor," *Esquire* (September 2009): 138.

13. John Roberts and Carl Kjellstrand, "Jack Kevorkian: A Medical Hero," *British Medical Journal* 312 (June 8, 1996): 1434.

14. Lifton, *Nazi Doctors*, 72.

15. Gunther Schwarberg, *The Murders at Bullenhuser Damm: The SS Doctor and the Children*, trans. Erna Barber Rosenfeld with Alvin H. Rosenfeld (Bloomington: University of Indiana Press, 1984), 100.

16. Henry V. Dicks, *Licensed Mass Murder: A Socio-Psychological Study of Some SS Killers* (New York: Basic Books, 1972), 147.

17. "Extracts from the Closing Brief of Defendant Karl Brandt," in *Trials of War Criminals before the Nuernberg Military Tribunals*, 15 vols. (Washington, DC: US Government Printing Office, 1949), 1:834 (hereafter cited as *War Crimes Trials*).

18. "Extracts from the Testimony of Defendant Brack," in *War Crimes Trials*, 1:878.

19. Zigmond M. Lebensohn, "Abortion, Psychiatry and the Quality of Life," *American Journal of Psychiatry* 128 (February 1972): 950.

20. Michael S. Burnhill, "Humane Abortion Services: A Revolution in Human Rights and the Delivery of a Medical Service," *Mount Sinai Journal of Medicine* 42 (September-October 1975): 438.

21. National Abortion Federation v. Ashcroft, 330 F. Supp. 2d 436 (S.D.N.Y. 2004).

22. Howard Caplan, "It's Time We Helped Patients Die," *Medical Economics*, June 8, 1987, 214, 216.

23. Sidney H. Wanzer et al., "The Physician's Responsibility toward Hopelessly Ill Patients," *New England Journal of Medicine* 310 (April 12, 1984): 956, 958–59.

24. Karl Binding and Alfred Hoche, *Permitting the Destruction of Unworthy Life: Its Extent and Form*, trans. Walter E. Wright (Leipzig: Felix Meiner, 1920). [Reprinted in *Issues in Law and Medicine* 8 (February 1992): 246–49, 252, 254.]

25. Earl W. Kintner, ed., *The Hadamar Trial: Trial of Alfons Klein and Others* (London: William Hodge, 1949), 102, 167.

26. Susan Benedict and Jochen Kuhla, "Nurses' Participation in the Euthanasia Programs of Nazi Germany," *Western Journal of Nursing Research* 21 (April 1999): 246–62.

27. "Letters," *American Journal of Nursing* 72 (February 1972): 240.

28. "Post-Abortion Fetal Study Stirs Storm," *Medical World News*, June 8, 1973, 21.

29. For a report on Dr. Anand's academic background and qualifications, university affiliations, research and other awards, and extensive publications in leading medical journals, see "Expert Report of Kanwaljeet S. Anand, M.B.B.S., D.Phil.," National Right to Life, January 15, 2004, https://www.nrlc.org/archive/abortion/Fetal_Pain/AnandPainReport.pdf.

30. "Mercy Death Law Proposed in State," *New York Times*, January 27, 1939, 21.

31. Charles E. Nixdorff, "Explaining Euthanasia," *New York Times*, January 30, 1939, 12.

32. John Wrable, "Euthanasia Would Be a Humane Way to End Suffering," *American Medical News*, January 20, 1989, 31.

33. Timothy Egan, "As Memory and Music Faded, Alzheimer Patient Met Death," *New York Times*, June 7, 1990, A13.

34. Gregory Crouch, "A Crusade Born of a Suffering Infant's Cry," *New York Times*, March 19, 2005, A4.

35. David Sommer, "After Quiet Moments of Mourning, Debate Refires over End-of-Life Choices," *Tampa Tribune*, April 1, 2005, Nation/World: 1.

36. "George Felos, Michael Schiavo's Attorney, Discusses the Death of Terri Schiavo," *Today*, April 1, 2005.

37. Michael Burleigh, *Death and Deliverance: "Euthanasia" in Germany, 1900–1945* (Cambridge: Cambridge University Press, 1994), 151.

38. Henry Friedlander, *The Origins of Nazi Genocide: From Euthanasia to the Final Solution* (Chapel Hill: University of North Carolina Press, 1995), 104.

39. Burleigh, *Death and Deliverance*, 201–2.

40. "Final Statement of Defendant Karl Brandt," in *War Crimes Trials*, 2:139–40.

41. See Dr. Carlson's letter to Representative Patricia Schroeder opposing the legal banning of partial-birth abortion in House Committee on the Judiciary, *The Report together with Dissenting Views on the Partial-Birth Abortion Ban Act of 1995*, 104th Cong., 1st. sess. (1995), 31–35.

42. "Shall This Child Die?," *Newsweek*, November 12, 1973, 70.

43. Diane M. Gianelli, "Inside a Hemlock 'How to Do It' Session," *American Medical News*, December 9, 1996, 25.

44. Mark Rust, "AMA Policy Cited in Coma Decisions," *American Medical News*, May 2, 1986, 1, 10.

45. Raul Hilberg, *The Destruction of the European Jews*, 3rd ed., 3 vols. (New Haven, CT: Yale University Press, 2003), 3:1083.

46. Steven Ertelt, "Pro-Abortion Attorney Tells Congress a Dismemberment Abortion is a 'Humane Procedure,'" LifeNews.com, September 9, 2015, http://www.lifenews.com/2015/09/09/pro-abortion-attorney-tells-congress-a-dismemberment-abortion-is-a-humane-procedure/.

Chapter 15. Graphic Exposures of Mass Destruction

1. Oron J. Hale, *The Captive Press in the Third Reich* (Princeton, NJ: Princeton University Press, 1973), 1–14.

2. Walter Laqueur, *The Terrible Secret: Suppression of the Truth about Hitler's "Final Solution"* (Boston: Little, Brown, 1980), 152–53.

3. Leon Poliakov, *Harvest of Hate: The Nazi Program for the Destruction of the Jews of Europe*, rev. ed. (New York: Schocken Books, Holocaust Library, 1979), 175.

4. Laqueur, *Terrible Secret*, 3, 106.

5. Laqueur, *Terrible Secret*, 8–9.

6. John Leo, "Is the Press Straight on Abortion?," *US News and World Report*, July 16, 1990, 17; David Shaw, "Abortion Bias Seeps into News," *Los Angeles Times*, July 1, 1990, A1, A50–A51; S. Robert Lichter and Stanley Rothman, "Media Bias and Business Elites," *Public Opinion* (October/November 1981): 42–46, 59–60.

7. Paul Berg, "Battle Lines in a Moral and Legal Dispute," *Sunday Pictures—St. Louis Post-Dispatch*, May 20, 1973, 1–15.

8. Robert H. Abzug, *Inside the Vicious Heart: Americans and the Liberation of Nazi Concentration Camps* (New York: Oxford University Press, 1985), 92.

9. Gene Currivan, "Nazi Death Factory Shocks Germans on a Forced Tour," *New York Times*, April 18, 1945, 1, 8.

10. Ulrike Weckel, "Does Gender Matter: Filmic Representations of Liberated Nazi Concentration Camps, 1945–46," *Gender and History* 17 (November 2005): 552.

11. Teresa Swiebocha, ed., *Auschwitz: A History in Photographs*, English ed. prepared by Jonathan Webber and Connie Wilsack (Bloomington: University of Indiana Press, 1993), 194, 196–201.

12. "Press Exposure of German Horror Camps," *Newspaper World*, April 28, 1945, 1, 14.

13. Editor, "Indisputable Proof," *News Chronicle*, April 19, 1945, 1.

14. "Atrocity Pictures," *Editor and Publisher*, May 5, 1945, 40.

15. Center for the Documentation of the American Holocaust, *The American Holocaust* (Palm Springs: Center for the Documentation of the American Holocaust, 1983).

16. Jane Floerchinger and Brian Levinson, "Wichita City Order Stuns Officials," *Wichita Eagle-Beacon*, August 8, 1983, 1C, 16C.

17. Monica Migliorino Miller, *Abandoned: The Untold Story of the Abortion Wars* (Charlotte, NC: Saint Benedict Press, 2012), 5, 8.

18. "Unborn Babies Found in Trash," Clinic Quotes, August 31, 2012, http://clinic quotes.com/unborn-babies-found-in-trash-from-mine-eyes-have-seen-the-glory/.

19. "Requiem for the Disappeared," Citizens for a Pro-Life Society, accessed September 28, 2020, http://www.prolifesociety.net/archives/2008/Sharpe/Requiem-ForTheDisappeared.aspx.

20. T. W. McGarry, "Fetuses Buried—With Hymns, Prayers," *Los Angeles Times*, October 7, 1985, Section 1:3.

21. Albert Oetgen, "'I Know What It's Like': The Emotion of Abortion Surfaces at Protest Rally," *Tallahassee Democrat*, August 6, 1988, 1A.

22. "Planned Parenthood VP Says Fetuses May Come Out Intact, Agrees Payments Specific to the Specimen," Center for Medical Progress, July 30, 2015, http://www.centerformedicalprogress.org/2015/07/planned-parenthood-vp-says-fetuses-may-come-out-intact-agrees-payments-specific-to-the-specimen/.

23. Charles E. Egan, "All Reich to See Camp Atrocities," *New York Times*, April 24, 1945, 6.

24. "Public Crowd for Pictures of Atrocities," *World's Press News* (London), April 26, 1945, 1.

25. Janina Struk, *Photographing the Holocaust* (London: I. B. Tauris, 2004), 125.

26. "Thousands See Life-Size Photos of Nazi Prison Camp Atrocities," *St. Louis Post-Dispatch*, May 30, 1945, 3.

27. "Atrocity Pictures Seen by 10,814 at Capital in 2 Days," *St. Louis Post-Dispatch*, July 2, 1945, 3A.

28. "Washington News," *Washington Sunday Star*, July 1, 1945, Section B.

29. "About the Pro-Life Action League," Pro-Life Action League, accessed July 7, 2020, http://prolifeaction.org/about/.

30. Pro-Life Action League, *Action News* 28, no. 2 (July 15, 2009): 1, 2.

31. *Center for Bio-Ethical Reform Newsletter* (June 2009).

32. *Center for Bio-Ethical Reform Communique* (June 2005).

33. *Center for Bio-Ethical Reform Communique* (October 2005).

34. Lucy S. Dawidowicz, "Lies about the Holocaust," *Commentary* (December 1980): 36.

35. Nazila Fathi, "Iran Opens Conference on Holocaust," *New York Times*, December 12, 2006, A3.

36. Udo Walendy, "Do Photographs Prove the NS Extermination of the Jews?," VHO.org, accessed July 7, 2020, http://www.vho.org/GB/Books/dth/fndgcffor.html.

37. "To Look at Horror," *Newsweek*, May 28, 1945, 34–35.

38. *Hearing on Partial-Birth Abortion, Before the Subcommittee on the Judiciary, House of Representatives*, 104th Cong., 1st Sess. 7 (June 15, 1995).

39. 104 Cong. Rec. H11609, H11613 (November 1, 1995).

40. Watson Bowes, MD, to Representative Charles Canady, July 11, 1995, reprinted in the Appendix to *Hearing on Partial-Birth Abortion*, 106.

41. Diane M. Gianelli, "Shock-Tactic Ads Target Late-Term Abortion Procedure," *American Medical News*, July 5, 1993, 21.

42. *Center for Bio-Ethical Reform Communique* (July 2007).

43. Gregg Cunningham, "Verifying Photograph Authenticity," AbortionNo.org, accessed July 7, 2020, https://www.abortionno.org/lawsuits/verifying-photograph-authenticity/.

44. *Trial of War Criminals before the Nuremberg Tribunal under Control Council Law*, 14 vols., Green Series 10 (Washington, DC: Government Printing Office, 1950–52), 10:1209 (Nuremberg Document NOKW 2523: letter of July 22, 1941, from 11th Army, signed by Woehler, Concerning Photographs and Reports of Executions).

45. "Press Exposure of German Horror Camps," *Newspaper World*, April 28, 1945, 14.

46. "Atrocity Pictures," *Editor and Publisher*, May 5, 1945, 40.

47. 104 Cong. Rec. S8863, S8865 (June 22, 1995).

48. 104 Cong. Rec. H11605 (1995).

49. *Center for Bio-Ethical Reform Communique* (November 2005).

50. *Center for Bio-Ethical Reform Communique* (April 2008).

51. *Center for Bio-Ethical Reform Communique* (March 2006); (August 2006).

52. *Center for Bio-Ethical Reform Newsletter* (March 2006).

Chapter 16. The Urgency of a Full-Scale Physicians' Crusade against Killing before and after Birth

1. Horatio R. Storer et al., "Report on Criminal Abortion," *Transactions of the American Medical Association* 12 (1859): 76, 78.

2. Storer et al., "Report on Criminal Abortion," 77.

3. Storer et al., "Report on Criminal Abortion," 75, 76.

4. In 1847, the distinguished histologist Dr. Albert von Kolliker "first demonstrated the true development of the spermatozoa, showing that they are not extraneous bodies, but originate testicular cells, and fertilize the ovum." Fielding H. Garrison, *An Introduction to the History of Medicine*, 4th ed., reprint (Philadelphia: W. B. Saunders, 1929), 461.

5. Storer et al., "Report on Criminal Abortion," 77.

6. Storer et al., "Report on Criminal Abortion," 77–78.

7. D. A. O'Donnell and W. L. Atlee, "Report on Criminal Abortion," *Transactions of the American Medical Association* 22 (1871): 250.

8. O'Donnell and Atlee, "Report on Criminal Abortion," 251, 253.

9. O'Donnell and Atlee, "Report on Criminal Abortion," 240, 241, 251, 252.

10. O'Donnell and Atlee, "Report on Criminal Abortion," 244, 247, 248, 250, 254.

11. O'Donnell and Atlee, "Report on Criminal Abortion," 240, 251, 257.

12. O'Donnell and Atlee, "Report on Criminal Abortion," 257.

13. O'Donnell and Atlee, "Report on Criminal Abortion," 258.

14. O'Donnell and Atlee, "Report on Criminal Abortion," 257–58.

15. James C. Mohr, *Abortion in America: The Origins and Evolution of National Policy, 1800–1900* (New York: Oxford University Press, 1978), 147, 200.

16. "AMA Policy on Therapeutic Abortion," *Journal of the American Medical Association* 201 (August 14, 1967): 544.

17. "Therapeutic Abortion," *Proceedings of the House of Delegates, the American Medical Association* (June 1967): 42.

18. Storer et al., "Report on Criminal Abortion," 77.

19. O'Donnell and Atlee, "Report on Criminal Abortion," 248, 251, 257.

20. "Therapeutic Abortion," 42–43, 49.

21. "Obstetricians Back Liberal Abortions," *New York Times*, May 10, 1968, 21.

22. C. Gerald Fraser, "Reuther Asks National Health System," *New York Times*, November 15, 1968, 28.

23. "Therapeutic Abortion," *Proceedings of the House of Delegates, the American Medical Association* (June 1970): 221.

Chapter 17. Toward a Revitalization of the Hippocratic Ethic in the Face of Widespread Assaults on the Hippocratic Oath

1. Margaret Mead, quoted in Maurice Levine, *Psychiatry and Ethics* (New York: George Braziller, 1972), 324–25.

2. Francis Adams, trans. *The Genuine Works of Hippocrates* (Baltimore: Williams & Wilkins, 1939), 347–60.

3. Arturo Castiglioni, *A History of Medicine*, trans. E. B. Krumbhaar, 2nd ed. (New York: Alfred A. Knopf, 1958), 148.

4. Ludwig Edelstein, trans., *The Hippocratic Oath: Text, Translation, and Interpretation* (Baltimore: Johns Hopkins Press, 1943), 3.

5. Mead, in Levine, *Psychiatry and Ethics*, 324.

6. Mead, in Levine, *Psychiatry and Ethics*, 325.

7. Mead, in Levine, *Psychiatry and Ethics*, 325.

8. Herbert Ratner, "The Hippocratic Oath," *Child and Family* 11, no. 2 (1972): 99.

9. Herbert Ratner, "The Oath—III. Why?," *Child and Family* 10, no. 2 (1971): 100.

10. Karl Binding and Alfred Hoche, *Permitting the Destruction of Unworthy Life: Its Extent and Form*, trans. Walter E. Wright (Leipzig: Felix Meiner, 1920). [Reprinted in *Issues in Law and Medicine* 8 (February 1992): 255.]

11. "Opening Statement of the Prosecution by Brigadier General Telford Taylor, December 9, 1946," in *Trials of War Criminals before the Nuernberg Military Tribunals*, 15 vols. (Washington, DC: US Government Printing Office, 1950), 1:68 (hereafter cited as *War Crimes Trials*).

12. "Transcript of the Proceedings in Case 1," in *The Medical Case*, vol. 1 of *War Crimes Trials*, 1:7130–32 (testimony of Gregor Welz).

13. "Transcript of the Proceedings in Case 1," in *The Medical Case*, 1:2434–35 (testimony of Karl Brandt).

14. A definitive, in–depth analysis of this and other pro-abortion decrees imposed on the countries in the Eastern Territories under Nazi occupation can be found in Jeffrey C. Tuomala, "Nuremberg and the Crime of Abortion," *University of Toledo Law Review* 42 (Winter 2011): 288, 343, 386.

15. Tuomala, "Nuremberg and the Crime of Abortion," 320, 327.

16. "I. Indictment: Count Two—War Crimes," in *War Crimes Trials*, 1:11.

17. "I. Indictment: Count Three—Crimes against Humanity," in *War Crimes Trials*, 1:16–17.

18. "I. Indictment: Count One—Crimes against Humanity," in *War Crimes Trials*, 8:610.

19. Prosecutor, *The Nuremberg RuSHA (Race and Resettlement Office) Trial*, March 1948, Microfilm 894, roll 31, 13–14, National Archives and Records Administration, College Park, MD.

20. "The World Medical Association Declaration of Geneva (1948) Physician's Oath," Circumcision Information and Resource Pages, accessed July 7, 2020, http://www.cirp.org/library/ethics/geneva/.

21. "International Code of Medical Ethics of the World Medical Association—1949," Circumcision Information and Resource Pages, accessed July 7, 2020, http://www.cirp.org/library/ethics/intlcode/.

22. Albert Deutsch, "A Note on Medical Ethics (Including the New Hippocratic Oath of the World Medical Association)," in *Doctors of Infamy: The Story of the Nazi Medical Crimes*, ed. Alexander Mitscherlich and Fred Mielke (New York: Henry Schuman, 1949), xxxvii–xxxix.

23. Roe v. Wade, 410 U.S. 131 (1973).

24. Bolivar M. Escobedo, "More on When Life Begins," *St. Louis Post-Dispatch*, January 17, 1979, 4C.

25. Thomas G. Gulick, "Even Abortionists Having Second Thoughts," *Human Events*, April 12, 1980, 18.

26. Derek Humphry, "Inquiry, Topic Euthanasia," *USA Today*, January 17, 1986, 11A.

27. Ralph E. Thompson, "I Swear by Apollo, the Hippocratic Oath Is Obsolete," *Physician Executive* 30 (March-April 2004): 60.

28. Ricard Momeyer, "Does Physician-Assisted Suicide Violate the Integrity of Medicine?," *Journal of Medicine and Philosophy* 20 (1995): 23.

29. Sherwin B. Nuland, "Physician-Assisted Suicide and Euthanasia in Practice," *New England Journal of Medicine* 342 (February 24, 2000): 584.

30. Robert D. Orr et al., "Use of the Hippocratic Oath: A Review of Twentieth Century Practice and a Content Analysis of Oaths Administered in Medical Schools in the U.S. and Canada in 1993," *Journal of Clinical Issues* 8 (Winter 1997): 380–81, 386.

31. Erich H. Loewy, "Oaths for Physicians—Protection or Hoax," *Medscape General Medicine* 9 (January 10, 2007): 2.

32. Imre Loefler, "Why the Hippocratic Ideals Are Dead," *British Medical Journal* 324 (June 15, 2002): 1463.

33. Deutsch, "Note on Medical Ethics," xxxvii–xxxix.

34. Nigel M. de S. Cameron, *The New Medicine: Life and Death after Hippocrates* (Wheaton, IL: Crossway Books, 1992), 84–89.

35. Mary Arneson, "The Hippocratic Oath," *CA1—A Cancer Journal for Clinicians* 40 (March-April 1990): 126.

36. Louis Weinstein, "The Oath of the Healer," *Journal of the American Medical Journal* 265 (May 15, 1991): 2484.

37. "Declaration of Geneva 1994," World Medical Association, September 1994, https://www.wma.net/what-we-do/medical-ethics/declaration-of-geneva/decl-of-geneva-v1994/.

38. William J. Curran and Ward Casscells, "The Ethics of Medical Participation in Capital Punishment by Intravenous Drug Injection," *New England Journal of Medicine* 302 (January 24, 1980): 230.

39. Curran and Casscells, "Ethics of Medical Participation," 227.

40. "Position Statement on Medical Participation in Capital Punishment," *American Journal of Psychiatry* 137 (November 1980): 1487.

41. Council on Ethical and Judicial Affairs, American Medical Association, "Physician Participation in Capital Punishment," *Journal of the American Medical Association* 270 (July 21, 1993): 365.

42. Atul Gaeande, "When Law and Ethics Collide—Why Physicians Participate in Executions," *New England Journal of Medicine* 354 (March 23, 2006): 1223.

43. Judicial Council, "Terminal Illness," in *Proceedings of the House of Delegates, June 1977, 26th Annual Convention* (Chicago: American Medical Association), 106–10.

44. Council on Ethical and Judicial Affairs, American Medical Association, "Decisions Near the End of Life," *Journal of the American Medical Association* 267 (April 22/29, 1992): 2232–33.

45. Lonnie R. Bristol, "Assisted Suicide Is Not an Ethically Acceptable Practice of Physicians," in *Euthanasia: Opposing Viewpoints* (San Diego, CA: Greenhaven Press, 2000), 167.

46. Washington et al. v. Glucksberg et al., 521 U.S. 702 (1997).

47. Leon Kass, "Neither for Love Nor Money: Why Doctors Must Not Kill," *Public Interest* 94 (Winter 1989): 39.

48. Leon Kass, *Toward a More Natural Science: Biology and Human Affairs* (New York: Free Press, 1985), 234–35.

49. Joseph R. Stanton, E. Joanne Angelo, and Marianne Rea-Lethin, "Swearing to Life," *First Things* (January 1996): 13.

50. "The Hippocratic Oath and Abortion," American Right to Life, accessed September 28, 2020, https://americanrtl.org/Hippocratic-Oath-and-Abortion.

51. Jonathan Imbody, "Abortion and Doctors," *Los Angeles Times*, May 24, 2007, A24.

52. "Mission and Vision," website of the American Association of Pro-Life Obstetricians and Gynecologists, accessed July 7, 2020, http://www.aaplog.org/about-2/our-mission-statement/.

53. "March 27–29, 2020, Online Conference," website of the American Association of Pro-Life Obstetricians and Gynecologists, accessed July 7, 2020, http://conference.aaplog.org/.

54. "Extracts from the Testimony of Dr. Andrew Ivy," in *War Crimes Trials*, 2:86.

55. A. C. Ivy, "Nazi Crimes of a Medical Nature," *Journal of the American Medical Association* 139 (January 15, 1949): 133.

Conclusion

1. "A Statement on Abortion by One Hundred Professors of Obstetrics," *American Journal of Obstetrics and Gynecology* 112 (April 1, 1972): 992.

2. Herbert Ratner, "Editor's Comments," *Child and Family* 12, no. 3 (1973): 286.

3. World Health Organization, *Safe Abortion: Technical and Policy Guidance for Health Systems*, 2nd ed. (Geneva: WHO Press, 2012), 7, 8, 10, 12, 36, 38–48.

4. Steve Doughty, "Belgian GPs 'Killing Patients Who Have Not Asked to Die': Report Says Thousands Have Been Killed Despite Not Asking Their Doctor," *Daily Mail*, June 11, 2015.

5. Wesley J. Smith, *Assisted Suicide Is Not Compassion* (Washington, DC: Charlotte Lozier Institute, 2015), 3.

6. For Operation Rescue's extensive collection of data on surgical abortion clinics, abortion pill clinics, and physician abortionists, see AbortionDocs.org, accessed July 7, 2020.

7. D. A. O'Donnell and W. L. Atlee, "Report on Criminal Abortion," *Transactions of the American Medical Association* 22 (1871): 258.

8. George Orwell, *The Orwell Reader: Fiction, Essays, and Reportage by George Orwell*, introduction by Richard H. Rovere (New York: Harcourt Brace Jovanovich, 1956), 355–66.